The Single Market for Pharmaceuticals

Rhodri Thompson, M.A., B.Phil.
Barrister, London and Brussels

Butterworths
London, Dublin, Edinburgh
1994

United Kingdom	Butterworth & Co (Publishers) Ltd, Halsbury House, 35 Chancery Lane, LONDON WC2A 1EL and 4 Hill Street, EDINBURGH EH2 3JZ
Australia	Butterworths, SYDNEY, MELBOURNE, BRISBANE, ADELAIDE, PERTH, CANBERRA and HOBART
Canada	Butterworth Canada Ltd, TORONTO and VANCOUVER
Ireland	Butterworth (Ireland) Ltd, DUBLIN
Malaysia	Malayan Law Journal Sdn Bhd, KUALA LUMPUR
New Zealand	Butterworths of New Zealand Ltd, WELLINGTON and AUCKLAND
Puerto Rico	Butterworth of Puerto Rico, Inc, SAN JUAN
Singapore	Butterworths Asia, SINGAPORE
South Africa	Butterworth Publishers (Pty) Ltd, DURBAN
USA	Butterworth Legal Publishers, CARLSBAD, California; SALEM, New Hampshire

Publications and Information Manager
Sandra Dutczak, LL.B.

Editors
Katy Sadat, B.A., Barrister, Joe Nixon, B.A.

Editorial Assistants
Maria D'Souza
Lorna Sullivan

Printed in Great Britain by Ashford Colour Press Ltd, Gosport, Hampshire

Publisher's Note

With the momentum of change within the Community gathering pace it is hard to keep abreast of developments and obtain expert opinion and analysis together with original texts of legislation or cases as and when such events occur.

The *Current EC Legal Developments Series* is designed to provide the lawyer, consultant, researcher etc with commentary and source materials of relevant practical interest on fundamental changes in Community law.

Each title in the series has a similar format presenting the full text of proposed or enacted legislation or judicial decisions under review and provides analysis and comment written by leading practitioners in the subject area under consideration.

The views expressed by the author are personal and are not intended to be applied to particular situations.

Any queries as to the nature or content of the *Current EC Legal Developments Series* or in respect of this title in the *Series* should be directed to the Managing Editor, Butterworths European Law Group, Halsbury House, 35 Chancery Lane, LONDON WC2A 1EL.

Butterworth & Co (Publishers) Ltd

Current EC Legal Developments Series

Consultant Editor for the Series
DAVID VAUGHAN, QC

Titles already published in this Series :

ACKNOWLEDGEMENTS

I have received considerable assistance from Eduardo Pisani and Paul Adamson, formerly and currently of Adamson Associates, Brussels; from Tony Willis of the Association of the British Pharmaceutical Industry; and from Karen Knufmann of Directorate-General III of the European Commission. Philippa Watson originally suggested that I write this book but my principal debt is to my wife, Paula Thompson, who gave me a great deal of help and who endured the disruption necessarily involved in completing the job.

The Single Market for Pharmaceuticals

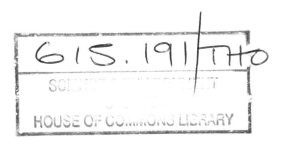

This book is dedicated to my mother, my wife and my daughter, each of whom has made a unique contribution to its completion.

Table of Contents

Tables

CASES BEFORE THE COURT OF JUSTICE AND COURT OF FIRST INSTANCE

PART I : THE SCOPE OF COMMUNITY
PHARMACEUTICAL REGULATION

Chapter 1 : Introduction

1.1   Scope of this work

There are three main ways in which European Community law[1] can affect a major industrial sector such as the pharmaceutical industry:

(1) harmonisation measures adopted by the Community may either lead to implementing legislation by the Member States of the Community or may create directly enforceable rights under Community law (often because the measures take the form of a Directive addressed to the Member States and the Member States have failed to implement the legislation correctly or at all by the time specified in the Directive, but sometimes because the Community measures take the form of a Regulation : see article 189 of the EC Treaty);

(2) the general Community rules on the free movement of goods within the Community, in particular articles 30 and 36 of the EC Treaty, may alter the trading conditions within the different Member States by facilitating the movement of goods across national boundaries;

(3) the general Community rules on competition, articles 85 to 94 of the Treaty, control restrictive practices, market dominance, the conduct of undertakings performing a national public service and the grant of state aids to industry; Council Regulation (EEC) 4064/89[2] now also enables the Commission to regulate significant structural change within the Community; those rules apply to a very wide range of sectors of the Community economy and can lead to the intervention of the EC Commission to regulate the pharmaceutical industry, among others, and to penalise infringements of the competition rules by individual undertakings.

The scope of this work is limited to an attempt to deal in some detail with the way in which the first of those issues has materially affected the operation of the Community pharmaceutical market. The second and third issues are dealt with in a number of textbooks and practitioners' works and readers should consult such works for analysis and materials[3]. The general principles in relation to free

---

1.   Despite the fact that nationals of the Member States of the European Economic Community became citizens of the European Union on 1 November 1993 - with the coming into force of the Treaty on European Union, and thus of article 8 of the newly amended and renamed European Community Treaty (formerly the European Economic Community) - this work is concerned only with the "first pillar" of the new tripartite structure of the Union, the pre-existing Communities and, of those, only with the renamed European Community. Explanation of the complexities and absurdities of the new constitutional framework falls outside the scope of the present work.

2.   OJ L395 30.12.89 p1.

3.   For example, on competition law, Bellamy and Child *Common Market Law of Competition* (4th edn, 1993) Sweet & Maxwell; Whish *Competition Law* (3rd edn, 1993) Butterworths; Freeman and Whish Eds. *Competition Law* (looseleaf) Butterworths; *Competition Law Handbook* (3rd edn, 1993) Butterworths, which provides a comprehensive selection of materials (subordinate legislation,

movement of goods and competition law vary in their application depending on the nature of the goods or economic activities to which the rules are applied. Because of the very unusual characteristics of the pharmaceutical market, those rules have operated in quite particular ways in respect of that market. The most striking instances of those applications are briefly described at section 1.4 post but detailed analysis of the relevant principles and case law falls outside the scope of this work.

1.2 Harmonisation of the pharmaceutical market

The unique characteristics of the pharmaceutical industry have invited the attention of regulators throughout the world, not just those of the Community[1]. The Community's own attempts to regulate the industry, and to harmonise national controls, have a long history, but the recent legislative programme for pharmaceuticals has been particularly ambitious and wide-ranging[2].

The recent pharmaceutical legislation formed a significant part of the Community's attempt to create the single or internal market, announced by the Commission White Paper of 1985[3] and made possible by the alterations to the EC Treaty (then the EEC Treaty) made by the Single European Act of 1986. The Commission White Paper and the Single European Act were designed to provide a focus for European integration by announcing and facilitating a programme of legislation across a wide range of economic sectors of the Community, with a view to achieving a significant degree of harmonisation in each sector and thus creating the single or internal market. That programme was intended to be in effect by 31 December 1992 and is referred to in this work as "the 1992 Programme".

The details of the legislative procedures introduced by the Single European Act are beyond the scope of this work, but it emerges from the preambles to the various Directives and Regulations discussed in this work that the majority of the recent pharmaceutical legislation adopted by the Community institutions has been adopted under article 100a of the EC Treaty, introduced by the Single European Act, which permitted harmonisation measures to be introduced by a qualified majority of the Member States rather than by unanimity. Article 100a thus enabled the internal market legislation to be adopted even where individual Member States had reservations about its contents. The insuperable difficulties which would have faced the 1992 Programme if unanimity had been required for each item of legislation were well illustrated by the protracted difficulties faced by the

---

Commission notices, etc); on free movement of goods, see Oliver *Free Movement of Goods in the EEC* (2nd edn, 1988) Sweet & Maxwell (3rd edition in preparation).

1.   "Of all industrial sectors, it is perhaps the pharmaceutical industry which is subject to the greatest level of regulation and control by the public authorities" : the Director-General for Internal Market and Industrial Affairs, Introduction to Volume I of EC Commission *The Rules Governing Medicinal Products in the European Community* (1989) Office for Official Publications of the European Communities; see also Hancher *Regulating for Competition* (1990) Clarendon Press, for a detailed comparative study of regulatory strategies for the industry in the United Kingdom and France.

2.   There is an interesting story to be told of political compromise and negotiation, not only between the Member States and the Community but also involving the industry itself. The present work aims to clarify the current position rather than to give a history of regulatory strategies and counter-strategies, but see Hancher's works for a detailed account of the historical and strategic background : in particular, Chapter 5 of *Regulating for Competition* (1990) Clarendon Press; and 'The European Pharmaceutical Market - Problems of Partial Harmonisation' (1990) 15 ELR 9, at pp11-18.

3.   *White Paper on the Completion of the Internal Market* COM(85) 310, in particular Annexes 17 and 18.

Community in passing Regulation (EEC) 2309/93[1], the most important single piece of legislation in the 1992 Programme for pharmaceuticals. Because the Regulation provided for central Community authorisation procedures and for the creation of a new Community institution, the European Agency for the Evaluation of Medicinal Products, it could not be adopted under article 100a. Unanimity was therefore required for its adoption, leading to severe difficulties in the Council in persuading each Member State to vote for the Regulation.

The 1992 Programme for pharmaceuticals was not in fact concluded until 14 June and 22 July 1993, with the adoption on those dates of the principal texts of the Future System legislation discussed in Chapters 7 and 8 of this work. Various matters remained outstanding even then, notably the location of the European Agency for the Evaluation of Medicinal Products. That issue was resolved in favour of London on 29 October 1993 but the financial and administrative arrangements for the Agency remained to be finally resolved at the start of 1994. The Future System is scheduled to come into effect on 1 January 1995, two years after the proposed creation of the single market for pharmaceuticals, and one important element in the package does not come into effect until 1 January 1998[2].

This work attempts to describe the legislative position that has emerged as a result of the 1992 Programme. The legislation in respect of market authorisation will only gradually come into complete effect so that it has been necessary to describe not only the present position (Chapters 3 to 6) but also the future arrangements (Chapters 7 to 9).

A final twist should be noted. The legislation described in this work is extremely complex and fragmented in its structure; topics are interwoven in different pieces of legislation and individual Directives contain disparate elements. On 24 November 1993, the Commission produced a draft report to the European Council on the adaptation of existing legislation to the principle of subsidiarity[3]. That report proposed, at pages 6 and 11, that the pharmaceutical legislation might be "recast" :

> "In this connection recasting would increase the degree of consistency and help put the main ideas behind subsidiarity into practice by :
>
> — clarifying - particularly with regard to authorisation and withdrawal - the difference between Commission decisions based on the opinion of the Medicinal Products Agency and decisions made by the national authorities and ensuring better co-ordination and hence increased consistency between decisions taken at Community and national level; and
> — simplifying and updating basic concepts and clarifying terminology in the various Community languages, given the importance of terminology in this particular field, and eliminating needless repetitions of definitions and procedural overlaps, thus reducing the volume of regulations by more than a third.

> Its entry into force could be arranged to coincide with the setting-up of the Agency, ie towards the end of 1994 or the beginning of 1995."

---

1.   OJ L214 24.8.93 p1. See Appendix 5 post.
2.   The new article 7a of Directive (EEC) 75/319 (OJ L147 9.6.75 p13) will introduce a system of compulsory Community arbitration in respect of medicinal products to be marketed in more than one Member State of the Community whenever an authorisation of the product by one Member State is not accepted by the other Member States concerned : see section 8.4 post.
3.   COM(93) 545.

The report later peremptorily states that "[r]ecasting would make it possible to repeal 20-odd Council and Commission Directives". The idea behind the report is certainly praiseworthy and the complexity of the current legislative structure is a legitimate target for criticism. However, the Commission's proposal appears wildly optimistic, taking no account of the great practical difficulties that would face a draughtsman seeking to recast technical legislation occupying well over one hundred pages of the Official Journal; or of the constitutional implications of primary legislation, only agreed after lengthy negotiations between the Member States, being rewritten by a simple bureaucratic process (the timetable for the recasting exercise would clearly render it impossible for such a massive legislative package to be reconsidered by the Council and the Parliament).

In practice, the Commission's immediate plans appear to extend no further than to a further edition of consolidated texts of the kind found in the Appendices to this work and in Volume I of *The Rules Governing Medicinal Products in the European Community*, published by the Commission in 1989 and republished in 1991[1].

1.3   The structure of this work

This work falls into five parts. Part I (Chapters 1 and 2) comprises this introduction and an overview of the Community pharmaceutical regime, together with a discussion of the fundamental concept, "medicinal product", which links all the legislation considered in this work.

Part II (Chapters 3 to 6) describes the existing structure of regulation, which was established by Directive (EEC) 65/65[2] and has been in a gradual state of evolution since 1965. In 1965, the Community simply set out framework requirements in respect of the authorisation of marketing of medicinal products and laid down three fundamental criteria for such authorisation : quality, safety and efficacy. The substance of the tests to be applied and the procedures to be followed by the Member States in implementing Directive (EEC) 65/65 were made considerably more detailed in 1975 and mechanisms for discussion of national decisions were also introduced. Those procedures were further developed after 1975 and a new procedure was introduced in 1987, increasing the Community's involvement in the authorisation of certain high technology products. In substance, that legislative structure remains in place until 1 January 1995 in respect of the initial authorisation of medicinal products.

Part III (Chapters 7 to 9) describes the Future System legislation, which comes into force on 1 January 1995 and which replaces the existing system of marketing authorisations where more than one Member State of the Community is involved. The principal elements are : the introduction of compulsory Community procedures, both for arbitration between national authorities in respect of divergent national assessments and for unitary Community authorisations for, as yet, a limited class of products; and the creation of the European Agency for the Evaluation of Medicinal Products, to co-ordinate and administer the new regulatory structure.

Part IV (Chapters 10 to 12) deals with post-authorisation control of medicinal products. Since 1965, the Community's principal efforts in seeking to harmonise the national rules and procedures of the Member States have been directed to the issues of when and how initial authorisation to place a medicinal product on a national market should be given : see Parts II and III of this work. Initial authorisation has been and remains the "hub and linchpin of the whole system of

---

1.   See section 1.5 post.
2.   OJ No 22 9.2.65 p369/65. See Appendix 1 post.

rules"[1]. However, the detailed rules contained in Directive (EEC) 65/65 for the provision of information are intended to guarantee that a product for which marketing authorisation is granted satisfies the Community criteria of quality, safety and efficacy; it would clearly undermine the effectiveness of such rules if the product actually manufactured and marketed after authorisation had been granted did not conform to the information supplied to the national (or Community) authorities. Likewise, the natural correlative to initial marketing authorisation is continuing marketing supervision, and a central element of such supervision is adverse reaction monitoring, referred to in the newly revised Community legislation as "pharmacovigilance". Manufacture, supervision and pharmacovigilance are considered in Part IV of this work. Those areas of continuing control are currently (and will to a large extent remain) covered by Directives (EEC) 65/65, 75/318[2] and 75/319[3], as amended by Directive (EEC) 93/39[4]. Because the Community legislation deals with the issues in a highly fragmentary manner, it is necessary to consider a range of legislation in respect of each issue.

Part V deals with four other matters which, with the exception of labelling and package leaflets, had not been considered in the original legislation and which are now covered by four separate Directives. Those four Directives, the so-called Rational Use package of legislation, were adopted on 31 March 1992 and constitute the second major element of the 1992 programme for pharmaceutical products (along with the Future System legislation)[5]. The package dealt with four topics : wholesale distribution; classification for the purposes of supply; labelling and package leaflets; and advertising. Although all four Directives were adopted simultaneously and were published in a single volume of the Official Journal, they do not represent a single complex scheme in the manner of the Future System described in Part III : Directives (EEC) 92/25 and 92/26[6] represent minor but important further steps to harmonise the operation of the Community pharmaceutical market in respect of wholesale distribution and legal classification respectively; Directive (EEC) 92/27[7] is in essence a consolidating piece of legislation, repealing parts of Directives (EEC) 65/65 and 75/319 and laying down somewhat more detailed rules in respect of labelling and package leaflets than had previously been found necessary; while Directive (EEC) 92/28[8] is a specific measure forming part not only of the Community legislation on pharmaceuticals but also of the legislation dealing with the difficult issues of control over misleading or undesirable advertising. Looked at from another perspective, Directives (EEC) 92/26 and 92/27 add further elements to the already complex process of original marketing authorisation (each is referred to in the Future System legislation), whereas Directives (EEC) 92/25 and 92/28 set up distinct minor regimes controlling respectively the distribution and the advertising of medicinal products for human use.

---

1.   See the quotation from Advocate-General Lenz's Opinion in Case C-112/89 *Upjohn v Farzoo* [1991] ECR I-1703 cited at section 3.2 post.

2.   OJ L147 9.6.75 p1. See Appendix 2 post.

3.   OJ L147 9.6.75 p13. See Appendix 3 post.

4.   OJ L214 24.8.93 p22.

5.   The "extension" Directives 89/341, 89/342, 89/343 and 89/381, extending the scope of Directives (EEC) 65/65 and 75/319, were adopted in 1989 but they did not introduce a fundamentally new element into the Community regime. They are discussed briefly in Chapter 3. The other significant new element, the adoption of Directive (EEC) 92/73 in respect of homeopathic products, establishes a new regime for the initial authorisation of such products and therefore is considered in Chapter 9 post as part of the Future System legislation.

6.   OJ L113 30.4.92 pp1-4, 5-7. See Appendices 10 and 11 post.

7.   OJ L113 30.4.92 pp8-12. See Appendix 12 post.

8.   OJ L113 30.4.92 pp13-18. See Appendix 13 post.

1.4 Topics not covered in this work

As stated above, this work concentrates on the harmonisation measures introduced as part of the 1992 Programme. That approach accords with the purpose of the series of which this work forms part, to cover "current EC legal developments"[1]. The necessary consequence is that certain complex issues affecting the pharmaceutical sector are not here considered.

Two major areas of the greatest commercial significance are not considered in any detail in the main body of this work : intellectual property protection for pharmaceutical products; and harmonisation of price control and the conditions for reimbursement of such products. Each topic raises fundamental questions in respect of the free movement of goods and competition and also impinges on other issues of great importance to the development of a harmonised Community market : in the case of intellectual property protection, pharmaceutical products are paradigm instances of products enjoying patent, trade mark and copyright protection (patent protection in respect of the original formulation and manufacture of the product, trade mark protection in respect of the brand, and copyright in respect of the package leaflet and/or the design of the get up of the packaging); in the case of pricing and reimbursement, assertion of control by the Community over such issues is highly sensitive, challenging the autonomy of the Member States in respect of their management of the economic and social conditions prevailing in the national territory.

Neither area was subject to extensive harmonisation as part of the 1992 Programme, so that they fall substantially outside the scope of this work. However, given the importance of those two topics, two recent pieces of legislation, relevant to patent protection and transparency of price controls respectively, are included in the Appendices to this work and two Commission Communications are also included, setting out the Commission's understanding of two important areas : parallel imports of proprietary medicinal products for which marketing authorisations have already been granted; and the compatibility with article 30 of the EC Treaty of measures taken by Member States relating to price controls and reimbursement of medicinal products[2]. Given the importance of those four topics, they are described briefly below.

1.4.1 The supplementary protection certificate
The pharmaceutical industry depends very heavily on investment in research and development. The profitability of the leading pharmaceutical companies is to a large extent based on a relatively limited number of innovative products and depends crucially on the ability of those companies to market their products during the period in which they enjoy patent protection from generic competition. Because of the stringent demands imposed by the regulatory authorities in respect of the authorisation of new medicinal products, in particular under the rules introduced in accordance with Directive (EEC) 65/65, there is frequently a delay of several years between the filing of an application for a patent and the grant of a marketing authorisation in respect of a new product. That period of delay represents a major lost opportunity for the company concerned and the Community accepts that the effect of such delay is to disadvantage Community pharmaceutical companies by comparison with such companies outside the Community.

Council Regulation (EEC) 1768/92 concerning the creation of a supplementary protection certificate for medicinal products was introduced partially to remedy the situation by granting a period of supplementary protection beyond the expiry of ordinary patent protection where there was an extended period between the filing

---

1.   See section 1.1 ante.
2.   See Appendices 14 to 17 post.

of the original patent application and the grant of marketing authorisation. The most significant single article of the Regulation is article 13, which provides that the supplementary protection is :

(a) to take effect at the end of the lawful term of the basic patent;
(b) to last for a period equal to the difference between the date of filing for the basic patent and the date of marketing authorisation of the product in question, minus a period of five years (article 13(1)); and
(c) to last for a maximum period of five years (article 13(2)).

The effect is that no supplementary protection is granted unless the delay is more than five years (a delay of six years will give one year's supplementary protection, seven years two years' protection and so on); and that no further protection will be granted if the delay is greater than ten years (a delay of ten years will give five years' supplementary protection, as will any longer delay). Where normal patent protection is 20 years, the effect will be to grant a minimum period of protection of 15 years unless the delay is more than ten years, and a gradually declining period thereafter, in each case five years longer than the period of protection under the patent itself. The Regulation entered into force on 2 January 1993 and applies to products protected by a valid basic patent for which the first marketing authorisation within the Community was granted after 1 January 1985 (in Denmark and Germany, the relevant date is 1 January 1988; in Belgium and Italy, 1 January 1982)[1].

1.4.2 Transparency in pricing and reimbursement under national health insurance systems

The issue of health costs is not expressly provided for in the Treaty, but the European Court of Justice has accepted that measures adopted to contain costs do not infringe the rules on free movement of goods, subject to certain conditions[2]. At the time of publication of the Commission White Paper on completing the internal market, and in the light of the existing jurisprudence of the Court, the Commission issued a Communication on the compatibility with article 30 of the EC Treaty of measures taken by Member States relating to price controls and reimbursement of medicinal products[3]. That Communication sets out the Commission's understanding of the current legal position. The statutory position has now been clarified by Regulation (EEC) 2309/93[4] and Directive (EEC) 93/39, each of which contains express provisions preserving the rights of the Member States to refuse to pay for medicinal products even where they have obtained marketing authorisation either in that Member State or in the Community as a whole[5].

Council Directive (EEC) 89/105 relating to the transparency of measures regulating the pricing of medicinal products for human use and their inclusion in the scope of national health insurance systems[6] was intended to be a first step in the introduction of a harmonised regime for the imposition of price controls and restrictions of reimbursement by the national authorities. The Directive lays down

---

1.   Regulation (EEC) 1768/92 has been challenged by Spain in Case C-350/92 *Spain v Council* (for notification see OJ C260 9.10.92 p2) on the basis that it exceeds the Community's legal powers to extend intellectual property protection, that it is contrary to the Treaty provisions on the free movement of goods, and that the legal basis for such an extension should not in any event have been the harmonisation measure, article 100a of the EC Treaty. No further steps in the proceedings have as yet been taken.
2.   In particular Case C-181/82 *Roussel* [1983] ECR 3849, Case C-238/82 *Duphar* [1984] ECR 523.
3.   OJ C310 4.12.86 p7. See Appendix 17 post.
4.   OJ L214 24.8.93 p1. See Appendix 5 post.
5.   See Chapters 7 and 8 post.
6.   OJ L40 11.2.89. See Appendix 15 post.

minimum requirements to be followed by the Member States in respect of national systems : (a) requiring price approval prior to marketing (article 2); (b) requiring approval prior to price increases (article 3); (c) imposing price freezes on medicinal products (article 4); (d) controlling profitability of pharmaceutical companies (article 5); (e) reimbursing the costs of a medicinal product only if it is included on a list of approved products (article 6); (f) permitting the competent authorities to exclude medicinal products from reimbursement (article 7). The requirements did not fetter the discretion of the Member States to adopt such measures, but required that basic principles of good procedure should be observed and that the criteria for imposition of the various restrictions on price and/or reimbursement should be published. The Member States were required to adopt implementing measures by 31 December 1989 and the Commission was required to submit proposals by 31 December 1991 for further measures "leading towards the abolition of any remaining barriers to, or distortions of, the free movement of proprietary medicinal products, so as to bring this sector closer into line within the normal conditions of the internal market".

In practice, integration of the Community market is severely impeded by the unique characteristics of the pharmaceutical market, whereby price competition is fundamentally distorted by systematic intervention by the national social security systems and neither those who prescribe medicinal products nor those who consume them normally pay for those products themselves. Clearly, harmonisation of the national systems would at least create the same distortions in each national market and should therefore reduce the drastic variations in price between the national markets which currently exist. However, the Member States have widely divergent traditions in respect of these issues, from highly regulated markets relying on direct price controls to impose low prices entirely unrelated to market prices (for example, Portugal or Greece) to relatively unrestricted markets where controls over price or reimbursement operate either via reimbursement limited to reference prices set for products within a therapeutic category (for example, Germany and the Netherlands), or via controls over overall profitability of pharmaceutical companies (the United Kingdom). The national preference is of course related to varying national attitudes to the importance of the national pharmaceutical industry, the least regulated markets being in general those where the national industry is most successful.

The timetable for further progress on harmonisation of the pricing mechanisms of the Member States has now been abandoned. In a speech delivered on 1 December 1992 entitled "Making a reality of the single market : pharmaceutical pricing and the EEC", Sir Leon Brittan, Vice President of the Commission with responsibility for Competition, expressed the view that "at present, it is neither possible nor desirable to attempt widespread harmonisation in this sector"; he favoured "an evolutionary process leading to a gradual convergence of the national systems in so far as necessary to create a single market".

The result is that the Commission has now changed its tactics and on 2 March 1994, after extended discussions within Directorates III (responsible for industrial policy) and V (responsible for social policy) of the Commission and with the industry, the Commission issued a Communication to the Council and the European Parliament "on the outlines of an industrial policy for the pharmaceutical industry in the European Community"[1]. A Communication on such a topic, rather than on, for example, Community rules for pricing and reimbursement, indicates the extent to which the Commission has abandoned its earlier ambitions. In relation to price, the Commission now appears to favour the dismantling of direct price controls, which entirely nullify price competition, in favour of more general controls over cost on the German or British model. On the wider issue of the

---

1.   COM(93) 718 final.

industrial policy of the Community, the 1994 Communication is generally sympathetic to the interests of the pharmaceutical industry. However, the tension between industrial policy and the social function of the pharmaceutical industry has been central to the Community's interests in the sector since 1965[1] and will undoubtedly continue to be so.

1.4.3   Generic competitors and parallel importers

The most likely parties in any litigation concerning pharmaceutical products are (i) the manufacturer of an innovative product marketed under an original brand; (ii) a rival manufacturer seeking to market a similar or identical product on the expiry of relevant intellectual property protection; (iii) a distributor of the original product who wishes to "re-import" a product into the Member State where the original product was manufactured, to compete on price with the normal distribution channels for the product; (iv) a distributor of a product in substance identical to the original product, who wishes to import, whether or not in parallel to the normal distribution channels for the original product, the identical product into the Member State, to compete on price with the original product; and (v) the national regulator, who is very frequently caught in the cross-fire between the other parties, being accused by one or more of them of either refusing or granting authorisation, to parties (ii), (iii) or (iv), to market or distribute the products in question on a basis contrary to national or Community law.

It will be apparent that party (ii), the generic competitor, is a natural and inevitable feature of a market characterised by rapid innovation and therefore by elaborate intellectual property protection. By contrast, parties (iii) and (iv), normally classed together as "parallel importers", only exist because of price disparities between the Member States sufficient to justify the creation of new, and in many cases artificial, patterns of trade running in parallel to those of the normal distribution networks of the original manufacturer.

The extent to which an original manufacturer should be protected from generic competition, and the converse issue of the extent to which a generic competitor should be permitted to take advantage of the prior research and development efforts of the original manufacturer in obtaining authorisation to market his similar or identical product, are regulated by Regulation (EEC) 1768/92[2], and by special provisions in Directive (EEC) 65/65 in relation to so-called "abridged applications"[3].

The position of the parallel importer is more controversial. In May 1991, a report on "Impediments to Parallel Trade in Pharmaceuticals within the European Community" was prepared for Directorate-General IV of the Commission by REMIT Consultants, London[4]. The conclusions of the report were ambiguous : parallel trade is an entirely artificial economic phenomenon, resulting from price controls in one Member State driving down market prices so far that the parallel importer's costs and other disadvantages are less than the price difference between the price of the product in a low price and a high price market; facilitating parallel imports has certain obvious benefits in that it introduces a significant downward pressure on both costs and pricing by original manufacturers in high priced markets; but that effect can be argued to be counter-productive, in that it serves to align prices throughout the Community according to the artificially low prices imposed in the

---

1.   See Chapter 3 post.
2.   OJ L182 2.7.92 p1. See section 1.4.1 ante.
3.   See section 3.4.2 post.
4.   The REMIT report was published by the Commission in 1992 by the Office for Official Publications of the European Communities, Luxembourg. It contains a full description of the difficulties caused to original manufacturers by the parallel importer and of the impediments to parallel trade created by both the manufacturer and the national regulatory regimes.

most completely regulated markets. The report's final conclusion attacks the lack of market pricing that makes the parallel importer's trade possible :

> "Moreover, any measures aimed at facilitating or increasing parallel trade in pharmaceuticals while leaving in place the existing widely diverse and regulated national price regimes will not create a genuine single market in the Community. A market economy requires market pricing and market pricing creates the conditions under which prices converge to the point where parallel trade ceases to be profitable."[1]

Original manufacturers have sought to impede the activities of the parallel importer in every way open to them, leading to a series of legal confrontations. The original manufacturer has two principal weapons : intellectual property rights and the restrictive rules imposed by the Member States and the Community for marketing and manufacturing authorisations. National intellectual property rights have been upheld even where they impede trade between Member States, but they have been narrowly constrained by a series of judgments of the European Court of Justice under articles 30 and 85, so that in practice the parallel importer has frequently been able to evade such rights. Likewise, although article 36 of the EC Treaty itself provides for derogation from the principles of free movement of goods for "the protection of health and life of humans, animals or plants", the European Court of Justice has not been sympathetic to the argument that parallel imported products, in general substantially identical to those already marketed on the relevant market and significantly cheaper than the authorised product, should be excluded on such technical grounds[2].

A major difficulty potentially faced parallel importers, in that they were in general in no position, either commercially or technically, to satisfy the requirements of article 5 of Directive (EEC) 65/65, as implemented by national law, in relation to the detailed information required to be supplied for the purposes of marketing authorisation, and could also not in general satisfy the requirements of Directive (EEC) 75/319 in relation to the identification of the product[3]. Case C-104/75 *De Peijper*[4] in effect overruled the requirements of those Directives in such cases and, following the *De Peijper* ruling, the Commission issued a Communication on parallel imports of proprietary medicinal products for which marketing authorisations have already been granted[5], setting out its interpretation of the consequences of *De Peijper* (having been unable to obtain support for a Directive governing the issue). The *De Peijper* judgment and the Commission Communication have been followed by administrative changes in the practices of the Member States concerned (in practice, the United Kingdom, Germany, the Netherlands, Denmark and Ireland), enabling parallel importers to obtain product licences for the marketing of their products under certain less restrictive conditions than those ordinarily applied.

The *De Peijper* decision did not cater for every factual complication that may arise : other cases have followed[6], and there is every reason to suppose that test cases will

---

1. See p8 of the report, repeated at p84.
2. For a survey of recent case law, see Leigh Hancher, 'Creating the internal market for pharmaceutical medicines - an Echternach jumping procession?' (1991) 28 CMLRev 821; and 'The European Pharmaceutical Market : problems of partial harmonisation' (1990) 15 ELR 9.
3. See sections 3.2 and 10.2 post.
4. Case C-104/75 *De Peijper* [1976] ECR 613.
5. OJ C115 6.5.82 p5. See Appendix 16 post.
6. For example, Case C-347/89 *Freistaat Bayern v Eurim-Pharm* [1991] ECR I-1747 (products authorised in another Member State refused importation certificates into Germany because their labelling and package leaflet did not conform to German law, even though Eurim-Pharm was licensed in Germany to add such labelling and

continue to be brought in both the national and the Community courts by both manufacturers and parallel importers until such time as price levels in the Member States are harmonised. Likewise, generic suppliers will seek to impose pressure on the innovative manufacturer. As stated earlier, the relevant principles applicable to such cases are to be found in specialist works on competition law and the free movement of goods (and, even more specifically, on the protection of intellectual property rights).

1.4.4   Other issues

Apart from the major omissions of detailed discussions of the rules on competition and the free movement of goods, it should also be noted that the Community pharmaceutical legislation comprises not only the major texts discussed in this work but also a considerable body of technical material which does not raise difficulties of a legal kind but which is of the greatest importance to the industry, for example in preparation of technical dossiers for the national and Community authorities. In addition, the market for medicinal products for human use borders on a number of related areas and it should be borne in mind that those related areas are not considered in this work. The principal areas of omission are :

(1) Council Directive (EEC) 89/342 extending the scope of Directives (EEC) 65/65 and 75/319 and laying down additional provisions for immunological medicinal products consisting of vaccines, toxins or serums and allergens[1]; Council Directive (EEC) 89/343 extending the scope of Directives (EEC) 65/65 and 75/319 and laying down additional provisions for radiopharmaceuticals[2]; Council Directive (EEC) 89/381 extending the scope of Directives (EEC) 65/65 and 75/319 on the approximation of provisions laid down by law, regulation or administrative action relating to proprietary medicinal products and laying down special provisions for medicinal products derived from human blood or human plasma[3]; ("the extension Directives").

(2) Council Recommendations 83/571 and 87/176 concerning tests relating to the placing on the market of proprietary medicinal products[4]; those Recommendations set out very detailed guidelines for the application of the tests specified in the Annex to Directive (EEC) 75/318;

(3) Council Directive (EEC) 87/18 on the harmonisation of laws, regulations and administrative provisions relating to the application of the principles of good laboratory practice and the verification of their applications for tests on chemical substances[5]; and Council Directive (EEC) 88/320 on the inspection and verification of Good Laboratory Practice[6];

(4) Council Directive (EEC) 78/25 on the approximation of the laws of the Member States relating to the colouring matters which may be added to medicinal products[7];

---

package leaflets. The Bavarian authorities' conduct was held to be contrary to article 30 and unjustified under article 36). Compare Cases C-266 & 267/87 *R v Pharmaceutical Society of Great Britain, ex parte Association of Parallel Importers* [1989] ECR 1295 (national guidelines preventing the substitution of parallel imported products for prescribed products, even where the products were therapeutically identical, were upheld under article 36).

1.   OJ L142 25.5.89 p14.
2.   OJ L142 25.5.89 p16.
3.   OJ L189 28.6.89 p44.
4.   OJ L332 28.11.83 p11 and OJ L73 16.3.87 p1.
5.   OJ L15 17.1.87 p29.
6.   OJ L145 11.6.88 p35.
7.   OJ L11 14.11.78 p31.

(5) the numerous Guidelines issued by the Committee for Proprietary Medicinal Products on issues such as Quality, Safety, Efficacy, Good Manufacturing Practice, Good Clinical Practice, Biological and Biotechnology Products and on the Notice to Applicants; those guidelines are intended to give direct assistance to the pharmaceutical industry and to set out procedure to be followed by the national and Community regulatory bodies;

(6) veterinary medicinal products : the primary legislation is now Council Regulation (EEC) 2309/93[1], applying to veterinary medicines the rules discussed in Chapter 7 of this work; Council Directive (EEC) 81/851 on the approximation of the laws of the Member States relating to veterinary medicinal products[2]; and Directive (EEC) 81/852 on the approximation of the laws of the Member States relating to analytical, pharmaco-toxicological and clinical standards and protocols in respect of the testing of veterinary medicinal products[3]; the latter two Directives are now substantially amended, in parallel to the Future System legislation for products for human use, by Directive (EEC) 93/40 amending Directives (EEC) 81/851 and 81/852 on the approximation of the laws of the Member States relating to veterinary medicinal products[4];

(7) medical devices : these have recently become subject to Community rules; Council Directive (EEC) 90/385 on the approximation of the laws of the Member States relating to active implantable medical devices[5]; and Council Directive (EEC) 93/42 on the approximation of the law of the Member States relating to medical devices[6]; and

(8) the legal protection of biotechnological inventions : the Commission Communication on the outlines of an industrial policy for the pharmaceutical industry in the European Community[7] indicates that a Directive on this subject will be adopted in 1994.

In addition to the topics listed above, Chapter 2 makes it clear that other products, in particular foodstuffs and cosmetics, are not always easy to distinguish from medicinal products. Such products are again subject to specific rules that cannot be considered here.

1.5   Materials

The *Current EC Legal Developments Series* aspires to provide materials as well as analysis of recent legislation. In relation to pharmaceuticals, it is not possible to include everything within a single volume : the Commission published five volumes of such materials in 1989, and the number of volumes has now increased to seven (three of which concern veterinary products), even prior to the inclusion of the Future System legislation. *The Rules Governing Medicinal Products in the European Community*[8] are periodically updated and the latest versions available in May 1993 were, according to the latest Commission report on the operation of the Committee of Proprietary Medicinal Products, SEC(93) 771 :

---

1.   OJ L214 24.8.93 p1. See Appendix 5 post.
2.   OJ L317 6.11.81 p1.
3.   OJ L317 6.11.81 p16.
4.   OJ L214 24.8.93 p31.
5.   OJ L189 20.7.90 p17.
6.   OJ L169 12.7.93 p1.
7.   COM(93) 718 final, referred to at section 1.4.2 ante.
8.   EC Commission, Office for Official Publications of the European Communities, Luxembourg.

Volume I   The rules governing medicinal products for human use in the European Community (Principal legislation) 1991;

Volume II   Notice to applicants for marketing authorisations for medicinal products for human use in the Member States of the European Community (Second edition) 1989;

Volume III Guidelines on the quality, safety and efficacy of medicinal products for human use 1989; Addendum July 1990; Addendum 2 May 1992;

Volume IV   Good Manufacturing Practice 1991.

Volume IIA, replacing pages 1 to 47 of the existing Volume II, was published in July 1993; Volume IIB, replacing the remainder of the existing Volume II, will be produced in 1994 and Volume IIA will itself be replaced by a new Notice to Applicants for the purposes of the introduction of the Future System procedures on 1 January 1995. Volume IIB will remain valid under the Future System. Volume III in particular is continuously supplemented by CPMP guidelines on a wide variety of topics.

In the circumstances, I have attempted to provide sufficient materials for basic reference purposes and to make the more detailed analytical sections comprehensible but it has been necessary to be less than comprehensive in this respect as in others in order to produce a useful book of manageable size.

Chapter 2 : What is a "Medicinal Product" ?

2.1   The concept of "medicinal product" in Community law

Article 1(2) of Council Directive (EEC) 65/65[1] defines "medicinal product" as :

> "Any substance or combination of substances presented for preventing disease in human beings or animals.
>
> Any substance or combination of substances which may be administered to human beings or animals with a view to making a medical diagnosis or to restoring, correcting or modifying physiological functions in human beings or in animals is likewise considered a medicinal product."

Until 1 January 1992, the significance of this definition was limited in Community law by the fact that the substantive provisions of Directive (EEC) 65/65 in relation to product authorisation were limited by articles 2 and 3 of the Directive to "proprietary medicinal products", defined by article 1(1) as :

> "Any ready-prepared medicinal product placed on the market under a special name and in a special pack."

The effect was that other "medicinal products", as defined by article 1(2), as well as products falling outside the scope of the Community definition of "medicinal products" were not subject to the Community requirements in relation to authorisation. That has now been changed by Council Directive (EEC) 89/341[2], which provided that all new medicinal products (with only limited exceptions, set out in Chapter 3 below) should be subject to the Community rules from 1 January 1992 and that the rules should be progressively extended to existing medicinal products before 31 December 1992. The issue is considered in more detail in Chapter 3.

Nonetheless, even before 1 January 1992, the Community definition of medicinal product had acquired general importance from the fact that several Member States had used the Community definition as the basis for national definitions of products requiring authorisation before being marketed in that Member State or, more generally, of products subject to special conditions of supply (in particular in France the traditional pharmacists' monopoly over the supply of medicinal products had become based on the Community definition).

The European Court of Justice had therefore been asked to give rulings in a number of cases on the interpretation of article 1(2) of Directive (EEC) 65/65 :

—   Case C-227/82 *Van Bennekom* [1983] ECR 3883 (criminal proceedings in the Netherlands relating to the supply without registration as a medicinal product of vitamin and multi-vitamin tablets, pills and capsules)

---

1.   OJ No 22 9.2.65 p369/65. See Appendix 1 post.
2.   OJ L142 25.5.89 p11.

—   Case C-35/85 *Procureur de la République v Tissier* [1986] ECR 1207 (criminal proceedings in France relating to the manufacture and supply of "reagents" consisting of "carrier molecules" used in combination with a radioactive product for the purposes of medical diagnosis)

—   Case C-369/88 *Delattre* [1991] ECR I-1487 (criminal proceedings in France relating to breaches of the pharmacists' legal monopoly and rules on the advertising of medicinal products resulting from the supply of various slimming products, products to aid digestion and blood circulation, products to reduce itching and fatigue, and products to help customers stop smoking)

—   Case C-60/89 *Monteil and Samanni* [1991] ECR I-1547 (criminal proceedings in France in relation to breaches of the pharmacists' legal monopoly over the supply of medicinal products resulting from the supply of eosin and modified alcohol of a strength of 70 per cent used to clean the skin)

—   Case C-112/89 *Upjohn v Farzoo* [1991] ECR I-1703 (injunctive proceedings in the Netherlands relating to the supply without registration as a medicinal product of a product intended to counteract naturally occurring baldness in men)

Those rulings are now of general significance in relation to the application of the Community regulatory regime and the same principles have been applied and developed in subsequent cases :

—   Case C-290/90 *Commission v Germany* [1992] ECR I-3317 (article 169 proceedings against Germany for requiring authorisation as medicinal products for products imported from France and supplied for the cleansing of the eyes, in particular the removal of dust and chemical substances resulting from minor industrial accidents)

—   Case C-219/91 *Ter Voort* [1992] ECR I-5485 (penal proceedings in the Netherlands against an importer of herbal teas claimed, in brochures sent to purchasers, to have preventative or curative properties)

—   Case C-212/91 *Angelopharm v Freie und Manse Hamburg*[1] (proceedings for a declaration that a firm could lawfully produce and market another anti-baldness product, but under applicable EC and German *cosmetic* legislation; the Advocate-General considered the product in fact to be a medicinal product and the Court made its ruling subject to the principles established in *Upjohn*).

2.2   Difficulties of interpretation

The Community definition of "medicinal product" is complex. That complexity derives partly from the nature of the subject and partly from the approach adopted by the Community in drafting article 1(2) of Directive (EEC) 65/65.

Pharmaceutical products are in many cases scientifically sophisticated products and there are naturally difficulties in establishing legally satisfactory definitions in an area where scientific developments are frequently occurring; the concept "disease" is difficult to define precisely; the purpose of the Community legislation is necessarily complex, encompassing the protection of the consumer, the commercial and scientific interests of the Community in a strong pharmaceutical

---

1.   Not yet published in the ECR. (1994) Transcript 25 January, OJ C59 26.2.94 p2.

industry and the free movement of goods within the Community; finally, medicinal products are not clearly distinct from a number of other products, in particular from cosmetics, foodstuffs, various household products and medical devices. A useful discussion of the general issues of interpretation involved is to be found in the Opinions of the Advocates-General in the above cases, and in particular those of Advocate-General Lenz in the *Upjohn* case and Advocate-General Tesauro in the *Delattre* case.

In addition to those inevitable difficulties, the Community definition is itself complex in that it has two distinct elements whose interdependence is unclear and each of which uses distinct concepts to identify medicinal products from other products. The fact that there have now been eight cases where the Court has been obliged to consider the interpretation of article 1(2) of Directive (EEC) 65/65 is indicative of the complexity of the definitions.

2.3   The structure of article 1(2) of Directive (EEC) 65/65

2.3.1   The two definitions
The Court has repeatedly held that :

> "Directive 65/65 provides two definitions of the term "medicinal product" : one relating to presentation, the other to function. A product is medicinal if it falls within either of those definitions."[1]

Each of the two definitions is considered in more detail below but it is clear from the above quotation that each is independent of the other in the sense that it is sufficient, for a product to be classified as a medicinal product, that it satisfy either one of the definitions.

On the other hand, the Court has repeatedly stated that the two definitions are not wholly independent of one another :

> "It should be added that those two definitions cannot be regarded as strictly distinct from each other. As is stated in paragraph 22 of the judgment in Case C-227/82 *Van Bennekom* [1983] ECR 3883, a substance which is endowed with "properties for treating or preventing disease in human beings or animals" within the meaning of the first Community definition but is not "presented" as such falls within the scope of the second Community definition of a medicinal product."[2]

Strictly speaking, the Court's finding in *Van Bennekom* was simply to the effect that there is a class of products, namely those endowed with properties for treating or preventing disease but not "presented" as such (the component concepts of the two definitions are considered below), that falls outside the class of products captured by the first definition but within the class captured by the second definition. It does not follow from that fact that there is any overlap between the medicinal products identified under the first definition and those identified under the second definition. The connection derives rather from the fact that products that are *both* "presented" for the treatment or prevention of disease *and* "endowed" with such properties will be central examples of products captured by each of the definitions.

---

1.   *Upjohn* [1991] ECR I-1703, para 15 at I-1741; *Delattre* [1991] ECR I-1487, para 15 at I-1532; *Monteil* [1991] ECR I-1547, para 11 at I-1564; *Commission v Germany* [1992] ECR I-3317, para 9 at I-3345.
2.   *Delattre* [1991] ECR I-1487, para 16 at I-1532; *Monteil* [1991] ECR I-1547, para 12 at I-1564; *Upjohn* [1991] ECR I-1703, para 18 at I-1742 and *Commission v Germany* [1992] ECR I-3317, para 14 at 3346.

It is relatively straightforward to identify the category of products that is captured by the first definition but not by the second, namely products that are "presented" for the treatment or prevention of diseases but not "endowed" with such properties, ie "quack" products[1]. However, even that is not precisely correct. The second definition uses the concept of "administration" ... "with a view to making a medical diagnosis or to restoring, correcting or modifying physiological functions". There may well be products that are "presented" for the treatment or prevention of diseases which are *not* "endowed" with any such properties *but which are "endowed" with properties for the making of a medical diagnosis or the restoring, correcting or modifying of physiological functions*. Such products would be captured by both the first and second definitions. It is therefore only those products that are :

(1)   "presented" for the treatment or prevention of disease; and

(2)   *not* appropriate for "administration" with a view to making a medical diagnosis or to restoring, correcting or modifying physiological functions;

that will fall *within* the first definition *but outside* the second definition.

By contrast, there is a potentially very wide class of products that will fall outside the scope of the first definition but within the scope of the second definition. They include, using (in abbreviated form) the concepts of the two definitions :

—   products not presented as such but endowed with properties for the treatment or prevention of disease (the class identified by the Court in *Van Bennekom*);

—   products neither presented as such nor endowed with properties for the treatment or prevention of disease (if they fall within any of the other categories identified below);

—   products presented as suitable for administration for the purposes of medical diagnosis or to modify physiological functions (but not presented for the treatment or prevention of disease) and endowed with the appropriate properties;

—   products presented as suitable for administration for the purposes of medical diagnosis or to modify physiological functions (but not presented for the treatment or prevention of disease) but *not* in fact endowed with the appropriate properties (not all products in this category will necessarily be captured by the second definition but it seems probable that at least some will be);

—   products *not* presented as suitable for administration for the purposes of medical diagnosis or to modify physiological functions but in fact endowed with the appropriate properties (again it is not certain that all products in this category will be captured by the second definition but it again seems likely that at least some will be).

It is only those products that are *neither* presented as suitable for administration for the purposes of medical diagnosis or to modify physiological functions *nor* endowed with the appropriate properties that clearly fall outside the scope of the second definition. The likelihood of products falling within the various categories under the second definition is considered at 2.5 below.

---

1.   See *Van Bennekom* [1983] ECR 3883, para 2 of the Advocate-General's Opinion at 3910 : "[the first definition] aims to combat quackery".

2.3.2 The priority of the definition of "medicinal products" over other Community definitions

Although difficult questions may arise in determining whether or not a specific product is a medicinal product, a cosmetic or a foodstuff (or perhaps even a household material or a medical device), the Court is clear that the concept of medicinal product cannot be excluded by other definitions. The reasoning of the Court is contained in the *Delattre, Monteil* and *Upjohn* cases in relation to cosmetic products :

> "the legal rules applicable to proprietary medicinal products are stricter than those applicable to cosmetic products, in view of the particular risks to public health which the former may represent and which are not generally displayed by cosmetic products."[1]

The same reasoning would certainly apply in relation to foodstuffs and was implicit in both the *Van Bennekom* case, where the other possible classification of vitamin products was as foodstuffs, and the *Delattre* case, where it was arguable that at least some of the products were in fact foodstuffs.

The Community rules on medicinal products would clearly take precedence in general over the limited rules concerning domestic products (the only area where there might be doubt would be where there was an overlap between medicinal products and domestic products covered by consumer protection legislation or legislation covering toxic products or environmental assessment).

It is only the case of medical devices, where they are themselves subject to strict Community rules (recently updated by Council Directive (EEC) 93/42[2]) and where it is clear that the Community intends to lay down a clear division between the two classes of products and to subject each to an appropriate regulatory scheme, that there may be some doubt whether either scheme is *prior* to the other.

The difficulties that have arisen or likely to arise are considered in more detail at 2.7 below.

2.4 The presentation criterion

> "Any substance or combination of substances presented for treating or preventing disease in human beings or animals."

2.4.1 Substance

The concept of substance is defined at article 1(3) of Directive (EEC) 65/65 :

> "Any matter irrespective of origin which may be :
>
> — human, eg human blood and human blood products;
> — animal, eg micro-organisms, whole animals, parts of organs, animal secretions, toxins, extracts, blood products, etc;
> — vegetable, eg micro-organisms, plants, parts of plants, vegetable secretions, extracts, etc;
> — chemical, eg elements, naturally occurring chemical materials and chemical products obtained by chemical change or synthesis."

---

1. *Upjohn* [1991] ECR I-1703, para 31 at I-1744; *Delattre* [1991] ECR I-1487, para 21 at I-1533; *Monteil* [1991] ECR 1547, para 16 at I-1565; and Advocate-General Jacobs' Opinion in *Angelopharm*, para 5.
2. OJ L169 12.7.93 p1.

That definition has not been the subject of legal challenge or interpretation in the Community courts. It is, if taken literally, very broad in its terms (and could apparently include metal or wooden objects and even possibly intangible objects such as electricity - or money!) but the context of Directive (EEC) 65/65 strongly indicates that the Community legislator had two types of product in mind : those taken internally for the treatment or diagnosis of medical conditions (to use a neutral term); and those taken externally for the same purpose; more concretely, solid and liquid preparations taken orally or as suppositories, substances injected into the bloodstream, and substances applied to the surface of the body, normally in the form of creams or ointments. The examples given in article 1(3) are of substances that would naturally form part of such products and recital 3 of Directive (EEC) 65/65 refers to :

"medicinal products (excluding substances or combinations of substances which are food, animal feeding-stuffs or toilet preparations)".

That strongly suggests that the purpose of the definitions in article 1 is to distinguish medicinal products from foodstuffs and cosmetics, rather than from all other objects.

2.4.2 Presentation
The concept of presentation was considered by the Court in the *Van Bennekom* case :

"it should be observed that the directive, by basing itself, in the first Community definition of a medicinal product, on the criterion of the product's "presentation", is designed to cover not only medicinal products having a genuine therapeutic or medical effect but also those which are not sufficiently effective or which do not have the effect which consumers would be entitled to expect in view of their presentation. The directive thereby seeks to preserve consumers not only from harmful or toxic medicinal products as such but also from a variety of products used instead of the proper remedies. For that reason, the concept of the "presentation" of a product must be broadly construed.

It is therefore necessary to take the view that a product is "presented for treating or preventing disease" within the meaning of Directive 65/65 not only when it is expressly "indicated" or "recommended" as such, possibly by means of labels, leaflets or oral representation, but also whenever any averagely well-informed consumer gains the impression, which, provided it is definite, may even result from implication, that the product in question should, regard being had to its presentation, have an effect such as is described by the first part of the Community definition.

In particular, the external form given to the product in question - such as that of a tablet, pill or capsule - may in this connection serve as strong evidence of the seller's or manufacturer's intention to market that product as a medicinal product. Such evidence cannot, however, be the sole or conclusive evidence, since otherwise certain food products which are traditionally presented in a similar form to pharmaceutical products would also be covered."[1]

Van Bennekom was followed and developed in the *Delattre* and *Monteil* cases, in particular in relation to the external form given to the product :

"In the first place, form must be taken to mean not only the form of the product itself (tablets, pills or capsules) but also that of the packaging of the product, which may, for reasons of marketing policy, tend to make it resemble a

---

1.   Case-227/82 *Van Bennekom*, [1983] ECR 3883, paras 17 to 19 at 3900 to 3901.

medicinal product. In the second place, account must be taken of the attitude of an averagely well-informed consumer, in whom the form given to a product may inspire particular confidence similar to that normally inspired in him by a proprietary medicinal product, having regard to the safeguards normally associated with the manufacture and marketing of the latter type of product.

In those circumstances, a product may be regarded as a medicinal product by virtue of its presentation if its form and the manner in which it is packaged render it sufficiently similar to a medicinal product and, in particular, if on its packing and the information provided with it reference is made to research by pharmaceutical laboratories or to methods or substances developed by medical practitioners or even to testimonials from medical practitioners commending the qualities of the product in question. A statement that a product is not a medicinal product is persuasive evidence which the national court may take into consideration, but it is not in itself conclusive."[1]

These guidelines were further extended in the *Ter Voort* judgment. In that case, it was agreed that the herbal teas at issue were generally regarded as a foodstuff, that they had no known therapeutic effect and that the actual packaging of the products did not claim such properties. However, the Court considered that claims to preventative or curative properties in written material, sent on request to purchasers of the product, were sufficient to demonstrate an intention to market the products as medicines and thus to bring the products within the scope of article 1(2) of Directive (EEC) 65/65. It was only where such an assessment originated from a third party wholly independent of the manufacturer or vendor that such an intention could be excluded[2].

The Court has thus given relatively detailed guidance on what does and does not count as "presentation as a medicinal product". It is a matter of fact to be decided by a national court on a case by case basis[3] but relevant factors are :

— express assertions or denials that a product is a medicinal product, whether in leaflets, labelling, oral representations, or even written advice supplied on request after purchase;

— implied representations deriving from the external form of the product itself (for example, pills, tablets or capsules), from the packaging of the product, or from more specific aspects of its presentation such as references to pharmaceutical research, methods used or products produced by medical practitioners or even recommendations from medical practitioners;

— as one general test, whether the product is packaged or otherwise marketed sufficiently similarly to a medicinal product that a reasonably well-informed consumer would be inspired with that particular confidence in the product that he feels in a medicinal product in the light of the special safeguards covering the manufacture and marketing of such products;

— as another general test, whether in all the circumstances the seller or manufacturer intends to market the product as a medicinal product : see in particular *Van Bennekom* and *Ter Voort*.

1.   *Delattre* [1991] ECR I-1487, paras 40 and 41 at I-1536 to I-1537; *Monteil* [1991] ECR I-1547, paras 23 and 24 at I-1566 to 1567.
2.   *Ter Voort* [1992] ECR I-5485, in particular paras 28 to 31 at I-5511 to I-5512.
3.   See section 2.6 post.

It should be noted that those guidelines depend crucially on the idea of a "medicinal product" as part of the guidelines. That might appear to be a circular definition, but it is not in fact so. In that connection, a remark of Advocate-General Lenz in his Opinion in the *Upjohn* case is relevant (albeit that he was there discussing the application of the second definition) :

> "Even if that central core of products whose status as medicinal products is in no doubt cannot always be helpful as a standard of comparison where preparations with completely new effects are concerned, such a comparison should nevertheless at least facilitate classification for most products."[1]

The Court is using the concept of "medicinal product" in a similar way in its discussions of the "presentation criterion". It is legitimate and necessary to look at the normal case of a medicinal product - what it looks like, how it is marketed, what attitude to the product is held by a reasonably well-informed consumer - in order to assess whether a marginal case has or has not been "presented" on the market as another medicinal product. In the normal case, one is not relying solely or even principally on the "presentation" of the product, so no circularity is involved.

Such tests may clearly be very difficult for a court to apply in practice and there may be more subtle issues of marketing strategy than those as yet identified by the Court. An obvious example would be a selective distribution system used by a manufacturer of a product having no special therapeutic qualities but which the manufacturer attempts to sell only or predominantly through pharmacists (the converse of the French pharmacists' monopoly cases). If such a system was acceptable under the Community competition rules (a matter that falls outside the scope of this work) then that marketing strategy might be relevant to an assessment of whether a reasonably well-informed consumer would feel special confidence in the product.

2.4.3 Treatment or prevention of disease

The issues of treatment and prevention have not been separately considered by the Court in any of the cases in which it has interpreted the first definition. Those issues arise more naturally in relation to the second "functional" definition but the question naturally arises whether any particular modes of treatment or prevention of disease are intended to be included or excluded by the definition, in particular whether it is correct to assume that Directive (EEC) 65/65 is in fact limited to pharmaceutical products or whether products that are presented as achieving their ends by mechanical or psychological means might be included. Article 1(2) of the Directive is not helpful in this regard but the preamble expressly refers to the pharmaceutical industry at recital 2 and guidance is also obtained from the Directives on medical devices, where such devices are defined broadly but so as to limit the concept of medical device to a product :

> "which does not achieve its principal intended action in or on the human body by pharmacological, immunological or metabolic means, but which may be assisted in its function by such means"[2].

It is reasonably clear that a pair of crutches, an X-ray machine and a copper bracelet are none of them "presented for the treatment or prevention of disease" within the meaning of article 1(2). Condoms have been expressly stated to be medical devices within the scope of Directive (EEC) 93/42 in response to a question in the European Parliament[3].

---

1. *Upjohn* [1991] ECR I-1703, para 76 of the Opinion at I-1732.
2. Article 1(2)(a) of Directive (EEC) 93/42, OJ L169 12.7.93 p4.
3. OJ C232 5.9.91 p26.

On the other hand, it is equally clear, both from the wording of Directive (EEC) 93/42 and from the *Tissier* judgment, that pharmaceutical products used in combination with medical devices of a more or less mechanical kind are "medicinal products" : see article 1(3), (4) and (5) of the Directive, discussed in more detail below.

2.4.4 Disease

Until the judgment of the Court in *Delattre*, there was considerable room for doubt as to the meaning of the word "disease" as it appeared in article 1(2) of Directive (EEC) 65/65. Although the concept of "disease" is a familiar one, the precise limits of the medical or physiological conditions captured by that concept are not easy to draw. Are the symptoms of such conditions themselves diseases, for example pain or fatigue ? Is insomnia or baldness a disease ? Could infertility, or fertility, be a disease ? Could it be a disease to be physically underdeveloped, so that growth promoting products were captured by the first definition ? Could the mere capacity to feel pain be a disease, so that anaesthetics could come within the scope of the first definition (and therefore products *presented* as anaesthetics but in fact having no such properties) ?

Those difficult issues were considered by Advocate-General Tesauro in his Opinion in the *Delattre* case[1] and by Advocate-General Lenz in his Opinion in the *Upjohn* case[2]. Advocate-General Tesauro reached some tentative positive conclusions :

> "I shall rule out the possibility that there might be a precise and exhaustive Community, and in more general terms a legal, concept of illness, it being a term which is used in numerous Community instruments and doubtless has a similar meaning in all the Member States. Essentially, I do not think we can go far beyond the common meaning of the term and consider pathological conditions of the human organism, which for that very reason require medical treatment and recourse to products which provide a specific remedy.

> On the other hand, particular physiological conditions, such as mere tiredness (resulting from physical or mental effort) or bad digestion (due to bad eating habits) cannot reasonably - and I refer to common experience rather than common sense - be regarded intrinsically as illnesses. It seems to me that the question submitted by the national court on this point is almost rhetorical.

> It is indeed true that tiredness or indigestion may also be a symptom or effect of a pathological condition; however, in such cases products made from natural substances, which merely amount to a food supplement designed to promote the proper functioning of the body, will certainly not provide an adequate remedy for the pathological condition in question : the primary need will be for products - medicinal products - which treat the illness itself and do not merely provide relief from the tiredness which it causes."

The Court followed the Advocate-General's suggestions in the *Delattre* judgment. At paragraph 12 of the judgment, the Court merely points out that there is no definition of illness or disease laid down by Directive (EEC) 65/65 :

> "The only possible definitions for those terms are those most commonly accepted on the basis of scientific knowledge."[3]

---

1.   [1991] ECR I-1487, para 11 of the Opinion at I-1515 and I-1516.
2.   [1991] ECR I-1703, paras 25 to 28 of the Opinion at 1719 and 1720.
3.   [1991] ECR I-1487 at I-1531.

At paragraph 32, it states that the Member States must take account of "the results of international scientific research and, in particular, the work of specialised Community committees".

The Advocate-General does not make it clear, in the passage cited above, whether he considers that ambiguous symptoms such as tiredness or bad digestion can *never* be regarded as diseases (because of their ambiguity) so that products presented for the prevention or treatment of such symptoms could never fall within the scope of the first definition, and he was followed in this by the Court at paragraphs 33 and 34 of the judgment in *Delattre* :

> "The third point raised is whether a product presented as being intended to counteract certain sensations or states such as hunger, heaviness in the legs, tiredness or itching is a medicinal product within the meaning of Directive 65/65.
>
> Such states or sensations are in themselves ambiguous. They may be the symptoms of a disease or illness and, combined with other clinical signs, may reveal a pathological condition. Alternatively, as in the case of short-lived tiredness or a need for nourishment, they may have no pathological significance. A reference to such states or sensations in the presentation of a product is therefore not decisive."[1]

Advocate-General Lenz was more explicit in his Opinion in *Upjohn*. His discussion of the concept of "disease" occurs in his analysis of why there are two definitions of medicinal product in Directive (EEC) 65/65, responding to a suggestion that the second definition should itself be limited to products to be administered for the treatment or prevention of disease. Advocate-General Lenz's analysis was to the effect that the second definition is precisely intended to capture products for the treatment of conditions that could *not* be considered as diseases (as well as products not presented as such). He considers first the examples of hair restorers (the products at issue in *Upjohn* itself) and then contraceptive products :

> "The condition which such products are intended to avert - pregnancy - is not a disease (unless human reproduction is taken to be only the result of recurring illness)."[2]

He next considers products for the control of :

> "physiological functions or manifestations present in all human beings (among others, heartbeat, blood pressure, blood supply to organs and glandular function) ... The boundary between (still) "healthy" and (already) "diseased" is not always obvious. It is often not immediately possible to determine whether a product capable in such cases of correcting an impairment up to a certain degree but not covering the whole range of the disease, including the most serious forms, is a product for treating disease."[3]

He then considers pain relievers, which again may or may not be connected with anything that could reasonably be called "disease". Finally, he mentions products such as narcotics, which are clearly considered by the Community to be medicinal products in certain forms, but which the Advocate-General describes as performing "certain ancillary functions in a medical context, though they are not of direct use for treating or preventing disease". In all those cases, the Advocate-General's clear view is that the products presented as appropriate for the treatment of conditions

---

1.   [1991] ECR I-1487 at I-1535.
2.   *Upjohn* [1991] ECR I-1703, para 25 of the Opinion at I-1720.
3.   *Upjohn* [1991] ECR I-1703, para 26 of the Opinion at I-1720.

which are either clearly not diseases or which are ambiguous, should not be considered under the first definition but rather under the broader terms of the second definition.

The Court in *Upjohn* did not enter into any detailed discussion of the matters raised by Advocate-General Lenz, but it did apparently support his reasoning in that it decisively rejected any necessary connection between the concept of medicinal product and that of disease and specifically stated that the second definition could apply to products that did not treat or prevent "diseases" :

> "But products which alter physiological functions in the absence of disease, such as contraceptive substances, also fall within the scope of [the second] definition."[1]

2.5   The function criterion

> "Any substance or combination of substances which may be administered to human beings or animals with a view to making a medical diagnosis or to restoring, correcting or modifying physiological functions in human beings or in animals is likewise considered a medicinal product."

2.5.1   The status of the definition

The status of the second definition of medicinal product has been variously interpreted by the Court and in particular by the Advocates-General who have considered article 1(2) of Directive (EEC) 65/65. In the *Van Bennekom* case, Advocate-General Rozès described the second definition as "merely ancillary in character" considering only the case of products with toxic properties and therefore which posed a threat to health but which were not "presented as a medicine" ie the products identified at paragraph 22 of the *Van Bennekom* judgment as falling within the second definition[2]. Subsequent cases, in particular the *Tissier* and *Upjohn* cases, have greatly increased the importance of the second definition and, in *Commission v Germany*[3], Advocate-General Van Gerven went so far as to say that the second definition was logically prior to the first definition, it being necessary to decide on the meaning of "medicinal product" before one could decide whether something was "presented" as a medicinal product.

The wording of article 1(2) itself suggests that the original drafter of Directive (EEC) 65/65 may have intended the second definition to be subsidiary ("is likewise considered a medicinal product") but in practice the most likely area for legal dispute is precisely where the person responsible for putting the product on the market seeks to avoid the Community rules on medicinal products and therefore does not "present" the product as such a product. That was the case in each of the cases considered by the Court (in the *Commission v Germany* case, the issue arose in a slightly different context, of article 169 proceedings rather than national litigation, but the issue was in substance the same; a French company wished to market a product in Germany without being subject to the rules applicable to medicinal products). In practice, therefore, the first definition is only likely to apply to a limited class of cases where the supplier unintentionally "presents" the products in a way suitable for a medicinal product, whereas the second definition will apply in every case where a product has certain properties (to be defined) regardless of how it is marketed. It appears also that the second definition may also apply in a further limited class of case where the supplier claims unjustifiably that the product has certain properties (see below).

---

1.   *Upjohn* [1991] ECR I-1703, para 19 at I-1742.
2.   See section 2.3.1 ante.
3.   *Commission v Germany* [1992] ECR I-3317, para 6 of the Opinion at I-3335.

The current position is therefore that the second definition is potentially extremely broad in its application and the wording of the definition makes it difficult to limit its scope in any satisfactory way.

2.5.2 Substance
The definition of "substance" contained in article 1(3) of Directive (EEC) 65/65 was considered at section 2.4.1.

2.5.3 Administration
The wording of the second definition is different from that of the first definition and it was confirmed by the Court in *Upjohn* that the difference in wording was deliberate and significant[1] :

The concept of "substance or combination of substances" is the same as in the first definition but instead of the idea of "presentation" the second definition employs the idea of a product "which may be administered with a view to" achieving certain effects on human beings or animals. The concept of "administration" itself appears to be relatively straightforward : as with the ideas of treatment and prevention discussed at section 2.4.3, the concept of administration is naturally linked to the traditional modes of application of pharmaceutical products, namely swallowing or otherwise ingesting, injection into the bloodstream, application to the human body in the form of a cream or an ointment, etc. It does not mean irradiation or mechanical application.

Another possibility which can be discounted is *improper* administration, for example a child swallowing an antiseptic cream. That was considered by Advocate-General Lenz in *Upjohn* :

> "the only effects to be considered are those which the product has when applied to the part of the body to which, in the judgment of the average user, it is to be administered ... That limitation is clear, in the first place, from the wording of the second part of the definition in Directive 65/65, which focuses on the administration of the product, that is to say an act whereby its specific properties are to be intentionally rendered operative. There can, however, be no question that a product is administered if, contrary to its intended purpose - accidentally, for example - it is applied to a part of the human body other than that for which it is destined. That approach is borne out by article 5 of the directive, under which authorisation to market the product is to be refused if it is harmful "in the normal conditions of use"[2]. Effects which may arise when a product is applied to a part of the body other than the proper place should therefore not be taken into consideration. Otherwise, many products which are manifestly not medicinal products would have to be classified as such (nail varnishes, for example, which contain solvents)."[3]

Similar considerations apply to the words "may be" in the second definition. There are a number of products which *may be* administered to human beings and animals and which would have certain spectacular effects on their physiological functions but which would not be regarded by anyone as medicinal products. The most obvious examples are poisons. On the principles enunciated by Advocate-General Lenz, it is necessary to imply either into the concept of administration as it appears in the definition or into the words "may be" some idea of therapeutic intention :

---

1. See the discussion of the Court's judgment and of Advocate-General Lenz's analysis of article 1(2) at section 2.4.4 ante.
2. "That expression has, however, a rather wider meaning than the criterion of the proper place of application to be borne in mind here. It also covers, in particular, the frequency and duration of administration."
3. *Upjohn* [1991] ECR I-1703, para 63 of the Opinion at I-1729.

administration with an intention to kill or injure is not administration within the meaning of the definition. The point also arises in relation to the words "with a view to ..." discussed below.

The Court in *Upjohn* did not comment specifically on this issue; it simply used a form of words somewhat more explicit than those used in article 1(2) itself :

"The second definition, however refers to the function of medicinal products; it covers all products which are intended to restore, correct or modify physiological functions and which may thus have an effect on health in general."[1]

The words used by the Court telescope the words "may be administered with a view to" into the concept of intention. In the context of the legislation, with its primary aim of protecting public health, it can be assumed that the intention of the person administering the product can be broadly classified as "therapeutic". If that is correct then ill-informed and malicious administration as well as accidental administration of the product can be ignored. Advocate-General Lenz referred to article 5 of Directive (EEC) 65/65 in relation to "normal conditions of use" to justify a restrictive concept of true administration; article 5 also supports the idea that administration should be administration with a therapeutic intention, since authorisation for a medicinal product which lacks "therapeutic efficacy" must be refused.

2.5.4   Medical diagnosis

The *Tissier* judgment is important for two reasons in the interpretation of the second definition. First, it is the only judgment of the Court that concerned diagnostic pharmaceuticals. Secondly, it is the only judgment of the Court that concerned "non-active" medicinal products. That second point resolves an important question in relation to the scope of the Community pharmaceutical legislation; it is implicit in the requirements for authorisation of medicinal products under Directive (EEC) 65/65 that it is not only the active ingredients of a medicinal product which must be verified by the manufacturer but also the other ingredients used to compose the marketed product. In that regard, the essential question is not of course the therapeutic efficacy of the product, since it has none, but the quality of the product and its lack of harmful effects (see paragraph 27 of the judgment, cited below).

On the first point, the Court determined that although the first definition did not apply, the second definition, as a part of the whole definition set out in article 1(2) :

"may not be interpreted restrictively but must be construed as including substances which are not administered as they are to human beings or animals but which are manufactured separately and are intended to be used mixed with other substances, either as a simple combination of substances or after chemical transformation, or as a carrier substance.

In this regard it is also irrelevant whether such a substance is made available to the public or sold only to radiologists working in hospitals or in private practice; users should be able to rely on the quality of the substance without having to carry out checks when mixing it with other substances for administering to human beings or animals.

The answer to the question raised must therefore be that a substance which is not presented for treating or preventing disease in human beings or animals

---

1.   *Upjohn* [1991] ECR I-1703, para 17 at I-1741; see also para 32 at I-1745; *Delattre* [1991] ECR I-1487, para 22 at I-1533; and *Monteil* [1991] ECR I-1547, para 17 at I-1565.

but which is used for making medical diagnoses on them must be regarded as a medicinal product within the meaning of article 1 of Council Directive 65/65 of 26 January 1965 in so far as it is intended to be administered to human beings or animals, either on its own or mixed with other substances."[1]

The Court's ruling is not entirely satisfactory in that it might appear that water and many other common chemicals would thereby be classified as medicinal products (on the basis that water etc frequently form part of a product to be administered to human beings with the relevant intention) but the answer to the defect in the Court's definition must be to the effect that a product will only be a "medicinal product" where it is an intermediate product of some kind whose properties will have a significant impact on the characteristics of the end product. It should also be noted that the ruling again uses the concept of intention as the Court's interpretation of the words "may be" and "with a view to" in the second definition[2].

2.5.5   Restoration, correction or modification of physiological functions
The delineation of which products do and which products do not satisfy the last element of the second definition is an extremely difficult problem. Even if the difficulties of intention and administration discussed above at section 2.5.3 are dismissed and it can be assumed that the product is being administered correctly with a therapeutic intention, it is far from obvious that medicinal products are the only products that are so administered with a view to the restoration, correction or modification of physiological functions. Even if the more restrictive criterion of the first definition is used, it is not obvious that the correct products are uniquely identified :

> "Even if the inquiry is restricted to those products which may help to prevent or treat illness, the range of antiseptic and antibacterial products is still very extensive. It includes both ordinary soaps, which no-one classifies as medicinal products, and powerful antiseptics used in surgery which cannot be classified as anything other than medicinal products."[3]

The Court has made certain very general attempts to offer guidance to national courts and national authorities in their assessments on a case by case basis of whether a product satisfies the second criterion. In *Van Bennekom*[4], the Court distinguished between the consumption of vitamins in small quantities as "an essential part of the daily diet ... indispensable for the proper functioning of the body" and the use of vitamins "generally in large doses, for therapeutic purposes in combating certain diseases other than those of which the morbid cause is a vitamin deficiency". In the former case, vitamins were not generally medicinal products; in the latter they were. However, the Court was not prepared to offer any *definition* of medicinal products, in so far as the concept applied to vitamins, in terms of concentration alone, but merely gave the very general answer that :

> "the classification of a vitamin as a medicinal product within the meaning of the second part of the definition in Directive 65/65 must be carried out case by case, having regard to the pharmacological properties of each such vitamin to the extent to which they have been established in the present state of scientific knowledge."[5]

That approach has been followed and expanded in the *Monteil* and *Upjohn* cases. In his Opinion in the *Delattre* case, given on the same day as his Opinion in the

---

1.   *Tissier* [1986] ECR 1207, paras 26 to 28 at 1216 to 1217.
2.   See section 2.5.3 above.
3.   *Monteil* [1991] ECR 1547, para 25 at I-1567.
4.   [1983] ECR 3883, paras 25 to 29 at 3902 to 3903.
5.   *Van Bennekom* [1983] ECR 3883, para 29 at 3903.

Monteil case and referred to in the latter Opinion, Advocate-General Tesauro attempted to isolate medicinal products by reason of their action on "pathological" conditions as against the action of foodstuffs and cosmetics and to use the Community Directives applying to foodstuffs and cosmetics as guidelines in determining the somewhat arbitrary boundaries between the three concepts[1].

That approach was not followed by the Court except in so far as it allowed that the cosmetics legislation might be relevant "in dubious cases"[2]. The second definition was not considered in any detail in the *Delattre* judgment, and in *Monteil* the Court's clearest point was the negative one cited above, that in terms of function, "ordinary soaps" as well as "powerful antiseptics used in surgery" could be said to prevent or treat illness and thus to come within the scope of the functional definition of medicinal product.

The Court's only positive suggestion was to note that, according to the Member States, the products in question are :

> "known and used to varying extents, are used under diverse conditions and are supplemented by different adjuvants."[3]

The Court implies that it should be possible to distinguish between medicinal products and, in this context, household cleaning agents by reference to such background facts. That is confirmed in *Monteil* :

> "Consequently, it is for the national authorities to determine, subject to review by the courts, whether or not eosin of a strength of 2% and modified alcohol of a strength of 70% constitute medicinal products by virtue of their function within the meaning of the second subparagraph of article 1(2) of Directive 65/65. In that regard, account must be taken of the adjuvants also entering into the composition of the product, the manner in which it is used, the extent of its distribution, its familiarity to consumers and the risks which its use may entail."[4]

Those are clearly extremely general guidelines which give the national authorities a wide margin of appreciation and they are prefaced by remarks by the Court emphasising the extent to which the Member States do indeed retain the right to make differing classifications of products until harmonisation is more complete[5].

Both Advocate-General Tesauro in the *Delattre* and *Monteil* cases and Advocate-General Lenz in the *Upjohn* case attempted to give more detailed guidance to the national authorities. Advocate-General Lenz ultimately settled for the idea that :

> "a product is a medicinal product if it has an exceptional effect on physiological functions and therefore constitutes a risk to public health sufficient to justify the application of the authorisation system laid down in Directive 65/65."[6]

That is obviously a lame conclusion which the Advocate-General only felt able to supplement by the idea that reference should be made to central cases of both

---

1. See *Delattre* [1991] ECR I-1487, paras 7 to 11 of the Opinion at I-1512 to I-1517, and the discussion of foodstuffs and cosmetics below.
2. *Delattre*, para 20 at I-1533, *Monteil* [1991] ECR 1547, para 15 at I-1565.
3. *Monteil* [1991] ECR 1547, para 26, pI-1567.
4. [1991] ECR I-1547, para 29 at I-1568.
5. See section 2.6 post.
6. *Upjohn* [1991] ECR I-1703, para 86(2)(b) of the Opinion at I-1735; see also paras 66 to 70 at I-1729 to I-1731.

medicinal products and cosmetic products to provide guidance as to whether a borderline case should be considered to be one or the other[1]. That idea was considered in relation to the concept of "presentation" at section 2.4.2.

The Court in *Upjohn* attempted to be slightly more explicit at paragraphs 18 to 22 of the judgment :

> "a substance which is endowed with properties "for treating or preventing disease in human beings or animals" within the meaning of the first part of the Community definition, but which is not presented as such, falls within the scope of the second part of the Community definition of a medicinal product.
>
> But products which alter physiological functions in the absence of disease, such as contraceptive substances, also fall within the scope of that definition.
>
> Furthermore, the fact that the provision uses the expression "with a view to" means that the definition of a medicinal product may include not only products which have a real effect on physiological functions but also those which do not have the advertised effect, thereby enabling public authorities to prevent the marketing of such products in order to protect consumers.
>
> As regards the meaning of "restoring, correcting or modifying physiological functions", it is clear from the aim of health protection pursued by the Community legislature that the phrase must be given a sufficiently broad interpretation to cover all substances capable of having an effect on the actual functioning of the body.
>
> However, that criterion does not serve to include substances such as certain cosmetics which, while having an effect on the human body, do not significantly affect the metabolism and thus do not strictly modify the way in which it functions."[2]

Those final two paragraphs are the furthest the Court has been prepared to go in offering a *definition* of medicinal product in terms of function. The idea seems to be to give an extremely broad interpretation to the concept but to subject in to some sort of "de minimis" rule. It obviously leaves it open to the national courts and authorities to judge for themselves what degree of effect on "the actual functioning of the body" is sufficient to make a product a medicinal product. It equally clearly depends on strict application of the ideas discussed above in relation to "administration", that the product should be properly applied with a therapeutic purpose. Otherwise, many household products, carelessly or maliciously applied, could be said to affect the actual functioning of the body in a way that could not be dismissed as "de minimis".

The guidelines actually given to the national authorities by the Court in *Upjohn* are similar to those in *Monteil* :

> "It is for the national courts to determine on a case-by-case basis the classification of each product having regard to its pharmacological properties as they may be ascertained in the current state of scientific knowledge, to the way in which it is used, to the extent to which it is sold and to consumers' familiarity with it."[3]

---

1.   *Upjohn* [1991] ECR I-1703, paras 76 to 77 of the Opinion at I-1732.
2.   [1991] ECR I-1703 at I-1742.
3.   [1991] ECR I-1703, para 23 at I-1743.

Those factors again leave the national authorities, subject to review by the courts, with a wide margin of appreciation. However, helpful guidance in the application of the *Upjohn* criteria (in particular paragraph 23 above) is now available in the Opinion of Advocate-General Jacobs in *Angelopharm*, delivered on 16 June 1993. At paragraphs 22 to 28 he came to the clear conclusion, on the facts available to him, that :

> "a product which is used with a view to preventing hair loss, or restoring hair growth, by inhibiting the production or effects of a hormone occurring naturally in the tissue of the scalp, is a product which is intended to have an effect on the physiological functioning of the body."

He rejected any narrow construction of the words used in *Upjohn* ("significantly affect the metabolism"). The Court was content, at paragraphs 14 to 16 of its judgment, to refer to the *Upjohn* principles without discussing the facts of *Angelopharm* in any detail. If Advocate-General Jacobs' approach is followed in future, then it appears that the second limb of article 1(2) will indeed be wide in its scope.

2.5.6   "Presentation" under the second definition

It might be thought, given that the first definition exists and that it ties the concept of "presentation" to the relatively precise concepts of the treatment and prevention of disease, that it must have been the intention of the Community legislator to limit the products captured by the "presentation" criterion to those products captured by the first definition. If that was not the case, then it is hard to see why the first definition was not worded in the same broad way as the second definition, ie :

> "Any substance or combination of substances presented as capable of being administered to human beings or animals with a view to making a medical diagnosis or to restoring, correcting or modifying physiological functions in human beings or in animals."

However, once it has been accepted, as the Court has made clear in the recent cases on the second definition, that the second definition identifies a considerable group of products not identified by the first definition and not limited to products "endowed" with properties for the treatment and prevention of disease but not "presented" as such, it becomes obvious that there will be risks to public health from "quack" products which may not be caught by the first definition. For example, if contraceptive products are caught by the second but not the first definition then "quack" contraceptive products, products presented as effective contraceptives without in fact having the appropriate properties, would not be caught by the first definition.

The Court therefore made it clear at paragraph 20 of the *Upjohn* judgment, cited above, that the second definition captures :

> "not only products which have a real effect on physiological functions but also those which do not have the advertised effect, thereby enabling public authorities to prevent the marketing of such products in order to protect consumers".

This approach accords with the general approach of the Community legislator, enunciated in article 5 of Directive (EEC) 65/65, that protection of the consumer requires not only that products marketed as medicinal products should not be harmful when properly used but also that they should be efficacious in the way claimed by the supplier.

2.6   The role of the Member States

The Court has accepted that the Member States have two important roles in the definition of medicinal products : until such time as there is more complete harmonisation of the measures necessary to ensure the protection of health, the Member States will retain a margin of appreciation in their regulation of medicinal products and will not necessarily be limited to products falling with the terms of the Community definitions; in addition, it is a matter for the national authorities, under the primary control of the national courts, to establish whether or not any particular product is a medicinal product as defined by article 1(2) of Directive (EEC) 65/65 on a case by case basis. The basis for both those propositions is the *Van Bennekom* judgment.

2.6.1   National definitions of medicinal products before 1 January 1993
At paragraph 11 of the *Van Bennekom* judgment, the Court states that :

> "Directive 65/65 constitutes only the first stage in the harmonisation of national laws dealing with the production and distribution of pharmaceutical products."[1]

At the time of that judgment, the scope of the Community rules was limited to "proprietary medicinal products for human use intended to be placed on the market in Member States".[2]

At paragraphs 31 and following, the Court further states the relevant principles to be applied by a national court under articles 30 and 36 of the EEC Treaty relating to the free movement of goods :

> "it is apparent from the last recital in the preamble to Directive 65/65 that the directive aims to achieve only a progressive approximation of the relevant provisions laid down by law, regulation or administrative action. Therefore, whilst seeking to remove as far as possible obstacles to trade within the Community in respect of the products to which it relates, the directive does not preclude as such the possibility that products not covered by its provisions may be subjected by Member States to restrictions on their sale or marketing, provided always that the other provisions of Community law are complied with.

> Under article 30 of the Treaty quantitative restrictions on import and all measures having equivalent effects are prohibited in trade between Member States. According to a consistent line of decisions of the Court, any commercial legislation by Member States which is liable to hinder trade within the Community, whether directly or indirectly, actually or potentially, is to be regarded as a measure having an effect equivalent to quantitative restrictions.

> In that light it is clear that legislation which prohibits the marketing of vitamins and vitamin preparations without prior registration with the administrative authorities constitutes a measure having an effect equivalent to a quantitative restriction on imports within the meaning of article 30 of the EEC Treaty, since such a measure is liable to hinder trade between Member States.

> Under article 36 of the Treaty, however, "The provisions of article 30 to 34 shall not preclude prohibitions or restrictions on imports ... justified on grounds of ... the protection of health and life of humans ... ", unless they

---

1.   [1983] ECR 3883 at 3899.
2.   Article 2(1) of Directive (EEC) 65/65. See also para 12 of the *Van Bennekom* judgment at 3899 and 3900.

constitute "a means of arbitrary discrimination or a disguised restriction on trade between Member States."

It is only when Community directives, in pursuance of article 100 of the Treaty, make provision for the full harmonisation of all the measures needed to ensure the protection of human and animal life and institute Community procedures to monitor compliance therewith that recourse to article 36 ceases to be justified. It is, however not in dispute that such is not the case with the directives dealing with pharmaceutical products. It is therefore necessary to consider whether measures which restrict the marketing of vitamins may be justified by article 36 of the Treaty."[1]

As stated in Chapter 1, the principles underlying articles 30 and 36 of the Treaty fall outside the scope of this work. The significance of this passage for present purposes is that it states the Court's general perception, *in 1983*, of the state of harmonisation of the pharmaceutical market. That view was reiterated by the Court in the *Tissier* case :

"it should first be emphasised that, as Community law stands at present, the harmonisation of national legislation on medicinal products for human use covers only proprietary medicinal products, that is to say medicinal products placed on the market under a special name and in a special pack. Other medicinal products as well as pharmaceutical substances or combinations of pharmaceutical substances not meeting the Community definition of medicinal product are not therefore subject to controls and do not require prior marketing authorisation under the relevant Community rules. Secondly, subject to article 30 *et seq.* of the Treaty concerning products imported from other Member States, Community law does not affect the right of Member States to subject such substances to controls or to require prior authorisation in accordance with their own national law on medicinal products."[2]

The same view was expressed by the Court in the *Delattre* and *Monteil* cases, which were in turn followed in *Commission v Germany* :

"At the present stage of development of Community law, it is difficult to avoid the continued existence, for the time being and, doubtless, so long as harmonisation of the measures necessary to ensure the protection of health is not more complete, of differences in the classification of products as between Member States."[3]

2.6.2 The Member States' margin of appreciation after 1 January 1993
The purpose of this work is to set out the steps the Community has taken since those judgments to complete the harmonisation process. Although major changes have been made and will gradually come into effect over the next few years, it remains the case that the process is not complete.

On the other hand, it is now true to say that the principal area where the Court saw that harmonisation had not been completed has now disappeared. Since 31 December 1992 the Community authorisation rules have applied to virtually all medicinal products falling within the article 1(2) definition. Two questions potentially arise : is it legitimate for a Member State to continue to have its own definition of a "medicinal product" once the Community definition has become of general application ? and, independently of the answer to that first question, what

---

1.   *Van Bennekom* [1983] ECR 3883, paras 31 to 35 at 3903 and 3904.
2.   *Tissier* [1986] ECR 1207, para 22 at 1215.
3.   *Delattre* [1991] ECR I-1487, para 29 at I-1534; *Monteil* [1991] ECR I-1547, para 28 at I-1568; *Commission v Germany* [1992] ECR I-3317, para 16 at I-3347.

scope remains, under articles 30 and 36 of the EEC Treaty, for a Member State to demand that a product which falls outside the scope of the Community definition of "medicinal product" should be registered or authorised, or sold only under special conditions, on the grounds that it is necessary to impose such a requirement for the protection of public health.

The first question is unlikely in practice to be of any great significance. Whether or not a Member State continues to operate its own definition of "medicinal product" or of a closely analogous concept, the important question will be the second one, whether the Member State may legitimately impose extra marketing requirements, which may or may not be of the kind imposed by the Community on medicinal products as defined in article 1(2), on products which do not fall within the article 1(2) definition.

The second question will amount in practice to the question of what scope remains for the operation of article 30 and article 36 once the Community rules have been extended to cover all "medicinal products" identified by article 1(2). That issue has arisen four times : in *Tissier, Delattre, Monteil* and *Ter Voort*, and the Court has not been entirely consistent. In *Tissier* and *Ter Voort*, the Court restated the traditional position that, subject to articles 30 and 36, the Member States retained a general power to subject products falling outside the Community definition of medicinal product to (i) "prior authorisation"[1] or (ii) to "the regime applicable to medicinal products"[2].

However, an analogous issue was decided by the Court in the *Delattre* and *Monteil* cases in relation to the French pharmacists' monopoly, where the Court did indeed distinguish between products falling within and outside the article 1(2) definition :

> "In the absence of harmonisation of the rules on the distribution both of medicinal products and of "para-pharmaceutical" products, it is for the Member States to choose the level to which to ensure the protection of public health.
>
> In the case of medicinal products within the meaning of Directive 65/65, account must be taken of the very particular nature of the product and the market involved, which explains the fact that in all the Member States there are, albeit with differences of detail, rules restricting their marketing and, in particular, some form of monopoly on the retail sale of such products is granted to pharmacists by reason of the safeguards which pharmacists must provide and the information which they must be in a position to furnish to the consumer.
>
> ...
>
> It follows that although in principle the Member States may reserve to pharmacists the right to make retail sales of products that fall within the Community definition of medicinal products and although, in those circumstances, their monopoly over those products may be presumed to constitute an appropriate way of protecting public health, evidence to the contrary may be produced with respect to certain products whose use would not involve any serious danger to public health and whose inclusion within the pharmacists' monopoly would seem manifestly disproportionate, that is to say contrary to the principles laid down by the Court for the interpretation of articles 30 to 36 of the Treaty.

---

1.   *Tissier*, [1986] ECR 1207, para 22 at 1215.
2.   *Ter Voort*, [1992] ECR I-5485, para 42 at 5514.

If pharmacists are granted a monopoly of other products, such as "para-pharmaceutical" products, which may be of widely varying kinds, the need for such a monopoly in order to protect public health or consumers must, regardless of how the products concerned are classified under national law, be established in each individual case, and those two aims must not be attainable by measures less restrictive of intra-Community trade."[1]

From that reasoning one might deduce that the Member States will retain two powers to go beyond the Community rules for the foreseeable future. First, in the case of medicinal products within the scope of article 1(2) of Directive (EEC) 65/65, the Member States will have the power to impose certain restrictions on the marketing of the products *beyond* those required by the Community rules. Secondly, it will be open to the Member States to justify, on a case by case basis, restrictions imposed on the marketing of products other than those identified by article 1(2). It appears inevitable that further rulings from the Court will be needed to reconcile the different lines of authority in *Tissier/Ter Voort* and *Delattre/Monteil* but the *Delattre* and *Monteil* judgments are far more fully reasoned than the *Tissier* and *Ter Voort* judgments and represent a more imaginative development of Community law. The following paragraphs therefore assume that the reasoning in *Delattre* and *Monteil* will be followed.

With regard to *medicinal products falling within the scope of the Community definitions*, in *Delattre* and *Monteil* the issue concerned the pharmacists' monopoly over retail sales of such products but there seems no reason to restrict the Court's reasoning. Where a further reasonable requirement, at least where it is widespread among the Member States, is imposed, the Court accepts that such a requirement "may be presumed to constitute an appropriate way of protecting public health", subject to evidence to the contrary in relation to "certain products whose use would not involve any serious danger to public health", where the restriction would seem "manifestly disproportionate, that is to say contrary to the principles laid down by the Court for the interpretation of articles 30 to 36 of the Treaty".

It thus appears that, as a matter of law, there will be a limited, and rebuttable, presumption in favour of such restrictions with respect to products coming within the Community definition of medicinal product. As a matter of fact, the area of discretion available to the Member States has been further reduced by the Rational Use package of Directives described in Chapters 13 to 16. Those Directives lay down rules in relation to wholesale distribution, classification for the purpose of supply, labelling and packaging, and advertising of medicinal products as defined in article 1(2) of Directive (EEC) 65/65. The relevance of such Directives is confirmed by the *Delattre* and *Monteil* cases themselves, where the Court referred to the *lack* of "harmonisation of the rules on the marketing of medicinal products" to show that the Member States retained the power "to lay down rules on the distribution, in the strict sense of the term, of pharmaceutical products"[2]. That reasoning would no longer apply straightforwardly, though the Rational Use package is far from a complete harmonisation of the rules on distribution of pharmaceuticals, and does not, in particular, change any rules relevant to the pharmacists' monopoly[3].

---

1.   *Delattre* [1991] ECR I-1487, paras 53 to 57 at I-1540 and I-1541; *Monteil* [1991] ECR I-1547, paras 40 to 44 at I-1571.
2.   *Delattre* [1991] ECR I-1487, paras 47 and 48 at I-1539; *Monteil* [1991] ECR I-1547, paras 34 and 35 at I-1569.
3.   Directive (EEC) 92/26 does seek to harmonise rules on the classification of medicinal products as "prescription only". That does not in itself prevent a national rule preventing medicinal products being stocked by retail outlets other than pharmacies.

With regard to *products falling outside the scope of the Community definitions*, the burden of proof is reversed. Restrictions on the marketing of such products must be individually justified by the Member States on the grounds of the protection of public health or the health of consumers; further, it must not be possible to attain such aims by measures that are less restrictive of intra-Community trade[1].

One obvious distinction between the *Ter Voort/Tissier* line of authority and the *Delattre/Monteil* reasoning is that the former cases concerned initial marketing authorisation whereas the latter cases concerned subsequent restrictions on distribution. Refusal of initial authorisation is obviously more fundamental than imposition of marketing restrictions, so that one might have expected the Member States' discretion to impose the former to be more limited than its discretion to impose the latter. A similar issue potentially arose in the *Commission v Germany* case, where Germany sought to justify its requirement that the product in question in that case be authorised under article 36 of the EEC Treaty even if it was held by the Court that the product was not a medicinal product within the Community definitions. Given that both Advocate-General van Gerven and the Court considered that the Commission had not proved that the product was *not* a medicinal product, the issue did not arise for judgment by the Court but it was considered by the Advocate-General[2]. It is revealing that in the *Monteil* and *Commission v Germany* cases, the Advocates-General were clearly of the view that the Member States would *not* have been able to justify the restrictions in question under article 36 if the products were not medicinal products under the Community definitions, but that the restrictions were equally clearly *justified* if the products did fall within the definitions. In *Monteil*, the Advocate-General does not appear to have thought there was any real danger to public health :

> "[t]he products at issue are in fact very safe in use, are easily identifiable by consumers and are widely available for everyday use; accordingly there is no need for a pharmacist to be present when they are sold."[3]

In *Commission v Germany*, the Advocate-General was not satisfied that, if the product was not a medicinal product, the protection of the consumer could not have been achieved by less restrictive means than requiring full authorisation, as appears to have been the case in France in relation to the same product[4]. The reference to the situation in other Member States is of particular interest, given that in the case of medicinal products the Court has traditionally accepted that the different Member States may have different schemes of protection, unless the Community rules apply to the matter in issue.

Finally, the issue of discrimination under article 36 of the EEC Treaty has arisen both in relation to the definition of a medicinal product and in relation to the treatment of products as defined. It would be a clear infringement of the Treaty for imported products to be defined as medicinal products under the national law of a Member State where domestically produced but otherwise identical products were not subjected to the requirements imposed on medicinal products. It would equally be unacceptable to treat imported medicinal products differently from non-imported medicinal products, or imported products falling outside the Community definitions differently from non-imported products in that category. Those obvious points were raised by the Advocates-General in both *Delattre* and *Commission v*

---

1. More detailed discussions of the facts of *Delattre* and *Monteil* are contained in the Opinions of Advocate-General Tesauro, [1991] ECR at I-1508 to I-1524 and I-1556 to I-1560.
2. [1992] ECR I-3317, paras 12 to 14 at I-3339 to I-3341 of his Opinion.
3. *Monteil* [1991] ECR I-1547, para 5 of the Opinion at I-1560.
4. [1991] ECR I-3317 at I-3340.

Germany and considered briefly by the Court in the latter case. In *Delattre*, the Advocate-General was clearly suspicious that certain products of French origin falling outside the scope of the definition of medicinal products were being freely distributed, whereas imported goods were made subject to the pharmacists' monopoly[1]. In *Commission v Germany*, the Advocate-General and the Court were not satisfied that any discrimination had been proved either in the classification of products or restrictions resulting from those classifications[2].

2.6.3   The role of national courts

All of the eight cases considered in this Chapter apart from *Commission v Germany* arose under the article 177 procedure of reference from a national court for a preliminary ruling on a point of Community law. Under that procedure, it is for the national court to decide the case before it in the light of the guidance given by the Court[3].

In practice, the Court cannot hope to give precise answers to all the possible questions that may arise :

> "In view of the technicalities of the definition of medicinal products contained in Directive 65/65, the Court of Justice can do no more than provide a number of general guidelines enabling the dividing line to be drawn between medicinal products and foods."[4]

In the *Delattre, Monteil, Upjohn* and *Commission v Germany* cases, the Court expanded on that statement in virtually identical terms :

> "It is for the national courts to determine on a case-by-case basis the classification of each product having regard to its pharmacological properties as they may be ascertained in the current state of scientific knowledge, to the way in which it is used, to the extent to which it is sold and to consumers' familiarity with it."[5]

Delattre concerned primarily the "presentation" criterion whereas the passages cited from *Upjohn* and from *Monteil* concerned the "function" criterion. It is thus clear that the statement of principle applies equally to each of the Community definitions and that is confirmed in *Commission v Germany* where the statement is completely general and based on all three earlier judgments of the Court[6].

One further point arose in *Delattre*, whether the national authorities are obliged to consult the specialist committees advising the Commission (for example the CPMP or CVMP, as to which see Chapters 5 and 7 below) before adopting a divergent classification from that adopted by another Member State :

> "The second point raised is whether a product classified as a foodstuff in one Member State may nevertheless be classified as a medicinal product in another

---

1.   *Delattre* [1991] ECR I-1487, para 15 of the Opinion at I-1522.
2.   [1992] I-3317, para 14 of the Advocate-General's Opinion at I-3340 and I-3341; paras 21 to 23 of the judgment of the Court at I-3348.
3.   See *Van Bennekom* [1983] ECR 3883, para 10 at 3899.
4.   *Van Bennekom* [1983] ECR 3883, para 13 at 3900.
5.   *Upjohn* [1991] ECR I-1703, para 23 at I-1742; *Delattre* [1991] ECR I-1487, para 35 at I-1535; *Monteil* [1991] ECR I-1547, para 29 at I-1568; and *Commission v Germany* [1992] ECR I-3317, para 17 at I-3347.
6.   Whether the Court will in future be able to avoid giving specific answers is less certain: in the judgment in *Ter Voort*, and in the Advocate-General's Opinion in *Angelopharm* in particular, the facts of the case were considered in some detail.

Member State without prior consultation of the various committees which advise the Commission on such matters.

In applying the definition of medicinal product given in article 1(2) of Directive 65/65, the Member States must take account, as is the general rule in such matters, of the results of international scientific research and, in particular, the work of specialised Community committees (judgment in Case C-247/84 *Motte* [1985] ECR 3887). However, no legislation requires them to consult such committees before taking a decision concerning a particular product."[1]

The new rules laid down for the operation of the European Medical Agency for the Evaluation of Medicinal Products are described in Chapters 7 and 8. There will now be cases where the Member States *are* required to consult the CPMP or CVMP and to be bound by their decisions[2], but such cases will arise only where one Member State has already authorised a product *as a medicinal product* and the second Member State refuses to recognise that authorisation. No question arises of a difference of view as to the definition of medicinal product in such cases.

2.7   Products bordering on medicinal products

The four principal categories of products that could in principle be caught by the definitions of medicinal products but which are clearly not intended to be subject to the regulatory regime applicable to products so defined have been identified and discussed in earlier sections of this Chapter. In the interests of clarity, the principal points are summarised here. The first three categories - foodstuffs, cosmetics and household products - raise straightforward issues of definition. The risk of overlap between medicinal products, foodstuffs and cosmetics was recognised in the third recital to Directive (EEC) 65/65, with its express exclusion of "foods, animal feedingstuffs and toilet preparations" from the scope of the Directive. In broad terms, there is a demarcation problem between foods and medicinal products taken internally and between cosmetics and medicinal products applied externally. Household detergents etc would normally fall into the external category (discounting rat poison etc).

The fourth category - medical devices - is a parallel Community concept to that of medicinal product and the Community definition, which is more recent and in some respects more sophisticated than the definition of medicinal product, is set out and briefly discussed below.

Finally, a fifth category - excipients - is apparently subject to the Community rules on medicinal products; the way in which they are regulated emerges essentially from the detail of the authorisation process itself but the point is briefly discussed in the light of the *Tissier* judgment cited at section 2.5.4 ante.

2.7.1   Foodstuffs
The general problem of distinguishing foodstuffs from medicinal products arose in *Van Bennekom* (vitamins) and *Delattre* (various ordinary products such as garlic and guar gum presented in a "medicinal" form). The general passages concerning the identifying characteristics of medicinal as against food products have already been referred to : the idea accepted by the Court and the Advocates-General in the *Van Bennekom* and *Delattre* cases is that where the effect of the product is simply to restore a deficiency of the product itself which arises in an otherwise normally functioning body then the product is performing a "nutritional" function and should

---

1.   *Delattre* [1991] ECR I-1487, paras 31 and 32 at I-1535.
2.   See section 8.4 post.

be classified as a food; it is only where the product is being used to combat a physiological malfunction other than that of which the "morbid cause" is a deficiency of the product itself that the product should be treated as medicinal[1].

However, in *Delattre*, the Court was referred to a more or less obscure range of Community legislation relating to foodstuffs on which the national court required guidance on whether it might be relevant to the definition of medicinal products : Council Directive (EEC) 80/77 on the approximation of the laws of the Member States relating to the exploitation and marketing of natural mineral waters[2]; Council Directive (EEC) 77/436 on the approximation of the laws of the Member States relating to coffee extracts and chicory extracts[3]; and Council Directive (EEC) 74/329 on the approximation of the laws of the Member States relating to emulsifiers, stabilisers, thickeners and gelling agents for use in foodstuffs[4].

The references to the chicory and mineral waters legislation was merely to argue by analogy from certain claims and forms of presentation of the products expressly permitted by the Community legislation in the case of water and chicory products, that other products for which the same claims were made and which were presented in the same way could not therefore be regarded as medicinal products. The Court was unimpressed by such arguments, on the grounds that the mineral waters legislation was simply irrelevant because there was no risk of confusion between mineral waters and medicinal products[5] and that the provisions of the legislation on chicory products "cannot frustrate the application of the criteria relating to medicinal products laid down in Directive 65/65", more especially because the aspect relied on, "external form", was not in any event a decisive criterion for identifying medicinal products[6].

In relation to the legislation on emulsifiers etc, Directive (EEC) 74/329, neither the Court nor the Advocate-General ruled on whether the fact that guar gum was included in an Annex to the Directive proved that a product composed entirely of guar gum was a foodstuff rather than a medicinal product even if it was presented as a product that "creates a feeling of satiety which makes it possible to eat less". They merely reiterated the principles laid down under articles 30 and 36 in relation to products which were not medicinal products and stated that Directive (EEC) 74/329 did not affect the application of articles 30 or 36[7]. It might be deduced (from the fact that no mention was made of the position if guar gum was a medicinal product) that the Court was inclined to the view that guar gum was *not* a medicinal product but it did not confirm that the inclusion of a product in a list of products annexed to foodstuffs legislation was in any way conclusive evidence that the product could not be considered by a Member State to be a medicinal product, in at least certain forms and for certain uses.

It is therefore reasonably clear that the Community foodstuffs legislation will have no more than persuasive force in any proceedings concerned with borderline cases. Further, any overlap between foodstuffs and medicinal products must be resolved by classification as a medicinal product.

---

1.   See *Delattre* [1991] ECR I-1487, para 11 of the Opinion at I-1516 to I-1517; *Van Bennekom* [1983] ECR 3883, paras 26 and 27 at 3902.
2.   OJ L229 30.8.80 p1.
3.   OJ L172 12.7.77 p20.
4.   OJ L189 13.7.74 p1.
5.   See *Delattre* [1991] ECR I-1487, para 30 at p1-1534.
6.   See *Delattre* [1991] ECR I-1487, para 42 at p1-1537. See also 2.4.2 above for a discussion of "presentation" and external form.
7.   See *Delattre* [1991] ECR I-1487, paras 61 to 67 of the judgment, at I-1542 to I-1543 and para 16 of the Opinion at I-1522 to I-1523.

2.7.2   Cosmetics

Cosmetics differ from foodstuffs in that there is a specific Community definition of cosmetics, laid down by article 1(1) of Council Directive (EEC) 76/768 on the approximation of the laws of the Member States relating to cosmetic products :

> "any substance or preparation intended for placing in contact with the various external parts of the human body (epidermis, hair system, nails, lips and external genital organs) or with the teeth and mucous membranes of the oral cavity with a view exclusively or principally to cleaning them, perfuming them or protecting them in order to keep them in good condition, change their appearance or correct body odours."[1]

That definition is clearly much more specific than the definition of medicinal products at article 1(2) of Directive (EEC) 65/65 and there is therefore a strong temptation to use the more specific definition of cosmetics to determine the boundary between cosmetic products and medicinal products. The issue was considered in detail in the *Delattre, Monteil, Upjohn* and *Angelopharm* cases and the second question in the *Upjohn* case raised the issue directly :

> "how is the concept of "medicinal product" in Directive 65/65 to be delimited from that of "cosmetic product" in Directive 76/768 ?"

In *Delattre* and *Monteil*, although the point was not raised directly in either case, the Court dealt with the matter as a preliminary point in virtually identical terms to those used in *Upjohn* :

> "As stated in the fifth recital, which specifies that the directive "relates only to cosmetic products and not to pharmaceutical specialities and medicinal products", the rules laid down by Directive 76/768 concern only cosmetic products and not medicinal products.

> Consequently, while a comparison between the definitions of a cosmetic product and a medicinal product is not to be ruled out in doubtful cases before a product is classified functionally as a medicinal product, a product which has the characteristics of a medicinal product or a proprietary medicinal product still does not fall within the scope of Directive 76/768; it is subject only to the provisions of Directive 65/65 and the directives amending it."[2]

The only uncertainty is how the "doubtful cases" principle is to be applied in practice. The cosmetics definition can do no more than identify cosmetics, it cannot be used to exclude medicinal products and the Court has now decided that the definition of medicinal products will override what would otherwise be the operation of the cosmetics definition. The only use of the cosmetics definition will apparently be similar to that suggested by Advocate-General Lenz in *Upjohn*[3], to identify the "central core of cosmetic products established as such by general acceptance". It is questionable whether that type of general guidance will be of great assistance in "doubtful cases", where detailed consideration of the facts will be necessary : see Advocate-General Jacobs' Opinion in *Angelopharm* for an example of such an investigation.

---

1.   OJ L262 26.9.76 p169.
2.   *Upjohn* [1991] ECR I-1703, paras 29 and 30 at I-1744; *Delattre* [1991] ECR I-1487, paras 19 and 20 at I-1532 and I-1533; and *Monteil* [1991] ECR I-1547, paras 14 and 15 at I-1565.
3.   *Upjohn* [1191] ECR I-1704 at I-1732.

2.7.3   Household goods

Household goods such as bleach or soap could be regarded as falling within the scope of the second definition as endowed with properties for the prevention or treatment of disease[1]. The Court and the Community legislator have never felt there to be any serious difficulty of definition in this area. What is more likely to arise is that there will be an overlap between the increasing number of areas where harmonisation has been undertaken, so that medicinal products and other types of product will each fall under wider regulatory regimes : for an example, in a different area, see the references to Directive (EEC) 90/220 on the deliberate release into the environment of genetically modified organisms[2] at article 6 of Regulation (EEC) 2309/93, discussed at 7.3 below.

2.7.4   Medical devices

Article 1(2) of Council Directive (EEC) 93/42[3] defines "medical device" as :

> "any instrument, apparatus, appliance, material or other article, whether used alone or in combination, including the software necessary for its proper application intended by the manufacturer to be used for human beings for the purpose of :
>
> — diagnosis, prevention, monitoring, treatment or alleviation of disease,
> — diagnosis, monitoring, treatment, alleviation of or compensation for an injury or handicap,
> — investigation, replacement or modification of the anatomy or of a physiological process,
> — control of conception,
>
> and which does not achieve its principal intended action in or on the human body by pharmacological, immunological or metabolic means, but which may be assisted in its function by such means."

That definition is very similar to that contained at article 1(2)(a) of Council Directive (EEC) 90/385 on the approximation of the laws of the Member States relating to active implantable medical devices[4].

The regime applicable to medical devices is not the subject of this work, but the definition of medical device is clearly closely linked to the definition of medicinal product with which we are here concerned and is intended to set out a workable boundary between the two concepts which is wholly absent from Directive (EEC) 65/65. Article 1(3) to (8) of Directive (EEC) 93/42 set out specific rules in relation to a number of Directives in related areas. In relation to Directive (EEC) 65/65, article 1(3), (4) and (5)(c) provide :

> "3.   Where a device is intended to administer a medicinal product within the meaning of article 1 of Directive (EEC) 65/65, that device shall be governed by the present Directive, without prejudice to the provisions of Directive (EEC) 65/65 with regard to the medicinal product.
>
> If, however, such a device is placed on the market in such a way that the device and the medicinal product form a single integral product which is intended exclusively for use in the given combination and which is not reusable, that single product shall be governed by Directive (EEC) 65/65. The

1.   See *Van Bennekom* [1983] ECR 3883, para 22 at 3902; *Monteil* [1991] ECR I-1547, para 25 at I-1567, cited at section 2.5.5 ante.
2.   OJ L117 8.5.90 p15.
3.   OJ L169 12.7.93 p1.
4.   OJ L189 20.7.90 p17.

relevant essential requirements of Annex I to the present Directive shall apply as far as safety and performance related device features are concerned.

4.   Where a device incorporates, as an integral part, a substance which, if used separately, may be considered to be a medicinal product within the meaning of article 1 of Directive (EEC) 65/65 and which is liable to act upon the body with action ancillary to that of the device, that device must be assessed and authorised in accordance with this Directive.

5.   This Directive does not apply to :

   ...

   (c)   medicinal products covered by Directive (EEC) 65/65".

The intention of the legislator is sufficiently plain from article 1(5)(c) but it must remain doubtful whether all possible classification problems have been avoided between article 1(2) of Directive (EEC) 65/65 and article 1(2) of Directives (EEC) 90/835 and 93/42 (article 1(5)(b) of the later Directive excludes products covered by the earlier Directive from its scope).

Article 1(3) and 1(4) provide for three possibilities :

(1)   administration of a medicinal product by a medical device;

(2)   single integral and non-reusable medical devices incorporating a medicinal product; and

(3)   medical devices incorporating medicinal products whose action on the body is ancillary to that of the device.

In the case of (1), the device and the medicinal product are each regulated by their respective Directive : a typical example might be a syringe and a vaccine. In the case of (2), the product is to be regulated by Directive (EEC) 65/65 but subject to the provisions of Annex I to Directive (EEC) 93/42 as relevant to "safety and performance related device features". In the case of (3), the device falls under Directive (EEC) 93/42.

There are no cases on the interpretation of those provisions but it seems probable that there will be difficulties. In particular :

—   the division between category (2) and category (3) is far from clear; an obvious example of a category (3) product might be a condom containing spermicidal cream as an integral part of the whole, but that might equally be classified under (2); there is no guidance as to the meaning of "ancillary" in article 1(4);

—   which essential requirements laid down by Annex I to Directive (EEC) 93/42 may be "relevant" in any particular case is obviously open to argument;

—   article 1(4) makes no provision at all for assessment of the "ancillary" medicinal product incorporated within the device, despite the fact that the paragraph states that the product "if used separately, may be considered to be a medicinal product within the meaning of article 1 of Directive (EEC) 65/65"; if the product is not in fact ever used separately, there appears to be no requirement for the product to be authorised in any way; even if the product *is* subject to authorisation under Directive (EEC) 65/65 when used separately, there appears to be no requirement of any authorisation for the product itself where article 1(4) applies.

Given the technical complexity of the area, it seems inevitable that other difficult issues of fact and interpretation will arise.

2.7.5   Excipients

The relevant paragraphs from the Court's judgment in *Tissier* [1986] ECR 1207 were set out at 2.5.4 above. As there stated, there is a problem in making it generally the case that non-active ingredients of pharmaceutical products are to be subject to the authorisation process of Directive (EEC) 65/65 in that there is an obvious risk that ordinary chemicals will be caught by the definition.

The authorisation process laid down by Directive (EEC) 65/65 and its related legislation makes detailed provision for testing of every aspect of a product intended to be marketed as a medicinal product within the Community. A necessary element in that process is the testing of the product as it is actually to be used in therapeutic treatment of humans and/or animals. That necessarily involves testing and authorisation of the whole product, including any non-active ingredients : see article 4(3) of Directive (EEC) 65/65 and Part 2(A) of the Annex to Directive (EEC) 75/318 entitled "Qualitative and quantitative particulars of the constituents", in particular, paragraph 4.1 thereto :

> "An explanation should be provided with regard to the choice of composition, constituents and container and the intended function of the excipients in the finished product."

It might seem that this is a somewhat trivial or pedantic point but it is in fact a point of great practical and commercial significance : the Community rules are primarily rules relating to *marketing* authorisation and apply when a pharmaceutical product is intended to be marketed. There are certain rules relating to *manufacture* of medicinal products, but the authorisation process for manufacture is distinct from that laid down in Directive (EEC) 65/65[1]. For the purposes of marketing a product, the national and Community authorities are concerned with the product that is actually to be supplied to the medical practitioner or consumer, including all its non-active ingredients. For that purpose, the non-active ingredients of the product are of the highest importance : however beneficial the theoretical effects of a particular active ingredient may be, it will not be authorised as a medicinal product unless it can be successfully administered in a practical form.

---

1.   See Chapter 10 below. There are also generally applicable rules for Good Laboratory Practice and Good Clinical Practice : see section 1.4.4 ante.

PART II : MARKETING AUTHORISATION - THE CURRENT SYSTEM

Chapter 3 : Directive (EEC) 65/65¹ - The Original Framework Directive

3.1   The original principles : the recitals and the structure of the Directive

The five recitals to Council Directive (EEC) 65/65 on the approximation of provisions laid down by law, regulation or administrative action relating to medicinal products fall into three categories :

recital 1 states that :

> "the primary purpose of any rules concerning the production and distribution of medicinal products must be to safeguard public health";

recital 2 qualifies recital 1 :

> "this objective must be attained by means which will not hinder the development of the pharmaceutical industry or trade in medicinal products within the Community";

and recitals 3 to 5 concern the adverse effects on trade and on "the establishment and functioning of the common market" of :

> "disparities between certain national provisions, in particular between provisions relating to medicinal products (excluding substances or combinations of substances which are foods, animal feedingstuffs or toilet preparations)"

and state the need progressively to remove those hindrances, giving priority to those "liable to have the greatest effect on the functioning of the common market".

Those recitals have been referred to repeatedly in the cases cited in Chapter 2 above, in particular to show the two central purposes of the Community pharmaceutical legislation - to protect public health and to promote the free movement of goods - and to confirm that Directive (EEC) 65/65 "constitutes only the first stage in the harmonisation of national laws dealing with the production and distribution of pharmaceutical products"².

The main text of the Directive consists of five Chapters : I Definitions and scope; II Authorisation to place medicinal products on the market; III Suspension and revocation of authorisation to market medicinal products; IV Labelling of medicinal products; and V General and final provisions. Given the fundamental importance of Chapters I and II of the Directive to the entire legislative structure now in place and described in this work, the elements of those Chapters have been broken out in the following text (with reference back also to the discussion of a "medicinal product"

---

1.   OJ No 22 9.2.65 p369/65.
2.   *Van Bennekom [1983]* ECR 3883, para 11 at 3899; see also *Upjohn* [1991] ECR I-1703, para 10 of the Advocate-General's Opinion at 1-1716 and 1-1717; and section 2.6 ante.

in Chapter 2) rather than, as in the later chapters of this work, simply following the order of the Chapters and articles of the legislation.

3.2   The fundamental requirements : articles 3, 5 and 21

The fundamental requirements of Community law in relation to product authorisation were laid down in Council Directive (EEC) 65/65 and they have not changed, although the detail of the implications of those requirements has been in a continuous state of amendment since 1965 and the important changes introduced by Regulation (EEC) 2309/93[1] and Directive (EEC) 93/39[2] are described in Chapters 7 and 8. The principal articles are 3, 5 and 21[3] :

Article 3 provides that :

> "[n]o medicinal product may be placed on the market in a Member State unless an authorisation has been issued by the competent authority of that Member State".

All the powers and duties of the Member States, the Commission and the participant companies flow from the fundamental requirement of a marketing authorisation prior to placing a medicinal product on the market. As Advocate-General Lenz put the matter in his Opinion in *Upjohn* :

> "The requirement of an authorisation thus forms the hub and linchpin of the whole system of rules[4]."

The meaning of "placing a medicinal product on the market" is considered at section 3.3 below.

Article 5 provides that authorisation shall be refused if :

> "it proves that the medicinal product is harmful in the normal conditions of use, or that its therapeutic efficacy is lacking or is insufficiently substantiated by the applicant, or that its qualitative and quantitative composition is not as declared";

alternatively, if :

> "the particulars and documents submitted in support of the application do not comply with article 4";

as to article 4, see section 3.4 below.

Article 5 is not qualified in any way but it has in practice been subjected to two exceptions, one judicial and one statutory. The judicial exception derives from the ruling of the European Court of Justice in Case C-104/75 *De Peijper*[5], where the Court decided that it would infringe article 30, and could not be permitted under article 36, for national authorities to require a "parallel importer", of a product already authorised in the relevant Member State, to produce the documents relied on by the original applicant for authorisation so as to obtain what would be in

---

1. OJ L214 24.8.93 p1.
2. OJ L214 24.8.93 p22.
3. Article 11, relating to suspension and revocation of an authorisation, is considered in Chapter 11. That article is clearly of great practical importance.
4. *Upjohn* [1991] ECR I-1702, para 14 of the Opinion at I-1717.
5. Case C-104/75 *De Peijper* [1976] ECR 613.

effect a duplicate authorisation in respect of the parallel imported product. The Court did not address the issue of article 5 of Directive (EEC) 65/65 directly, though it had been raised by the British Government[1] and appeared to treat the case as concerning only the scope of article 36. The facts, of course, were in practice determinative, the Court deciding that it was contrary to Community policy for manufacturers of pharmaceutical products to frustrate the efforts of parallel importers by the simple expedient of refusing to give the parallel importers access to the materials relied on in the application for original authorisation.

The *De Peijper* exception has been developed and clarified in the Commission's Communication on parallel imports of proprietary medicinal products for which marketing authorisations have already been granted[2]. In the Communication, the Commission, which had been unable to obtain support for a Directive governing parallel imports, nonetheless gave detailed guidance as to its interpretation of the effect of the *De Peijper* judgment.

The statutory "exception" to article 5 is contained in Directive (EEC) 65/65, article 4, point 8, in a passage introduced by Directive (EEC) 87/21[3]. Of course, that is not strictly an exception to article 5, in that article 4 is applied in such cases. However, such "abridged applications", considered at 3.4.2 below, do benefit from waiver of the normal strict requirements of article 4 in certain important respects.

The question arises as to the relationship between *De Peijper* and article 4, point 8, of Directive (EEC) 65/65. The primary purpose of article 4, point 8, is plainly to benefit generic suppliers of products similar to the original proprietary product but its terms would be wide enough to include the case of parallel importers seeking authorisation. The matter has not been tested judicially, but it seems safe to assume that the rules laid down by the Commission in the light of *De Peijper* continue to represent Community law on the issue.

Article 21 provides that :

> "[a]n authorisation to market a medicinal product shall not be refused, suspended or revoked except on the grounds set out in this Directive."[4]

The meaning and effect of article 21 were considered by the European Court of Justice in Case C-301/82 *Clin-Midy and Others v Belgium*[5], where the Court determined : that article 21 was of direct effect (paragraph 4 of the judgment); that the scope of Directive (EEC) 65/65 was limited to the protection of public health and did not include, in particular, "any provision aimed at limiting the power of the Member States to regulate the prices of [medicinal] products" (paragraph 6 of the judgment); but that, article 21 did prevent the Member States refusing, suspending or revoking an authorisation to market on a ground other than that referred to by Directive (EEC) 65/65, that is to say a ground other than those laid down in articles

---

1.   See [1976] ECR 613 at p625.
2.   OJ C115 6.5.82 p5. See Appendix 16 post.
3.   OJ L15 17.1.87 p36.
4.   Article 6 makes special provision for those Member States where contraceptive products are banned, that they can also refuse to authorise such products: see 3.5 below. In addition, article 10(2) of Directive (EEC) 92/27 requires the competent authorities to refuse authorisation where labelling or the package leaflet of a product fails to comply with the requirements of that Directive and article 11(1) of the same Directive permits the Member States to suspend the authorisation in certain circumstances; this is considered further in Chapter 15.
5.   Case C-301/82 *Clin-Midy and Others v Belgium* [1984] ECR 251. See also Case C-83/92 *Pierrel v Ministero della Sanita*, judgment of 7 December 1993 (not yet reported in the ECR; (1993) Transcript 7 December, OJ C18 21.1.94 p3), discussed at section 11.1 post in relation to article 11 and article 21.

5 and 11 for the protection of public health (paragraph 11 and point 2 of the operative part of the judgment). However, the Court further held that in one very important respect, article 21 did not fetter the powers of the Member States in that the interpretation of the article favoured by the Court did not :

> "prevent Member States which introduce a price control system for [medicinal products] from ensuring that it is complied with by means which are appropriate to that system and compatible with the Treaty, in particular article 30 thereof"[1].

It should be noted that at paragraph 9 of the judgment, the Court reached a more general finding that the existence of a marketing authorisation granted in accordance with Directive (EEC) 65/65 "does not imply that the other requirements which a product must meet in order to be lawfully marketed are satisfied". It is doubtful whether, in the light of the new, much more comprehensive, legislation discussed in later Chapters, the Court would now maintain that general position, which is naturally linked to its finding that Directive (EEC) 65/65 was "only the first stage of harmonisation"[2]. However, article 1 of Regulation (EEC) 2309/93 and article 1 of Directive (EEC) 65/65, as amended by Directive (EEC) 93/39, make it clear that the new Future System rules do not affect the Member States' powers over price and reimbursement [3].

In summary, the framework for authorisation within the Community is that every medicinal product must have authorisation from a competent Member State authority and that the *sole* criteria for granting such an authorisation are the harmfulness of the product, its "therapeutic efficacy" and the conformity of its "qualitative and quantitative composition" to the description of the product in the application for authorisation (which must itself conform to the requirements of article 4 of Directive (EEC) 65/65). Of the three criteria, the third is clearly a "formal" criterion, the product must be as the applicant for authorisation says it to be, whereas the first two are "substantive", the product must not be "harmful" and it must not lack "therapeutic efficacy". That is not to say that the third criterion is trivial or easy to satisfy. Much of the detailed work involved in the authorisation process, as set out in the Community Directives and the accompanying Recommendations and guidelines, concerns the maintenance of high standards of performance at every stage of manufacture and distribution[4].

3.3   Placing medicinal products on the market : Chapter I, articles 1 and 2

The definition of "medicinal products" at article 1(2) was considered in detail in Chapter 2. Until 1989, the scope of the sections of Directive (EEC) 65/65 relating to authorisation was limited to "proprietary medicinal products" as defined at article 1(1) :

> "Any ready-prepared medicinal product placed on the market under a special name and in a special pack."

Directive (EEC) 89/341[5] removed that limitation, so that in principle *all* medicinal products are within the scope of Directive (EEC) 65/65, subject only to the

---

1.   *Clin-Midy and Others v Belgium* [1984] ECR 251, para 12 at 259.
2.   Ibid, para 5 at 258.
3.   See Chapters 7 and 8 post. The reservation in the text does not of course relate to the enforcement of intellectual property rights where such enforcement is consistent with the general Community rules on competition and free movement.
4.   For a slightly different analysis of article 5, see Advocate-General Lenz's Opinion in the *Upjohn* case at paras 16 to 20, [1991] ECR I-1703 at ppI-1717 and I-1718.
5.   OJ L142 25.5.89 p11.

qualifications introduced by Directive (EEC) 89/341 itself to the new paragraphs 1(4), 1(5), 2(3) and 2(4) of Directive (EEC) 65/65[1]. Those new paragraphs exclude medicinal products prepared in a pharmacy according to an individual prescription (article 1(4)), entitled "Magistral formula") or in accordance with the prescriptions of a pharmacopoeia for direct supply to patients (article 1(5), entitled "Officinal formula"), those intended for research and development trials and those intended for further processing by an authorised manufacturer (article 2(3); for manufacturing authorisation, see Chapter 10). They also give any Member State the option to exclude medicinal products which are :

> "supplied in response to a *bona fide* unsolicited order, formulated in accordance with the specifications of an authorised health care professional and for use by his individual patients on his direct personal responsibility" (article 2(4)).

Both articles 2 and 3 make use of the concept of "placing on the market" but there is no definition of the term in Directive (EEC) 65/65. In Directive (EEC) 93/42[2] article 1(2)(h), "placing on the market" is said to mean "the first making available in return for payment or free of charge ... with a view to distribution and/or use on the Community market". It thus includes supply to wholesalers as well as to end users, though it does not include the "individual" supplies of products described at article 2(3) and 2(4) of Directive (EEC) 65/65. The idea appears to be the offer of some sort of commercial or quasi-commercial transaction and, perhaps, of the passing of title to the goods from the "person responsible for placing that product on the market" to another person, whether a wholesaler, a retailer or a national health purchaser. Given the close relationship between "medicinal products" and "medical devices"[3] there seems no reason to take "placing on the market" in any different sense in Directive (EEC) 65/65.

The idea of industrial or commercial supply is confirmed by the provisions of article 2(2), which requires the Member States to apply the rules laid down by Chapters II to V where it "authorises the placing on the market of industrially produced medicinal products which do not comply with the definition of proprietary medicinal product". That provision, introduced by Directive (EEC) 89/341, indicates that the scope of the Directive is intended to be "industrially produced" rather than individually supplied products and the concept of "placing on the market" must roughly correspond to the idea of the first supply within a Member State of such a product.

3.4   Obtaining marketing authorisation : article 4

The procedure for obtaining authorisation for a new pharmaceutical product is necessarily complex. Modern pharmaceutical products take years to research and test and the results of the tests are technical and detailed, requiring sophistication

---

1.   Until 1989, the scope of Directive (EEC) 65/65 had also been limited by article 34 of Directive (EEC) 75/319, which excluded "proprietary medicinal products" which: (i) consisted of vaccines, toxins or serums; (ii) were based on blood or blood constituents or radioactive isotopes; or (iii) were homeopathic medicines. Directives (EEC) 89/342, 89/343 and 89/381 (OJ L142 25.5.89 pp14-16 and OJ L181 28.6.89 p44) make provision for all except homeopathic products and Directive (EEC) 92/73 has now set out rules applicable to homeopathic products: see Chapter 9. The sole remaining exception is provided for by article 1(2) of Directive (EEC) 89/381 relating to products derived from human blood or human plasma : "[t]his Directive shall not apply to whole blood, to plasma or to blood cells of human origin." Those substances are still outside the scope of Directive (EEC) 65/65.
2.   OJ L169 12.7.93 p1.
3.   See section 2.7.4 ante.

both to prepare and to comprehend adequately for the purposes of assessment or approval. Directive (EEC) 65/65 again lays down framework requirements for the application and authorisation process, but those requirements have been regularly amended and updated since 1965; in addition, the Community has now gone well beyond the framework in its efforts to harmonise both the administrative process and the detailed criteria applied to products seeking authorisation, with the ultimate purpose of introducing a co-ordinated system of multinational if not Community-wide authorisation. The Annex to Directive (EEC) 75/318, Annex 2 hereto, sets out the detail of the requirements and refers to the associated Commission guidelines.

This work is concerned with the legislative regime applicable to medicinal products. The detail of the many guidelines issued to the industry are not therefore considered, but it should be stressed that in practice those guidelines, and in particular the Notice to Applicants, published by the Commission as Volume II of *The Rules Governing Medicinal Products in the European Community*, gives practical guidance as to the proper procedures to be followed by applicants for marketing authorisation.[1]

3.4.1 The framework requirements for authorisation

The framework requirements for authorisation are laid down by article 4 of Directive (EEC) 65/65. That article has also been repeatedly amended and the reader is referred to Appendix 1 hereto for the latest version (that is to say the version effective from 1 January 1995, with the rest effective until that date indicated by footnotes). The first two paragraphs state in substance that the person responsible for putting a medicinal product on the market in any particular Member State must make an application for authorisation to the competent authority of that Member State, accompanied by a number of specific "particulars and documents" set out in numbered paragraphs :

(1)   the names and addresses of the persons responsible for marketing and manufacturing the product;

(2)   the brand name, common name or scientific name, in the latter two cases accompanied by the trade mark or name of the manufacturer;

(3)   qualitative and quantitative details of the constituents of the product;

(4)   "[b]rief description of the method of preparation";

(5)   "[t]herapeutic indications, contra-indications and side effects";

(6)   "[p]osology, pharmaceutical form, method and route of administration and expected shelf life";

(7)   details of controls and tests conducted throughout the manufacturing process;

(8)   "[r]esults of :
—   physico-chemical, biological or microbiological tests,
—   pharmacological and toxicological tests,
—   clinical trials"[2];

---

1.   The Notice to Applicants, published in 1989 as Volume II of *The Rules Governing Medicinal Products in the European Community*, is in the process of revision. A new Volume IIA was issued in July 1993, replacing pages 1 to 47 of the 1989 version; a further Volume IIB will be issued in 1994/95 replacing the remainder of the 1989 text; and a final version setting out the procedures is in preparation for 1995, when the Future System will come into effect: see Chapters 7 and 8.

2.   See section 3.4.2 below for a major qualification to this requirement.

(9)   a summary of the product characteristics, at least one specimen of the "sales presentation" and package leaflet (if there is one) of the product : this requirement is set out much more fully in article 4a[1]; it has been further refined and developed in Directive (EEC) 92/27, considered in detail in Chapter 15.

(10)   documentary evidence that the manufacturer of the product is authorised to produce medicinal products "in his own country";

(11)   "[a]ny authorisation obtained in another Member State or in a third country to place the relevant product on the market".

3.4.2   Abridged applications

Article 4(8) was considerably amended and expanded by Directive (EEC) 87/21[2], qualifying the requirements imposed in relation to the results of certain tests and trials specified by article 4(8) : article 4(8)(a), limiting the applicant's obligation "to provide the results of pharmacological and toxicological tests or the results of clinical trials" in three specific cases; and article 4(8)(b), limiting that obligation where a new product contains "known constituents not hitherto used in combination for therapeutic purposes". The two sub-paragraphs are prefaced by the statement that they are to be "without prejudice to the law relating to the protection of industrial and commercial property" and article 4(8)(a) in particular was introduced to balance the interests of generic suppliers in obtaining access to the market for products which no longer enjoyed complete intellectual property protection (in particular on the expiry of relevant patents) with the interests of innovative firms in the reasonable protection of their investments in research and development.

Article 4(8)(a) provides :

"The applicant shall not be required to provide the results of pharmacological and toxicological tests or the results of clinical trials if he can demonstrate :

(i)   either that the proprietary medicinal product is essentially similar to a product authorised in the country concerned by the application and that the person responsible for the marketing of the original proprietary medicinal product has consented to the pharmacological, toxicological or clinical references contained in the file on the original proprietary medicinal product being used for the purpose of examining the application in question;

(ii)   or by detailed references to published scientific literature presented in accordance with the second paragraph of article 1 of Directive (EEC) 75/318 that the constituent or constituents of the proprietary medicinal product have a well established medicinal use, with recognised efficacy and an acceptable level of safety;

(iii)   or that the proprietary medicinal product is essentially similar to a product which has been authorised within the Community, in accordance with Community provisions in force, for not less than six years and is marketed in the Member State for which the application is made; this period shall be extended to 10 years in the case of high-technology medicinal products within the meaning of Part A in the Annex to Directive (EEC) 87/22 or of a medicinal product within the meaning of Part B in the Annex to that Directive for which the procedure laid down in article 2 thereof has been followed; furthermore, a Member State may also extend this period to 10 years by a single Decision

---

1.   See section 3.4.3 below
2.   OJ L15 17.1.87 p36.

covering all the products marketed on its territory where it considers this necessary in the interest of public health. Member States are at liberty not to apply the above-mentioned six-year period beyond the date of expiry of a patent protecting the original product.

However, where the proprietary medicinal product is intended for a different therapeutic use from that of the other proprietary medicinal products marketed or is to be administered by different routes or in different doses, the results of appropriate pharmacological and toxicological tests and/or of appropriate clinical trials must be provided."

Sub-paragraphs (i) and (ii) do not cause any major difficulties of interpretation. Where the original supplier consents to the use of the material relied on in the original application for marketing authorisation in the country in question, the sole question for the national authority is the "essential similarity"[1] of the new product with the old. Where the original manufacturer consents to access to his original application that is unlikely to prove a major difficulty, in particular where the same active ingredient is shown to be present in each product. Likewise, there is no difficulty in understanding case (ii), where detailed references to the relevant medical literature are relied on. Prior to the adoption of Directive (EEC) 87/21, the Commission had expressed concern that some national authorities were too easily satisfied under this head, and the wording introduced by the Directive is considerably more restrictive[2].

Although cases (i) and (ii) are not hard to understand, they are of no practical assistance where the original manufacturer does *not* consent to use of his original file and where no sufficient scientific literature is available. That will often be the case. Where it is so, article 4(8)(iii) applies, exempting the second applicant from supplying the results of the specified tests and trials where he can demonstrate essential similarity to a product which (a) has been authorised within the Community according to Community provisions in force for at least six years (see below) and (b) is marketed within the relevant Member State. The period of six years is automatically extended to ten years for products within List A of Directive (EEC) 87/22[3] or where the "concertation" procedure has been followed for products on List B[4]. The Member States have two further discretions : (i) to extend the period to ten years for all products; or (ii) to limit the period to that of patent protection if such period is less than six years[5]. Article 13(4) of Regulation (EEC) 2309/93[6] contains an equivalent provision in respect of centrally authorised products under the new Future System procedures, granting those products ten years' protection.

Article 4(8)(a)(iii) therefore gives the original manufacturer extensive protection from generic competition, normally for six or ten years, but also releases the generic competitor from the requirements of article 4(8)(i) and (ii) once that period expires, provided that "essential similarity" can be shown to the product that is already authorised. The fundamental issue is therefore the second applicant's

---

1.   See post for the meaning of "essentially similar".
2.   For the Commission's views see its "explanatory memorandum", COM(84)437.
3.   OJ L15 17.1.87 p38. See Appendix 4 post.
4.   See Chapter 6 post for that procedure.
5.   Notice to Applicants IIA, states that Spain, Portugal, Greece, Denmark, Ireland and Luxembourg had opted for six years protection, whereas Belgium, France, Germany, Italy, the Netherlands and the United Kingdom had opted for ten years. In Denmark, Spain, Portugal and Greece, the period does not apply beyond the date of expiry of patent protection of the original product.
6.   See section 7.3 post.

ability to demonstrate the "essential similarity" of its product to the product that is already authorised[1].

The interpretation of article 4(8)(a)(iii) was considered by the House of Lords in *Smith Kline & French v Licensing Authority*[2] in the context of applications by Generics (UK) Ltd. and Harris Pharmaceuticals Ltd. to obtain product licences under the Medicines Act 1968 for products containing cimetidine, the sole active ingredient in a product originally marketed by Smith Kline as "Tagamet". Smith Kline, the original manufacturer and holder of the original UK marketing authorisation, sought to prevent generic competitors, who were seeking to demonstrate that their products were essentially similar to "Tagamet", from relying on material in the hands of the U.K. Licensing Authority. Smith Kline argued that such information (submitted by Smith Kline as part of their original application) was confidential and could only be used by the Authority for the purpose of assessment of the original application and supervision of the authorised product on the market. The House of Lords dismissed the original manufacturer's arguments, holding that the information had been given to the Authority for the purposes of the performance of its duties under the Medicines Act 1968 and that such duties included the evaluation of "essential similarity". The generic applicants were therefore entitled to rely on the information already submitted by the original manufacturer to demonstrate the essential similarity of their products with the originally authorised product.

The last sentence of article 8(a)(iii) prevents reliance on its terms "where the product is intended for a different therapeutic use from that of the other .. products marketed or is to be administered by different routes or in different doses". Notice for Applicants IIA calls such cases "Hybrid" applications and at pages 12 and 13 gives specific guidance as to the types of additional data required for specific differences between the original product and the second product for which authorisation is sought. (It should be noted that even where article 4(8)(a) can be relied on, it does not give general exemption from the requirements of article 4(8), but merely exempts a second applicant in respect of pharmacological and toxicological tests and clinical trials, the details of which are set out in the Annex to Directive (EEC) 75/318 and its associated Guidelines and Recommendations).

The overall effect of article 4(8)(a) is therefore to give considerable scope for the emergence of generic competition once (a) patent protection has expired and (b) the original product has been on the market for at least six, or ten, years. It should be noted that the Community rules only applied to "proprietary" products until 1 January 1992 so that the target of Directive (EEC) 87/21 was not pure generic competitors but rather rival branded products. That limitation has now disappeared.

Article 4(8)(b) simply provides that where "known constituents" are combined to form a new medicinal product, the tests which must be carried out and documented in the application can be limited to the new combination. The expression "known constituents" is not defined, and there is no guidance in Directive (EEC) 65/65 as to its meaning. However, in its 1989 Notice to Applicants for marketing authorisations the Commission states that :

---

1.   The CPMP note for guidance on "Abridged Applications", III/3879/90, states that the minutes of the Council in December 1986 recorded the definition of "essentially similar" to be: "(i) it has the same qualitative and quantitative composition in terms of active principles, and (ii) the pharmaceutical form is the same, and (iii) where necessary, appropriate bioavailability studies have been carried out in accordance with the principles set out in Annex X to [Council Recommendation (EEC) 87/176 (OJ L73 16.3.87 p1)]".

2.   *Smith Kline & French v Licensing Authority* [1990] 1 AC 64.

"The fact that in one Member State a given constituent is well-known does not necessarily imply that the same is true of all the other Member States. In certain Member States there may be no experience of the medicinal use of the constituent and complete documentation may therefore be required." (Chapter I(2), page 8).

The idea of "known constituents" thus appears to be relative to the state of knowledge of the individual Member State authorities.

3.4.3 The summary of product characteristics

Article 4a sets out, under six main headings, information which must be given of the product's characteristics for the purposes of the "summary of product characteristics" required at point 9 of article 4[1]. The summary (in particular the approved version described in article 4b) is a fundamental element of the authorisation process, providing a common focus not only for the applicant for authorisation and the relevant national authority but also for communication between the various national and Community bodies. A number of the headings in article 4a repeat requirements set out under the main headings of article 4, and the reader is referred to Appendix 1 for the precise wording. The six headings are :

(1) name of the product;

(2) qualitative and quantitative composition of the "excipients", that is to say the constituents other than the active ingredients;

(3) pharmaceutical form;

(4) pharmacological properties and, if useful, "pharmacokinetic particulars"[2];

(5) clinical particulars;

(6) pharmaceutical particulars.

Under (5), the applicant must give detailed information on a range of diverse but practically important issues, such as use during pregnancy or on children, overdosing and effects on the ability to drive a car or operate machinery. Under (6), details are required of such things as storage conditions, appropriate containers and any special care required over disposal. The applicant must also supply the "name, style and permanent address or registered place of business of the holder of the marketing authorisation". Those issues are further discussed in Chapter 15 below in respect of the detailed requirements now imposed on suppliers of medicinal products in respect of the package leaflets to be included in accordance with the requirements of Directive (EEC) 92/27[3]. Article 4a itself does not state that the information is intended as a prototype for requirements to be included on the

---

1.   The idea of a "summary of product characteristics" was introduced by Directive (EEC) 83/570 (OJ L332 28.11.83 p1). As a purely amending measure whose date for implementation is passed, the Directive is not reproduced here (except in the form of amendments) but recital 3 to the Directive states that the summary of product characteristics was introduced because "it is necessary from the point of view of public health and the free movement of medicinal products for the competent authorities to have at their disposal all useful information on authorised products, based in particular on summaries, adopted in other Member States, of the characteristics of products".

2.   "Pharmacokinetics means the study of the fate of the active substance within the organism, and covers the study of the absorption, distribution, biotransformation and excretion of the substance." Annex to Directive (EEC) 75/318, Part 3, section II, paragraph G.

3.   OJ L113 30.4.92 p8. See Appendix 12 post.

product's package leaflet, but article 4, point 9 and section B of Part 1 of the Annex to Directive (EEC) 75/318[1], entitled "Summary of product characteristics" makes it clear that the summary is so intended. That is confirmed and clarified by Directive (EEC) 92/27, in particular Chapter III and article 10(2) thereof, the latter of which states that authorisation is to be refused if the labelling or the package leaflet is :

"not in accordance with the particulars listed in the summary of the product characteristics referred to in article 4b of Directive (EEC) 65/65"[2].

Article 4b introduces a duty on the part of the competent authorities of the Member State, when they issue a marketing authorisation, to give the applicant :

"a summary of the product characteristics as approved by it. The competent authority shall take all necessary measures to ensure that the information given in the summary is in conformity with that accepted when the marketing authorisation is issued or subsequently."

In many cases the "summary" referred to in article 4b will be very similar if not identical to that referred to in article 4(9) and article 4a.

3.5   Contraceptive products : article 6

Article 6 provides :

"The competent authorities of Member States may refuse to authorise the placing of a medicinal product for use as a contraceptive where the sale of proprietary products intended principally for that purpose is prohibited under their laws.[3]"

This provision is clearly of considerable social and political significance, particularly in Ireland, and represents an isolated instance in the Community pharmaceutical legislation where a criterion other than "quality, safety and efficacy" is permitted in the authorisation process.

3.6   Administrative details : articles 7 to 10 and 12

Article 7 requires the Member States to take steps to ensure that the authorisation procedure "is completed within 120 days of the date of submitting the application", with provision for an extra 90 days in "exceptional" cases. The applicant is to be notified of the extension before the end of the initial period[4].

---

1.   OJ L147 9.6.75 p1. See Appendix 2 post.
2.   As discussed in Chapter 15, that provision is not apparently compatible with article 21 of Directive (EEC) 65/65 but a "purposive" construction of article 21 was adopted by the European Court of Justice in Case C-83/92 *Pierrel v Ministero della Sanita*, judgment of 7 December 1993 (not yet reported in the ECR; (1993) Transcript 7 December, OJ C18 21.1.94 p3).
3.   See Appendix 1 for text of article 6 effective as from 1 January 1995.
4.   The Commission stated, in its "Explanatory Memorandum on the Future System for the Free Movement of Medicinal Products in the European Community", COM(90) 283 final, pp3-45, at paragraph 6.1, that the 210 day extended period "has become the general rule" and that it should be accepted as the period within which authorisation should be granted in all cases. Directive (EEC) 93/39 amends article 7 to that effect.

Article 8 provides for the furnishing of proof that :

> "controls have been carried out on the finished product in accordance with the methods described by the applicant pursuant to item 7 of the second paragraph of article 4".

This provision is expanded and made more precise in Directives (EEC) 75/318 and 75/319.

Article 9 makes it clear that authorisation does not exempt the manufacturer or the person responsible for putting the product on the market from possible civil and criminal liability for the product.

Article 9a places the person responsible for marketing an authorised product under a continuing obligation to keep his control methods up to date to take account of technical progress and to do so in a way acceptable to the Member State authorities.

Article 10 provides that authorisation is for renewable periods of five years, renewal to be by application at least three months before expiry.

Article 12 is oddly positioned in Chapter III entitled "Suspension and revocation of authorisation to market medicinal products". In fact, it lays down general rules for the national authorities to follow in refusing, suspending or revoking marketing authorisations pursuant to articles 5, 6 or 11 of the Directive : only article 11 relates specifically to suspension and revocation.

The general requirement is to "state in detail the reasons" on which any such negative decision is based; to notify the "party concerned", either the applicant or the person responsible for marketing an initially authorised product, not only of the decision itself but also, and at the same time, "of the remedies available to him under the laws in force and of the time limit allowed for the exercise of such remedies". In practice, the appeal procedures open to the party concerned must be described to him by the national authority.

Finally, two types of decision, marketing authorisations and revocations of such authorisations, must be published "by each Member State in the appropriate official publication". That provision is ambiguous : it could naturally be read to mean that each Member State must publish every decision or revocation made by every Member State, for example, Greece is required to publish every Portuguese or Dutch decision; common sense dictates that it must only require Greece to publish Greek decisions and Portugal to publish Portuguese decisions.

The administrative requirements of Directive (EEC) 65/65 have been altered and developed by the new Future System legislation discussed in Chapters 7 and 8. However, they have also formed the basis for those developments and also for the various subsidiary regimes discussed in Chapters 9 to 16 below in respect of homeopathic products and the manufacture, wholesale distribution, labelling and advertising of medicinal products, introduced by Directives (EEC) 92/73, 75/319, 92/25, 92/27 and 92/28 respectively[1].

---

1.   OJ L297 13.10.92 p8; OJ L147 9.6.75 p13; OJ L113 30.4.92 pp1-4, 8-12, 13-18.

3.7   The suspension and revocation of a marketing authorisation : Chapter III, article 11

The suspension and revocation of marketing authorisations is considered in Chapter 11 below.

3.8   Labelling : articles 13 to 20

Articles 13 to 20, concerning labelling, were repealed by article 13 of Directive (EEC) 92/27, which is considered in Chapter 15.

3.9   Products already authorised : article 24

Chapter V of the Directive, articles 21 to 25, is entitled "General and final provisions" and is largely concerned with the implementation of the Directive almost thirty years ago. Only two articles remain of any relevance and of those, article 21 was considered above. The only other significant article, article 24, provides that :

> "Within the time limits and under the conditions laid down in article 39(2) and (3) of Directive (EEC) 75/319, the rules laid down in this Directive shall be applied progressively to medicinal products covered by an authorisation to place on the market by virtue of previous provisions".

Those provisions[1] gave the Member States in effect until May 1990 to apply the regime introduced by the two Directives to products which had already been authorised before the regime came into effect. It should not therefore be any longer relevant as all products covered by the two Directives are now subject to the Community rules[2].

---

1.   See further section 5.5 post.
2.   The exceptions were : the medicinal products other than "proprietary medicinal products" brought within the scope of Directive (EEC) 65/65 by Directive (EEC) 89/341; the products recently brought within the scope of the Community regime by the "extension Directives" (EEC) 89/342, 89/343 and 89/381 : and homeopathic products now covered by Directive (EEC) 92/73 : see Chapter 9. Article 24 remains relevant in 1994 only to the extent that a Member State is now clearly in breach of its obligations under the Directive in so far as it has failed to apply the requirements of the Directive to almost any medicinal products marketed within its territory.

Chapter 4 : Council Directive (EEC) 75/318[1] - The Substance of the Marketing Authorisation Process

4.1   The purpose of the Directive : the recitals

Recital 1 to Council Directive (EEC) 75/318 on the approximation of the laws of Member States relating to analytical, pharmaco-toxicological and clinical standards and protocols in respect of the testing of medicinal products states expressly that the Directive is intended to continue the harmonisation process begun by Directive (EEC) 65/65[2] and to ensure the implementation of the principles laid down in that Directive.

Recitals 2 to 5 set out the reasoning underlying the Directive, that the fundamental aims set out in the recitals to Directive (EEC) 65/65, the protection of public health and the free movement of medicinal products within the Community, are to be achieved by eliminating disparities between the Member States in the control of such products. Recital 2 draws particular attention to point 8 of article 4 of Directive (EEC) 65/65, which requires that the results of various tests and trials carried out on the product for which marketing authorisation is sought should be included in the particulars submitted with the application for authorisation. Recital 3 reasons that, because "standards and protocols for the performance of tests and trials on medicinal products are an effective means of control of these products", they are also an effective means of protecting public health; it further reasons that by laying down "uniform rules applicable to tests and trials, the compilation of dossiers and the examination of applications" the free movement of medicinal products will be facilitated. Recital 4 expands on the point by stating that the consequence of the Member States adopting common standards and protocols will be that the national competent authorities will reach (still independent) decisions "on the basis of uniform tests and by reference to uniform criteria"; that will in turn "help to avoid differences in evaluation". Recital 5 notes that the tests and trials to be described under point 8 of article 4 of Directive (EEC) 65/65 are closely linked to the particulars to be included under points 3, 4, 6 and 7 of the same article (the constituents of the product; the method of preparation; details of administration of the product; and manufacturer's control methods), with the result that it is necessary "to specify the data to be provided pursuant to these points"[3].

The hopes expressed in those recitals were to a large extent unfulfilled in that the continuing existence of independent national decision procedures, however similar in structure and in the criteria imposed by the national authorities, served to frustrate any major facilitation of movement of products between Member States. The major attempts to co-ordinate these national decision-making procedures are described in Chapters 5 to 8 below in the existing "multi-State" and "concertation" procedures introduced by Directives (EEC) 75/319[4] and 87/22[5], and in the soon to

---

1.   OJ L147 9.6.75 p1. See Appendix 2 post.
2.   OJ No 22 9.2.65 p369/65. See Appendix 1 post.
3.   For article 4 of Directive (EEC) 65/65, see section 3.4 ante.
4.   OJ L147 9.6.75 p13. See Appendix 3 post.
5.   OJ L15 17.1.87 p38. See Appendix 4 post.

be introduced "centralised" and "decentralised" procedures introduced by Regulation (EEC) 2309/93[1] and Directive (EEC) 93/39[2].

Recitals 6 to 8 make certain important observations concerning the three essential criteria of assessment introduced by article 5 of Directive (EEC) 65/65 : quality, safety and efficacy. Recital 6 states that setting out common standards for such tests in detail will guarantee the "quality" of those tests, thus helping to ensure that the Member State authorities all apply the third of the criteria[3] set out in article 5 of Directive (EEC) 65/65 in the same way :

> "Whereas the quality of the tests is the essential consideration; whereas therefore tests carried out in accordance with these provisions must be taken into consideration irrespective of the nationality of the experts who perform them or the country in which they are carried out".

Recitals 7 and 8 make important points about the other two "substantive" criteria, "harmfulness" and "therapeutic efficacy", set out in article 5 of Directive (EEC) 65/65. Recital 7 asserts that those two concepts :

> "can only be examined in relation to each other and have only a relative significance depending on the progress of scientific knowledge and the use for which the medicinal product is intended"

and that authorisation must be refused unless the application particulars and documents demonstrate that :

> "potential risks are outweighed by the therapeutic efficacy of the product".

Although it might be obvious in practice that the concept of "harmfulness" in this context must be a relative rather than absolute one, that was not clear from the wording of article 5 of Directive (EEC) 65/65. The balancing act required to be performed by the authorities is clearly of the greatest difficulty and sensitivity in those relatively common cases where a product combines significant therapeutic advances with substantial harmful side-effects.

Recital 8 emphasises the point made in recital 7 that the relativity is not only between the two concepts themselves, but also to the current state of scientific knowledge. As science advances, the balance between benefit and harm may shift significantly, and in either direction, for example as unwanted side-effects are revealed or nullified by scientific progress. As a result, the "standards and protocols" laid down by the Directive must be open to change.

4.2   The main text of the Directive

The main text of the Directive is short, consisting of only two significant articles and some additional material added on as articles 2a, 2b and 2c.

Article 1 simply states that the Member States must ensure that the "particulars and documents" listed at articles 4(3), 4(4), 4(6), 4(7) and 4(8) of Directive (EEC) 65/65 and provided by an applicant for product authorisation comply with the terms of the Annex to Directive (EEC) 75/318 (the "references to published data" permitted

---

1.   OJ L214 24.8.93 p1. See Appendix 5 post.
2.   OJ L214 24.8.93 p22. See Appendix 6 post.
3.   For the criteria, see section 3.2 ante.

under the special provisions of articles 4(8)(a) and 4(8)(b) are to be treated "in like manner"[1].

Article 2 requires the Member States to ensure that the assessment process is conducted in accordance with the Annex to the Directive.

Articles 2a, 2b and 2c lay down the procedure to be applied where it is necessary to amend the Annex in the light of technical progress. Article 2a states that the procedure is that laid down in article 2c and states that the procedure can be reviewed on application to the Council by the Commission :

"in connection with the detailed rules set for the exercise of the powers of implementation granted to the Commission";

(nothing in the Directive explains what this sentence means, but it apparently refers to the "comitology" rules provided for by Council Decision (EEC) 87/373 laying down the procedures for the exercise of implementing powers conferred on the Commission[2] : the procedures set out in article 2c of Directive (EEC) 75/318 are very similar to "variant (a)" of Procedure III laid down at article 2 of Decision (EEC) 87/373; articles 2a, 2b and 2c were introduced into Directive (EEC) 75/318 by Directive (EEC) 87/19 of 22 December 1986[3], whereas Decision (EEC) 87/373 was passed on 13 July 1987; the earlier rules are preserved by article 4 of Decision (EEC) 87/373, but the terms of article 2a appear to envisage that the procedures under article 2c should be reviewed at the same time as other procedural rules governed by Decision (EEC) 87/373; the Future System proposals in practice leave article 2c unchanged, although new articles 37a and 37b, in materially identical terms, have been inserted in Directive (EEC) 75/319 by article 4 of Directive (EEC) 93/39[4]).

Article 2b sets up a "Committee on the Adaptation to Technical Progress of the Directives on the Removal of Technical Barriers to Trade in the Medicinal Products Sector" consisting of representatives of the Member States and a representative of the Commission as chairman.

Article 2c sets out the procedure to be followed :

(a)   the chairman and the Member State representatives each have the power to have a matter referred to the Committee (article 2c(1));

(b)   the chairman submits draft measures to the Committee;

(c)   the Committee delivers an opinion on the draft according to a timetable set by the chairman to reflect the urgency of the matter;

(d)   the Member State representatives alone vote on the measures in accordance with the qualified majority procedure laid down by article 148(2) of the Treaty (article 2c(2));

(e)   where the Committee supports the measures, the Commission adopts them (article 2c(3)(a));

---

1.   See section 3.4.2 for discussion of those paragraphs.
2.   OJ L197 18.7.87 p33.
3.   OJ L15 17.1.87 p31.
4.   See section 8.3 post.

(f) where the Committee rejects the measures or fails to act, the Commission proposes the measures to the Council, which also acts by qualified majority (article 2c(3)(b));

(g) where the Council fails to act within three months of the proposal being made, the Commission adopts the measures.

Presumably, where both the Committee and the Council reject the Commission proposals, the Commission has to start again, though this possibility is not provided for by the Directive.

4.3   The Annex to the Directive

The Annex to Directive (EEC) 75/318 was replaced completely by Commission Directive (EEC) 91/507[1] adopted under the articles 2a, b and c procedure with the agreement of the Committee[2].

The Member States were required by article 2 of Directive (EEC) 91/507 to give effect to the new requirements by 1 January 1992[3]. The recitals to Directive (EEC) 91/507 make it clear that the principal reason for the new Annex is the coming into force of Directives (EEC) 89/342[4] (vaccines, toxins, serums, allergens), 89/343[5] (radiopharmaceuticals) and 89/381[6] (human blood or plasma) extending the scope of Directives (EEC) 65/65 and 75/319, though the second recital also refers to "technical progress" in relation to biotechnology and other high-technology products listed in the Annex to Directive (EEC) 87/22.

The Annex to Directive (EEC) 75/318 as amended is a detailed document directed to applicants for marketing authorisation for pharmaceutical products and to the Member State authorities that bear the responsibility for assessing such applications. The Introduction to the Annex refers expressly to two further documents issued by the Commission as guidelines to the industry in 1989 :

"The rules governing medicinal products in the European Community, Volume II : Notice to applicants for marketing authorisations for medicinal products for human use in the Member States of the European Community";

and

"The rules governing medicinal products in the European Community, Volume III and supplements : Guidelines on the quality, safety and efficacy of medicinal products for human use".

Although the Annex, as binding legislation of the Community, is included in Appendix 2 hereto, the details of the Annex and of these guidelines are beyond the scope of this work. Each of the three documents is precisely designed to give those applying for marketing authorisation and those assessing such applications the guidance they need.

---

1.   OJ L270 26.9.91 p32. The text of Council Directive (EEC) 75/318 as amended is set out in Appendix 2 post.

2.   See recital 7 to Directive (EEC) 91/507.

3.   With the exception of Part 2, para A, point 3.3, which does not have to be implemented until 1 January 1995. There were two minor corrections made subsequently to the text of Directive (EEC) 91/507 : see OJ L299 30.10.91 p52 and OJ L320 22.11.91 p35.

4.   OJ L142 25.5.89 p15.

5.   OJ L142 25.5.89 p16.

6.   OJ L181 28.6.89 p44.

Chapter 5 : Council Directive (EEC) 75/319[1] - Administrative Requirements and the Establishment of the Committee for Proprietary Medicinal Products - The "Multi-State" Procedure

5.1   The scope and structure of the Directive : the recitals

Council Directive (EEC) 75/319 has the same long title as Directive (EEC) 65/65[2] : "on the approximation of provisions laid down by law, regulation or administrative action relating to proprietary[3] medicinal products", and for that reason is entitled the "Second Council Directive" although it is the third of the major pharmaceutical Directives. Recital 1 of the Directive is in identical terms to recital 1 of Directive (EEC) 75/318[4] and makes it clear that the two Directives are intended jointly to extend the harmonisation process initiated by Directive (EEC) 65/65.

Recital 2 identifies the first main aim of the Directive : to lay down rules "on the control of [medicinal products] and the duties incumbent upon the Member States' competent authorities". Directive (EEC) 75/319 sets out procedural rules to be followed to complement the more detailed substantive rules set out in Directive (EEC) 75/318.

Recitals 3 to 5 announce a major initiative which has been greatly expanded and developed subsequently, in particular by Directives (EEC) 83/570[5], 87/22[6] and most recently by the Future System package of measures described in Chapters 7 to 9. As "one step" towards free movement of medicinal products, the Committee on Proprietary Medicinal Products ("the CPMP") is to be set up in order to facilitate "the issue of authorisations to place one and the same medicinal product on the market in two or more Member States". The CPMP is to consist of "representatives of the Member States and of the Commission" and is to be "responsible for giving an opinion as to whether a particular [medicinal product] complies with the requirements set out in Directive (EEC) 65/65". Recital 5 foresees that further such measures "will be necessary in the light of experience gained, particularly in the above-mentioned Committee".

The CPMP's role as the principal Community body responsible for the development of common procedures and standards throughout the Community is obviously crucial if the aims originally set out in the recitals to Directive (EEC) 65/65 are to be achieved. The importance of the CPMP will be further increased from 1 January 1995 with the coming into force of the Future System legislation described in

---

1.   OJ L147 9.6.75 p13. See Appendix 3 post.
2.   OJ No 22 9.2.65 p369/65. See Appendix 1 post.
3.   By an apparent oversight, the deletion of the word "proprietary" in Directive (EEC) 65/65 by Directive (EEC) 89/341 did not extend to the related provisions of (EEC) 75/319 with the result that certain absurdities remain in the wording of the later Directive. There is no conceivable reason why the scope of Directive (EEC) 75/319 should be more limited than that of Directive (EEC) 65/65. The convention has been adopted of writing "[medicinal products]" where the text of Directive (EEC) 75/319 is manifestly in need of amendment.
4.   OJ L147 9.6.75 p1. See Appendix 2 post.
5.   OJ L332 28.11.83 p1.
6.   OJ L15 17.1.87 p38.

Chapters 7 to 9 below but the CPMP's activities are described in detail in a series of reports by the Commission to date. There have been eight such reports issued since 1979, the latest of which was dated 12 May 1993[1]. The Reports contain some statistical analysis of the decisions taken by the national authorities and of the opinions issued by the CPMP pursuant to Directive (EEC) 75/319 and, more recently, Directive (EEC) 87/22[2] in addition to description of the activities of the CPMP and its working parties appointed to consider specific issues[3].

Recitals 6 and 7 state the need for minimum requirements for the authorisation and supervision of the manufacture of medicinal products in order to facilitate the movement of products and to prevent the controls carried out in one Member State being repeated in another, and also provides for the specification of minimum qualifications for a person responsible for the supervision and control of manufacture within a pharmaceutical manufacturing company. The provisions of Directive (EEC) 75/319 in respect of manufacture are considered in Chapter 10 below.

Recital 8 states that certain technically sophisticated products are beyond the scope of the Community rules "at the present time" (those products identified in article 34 of the Directive and now brought within the scope of the regime by Directives (EEC) 89/342, 89/343, 89/381 and 92/73[4]), while recital 9 notes that certain provisions are amending provisions in respect of Directive (EEC) 65/65 (as elsewhere in the Appendices to this work, amending provisions have been incorporated in the amended legislation and omitted from the text of the amending legislation).

The Directive is divided into seven Chapters : I Application for authorisation to place [medicinal products] on the market; II Examination of the application for authorisation to place [medicinal products] on the market; III Committee for Proprietary Medicinal Products; IV Manufacture and imports coming from third countries; V Supervision and sanctions; VI Miscellaneous provisions; VII Implementing provisions and transitional measures.

Chapter IV is considered in Chapter 10 hereto and Chapter V in Chapter 11. The important Chapters for present purposes are I, II and III : Chapter I further amplifies article 4 of Directive (EEC) 65/65 so as to require expert reports to be provided by applicants for market authorisation; Chapter II gives more detailed guidance to the Member State authorities in examining applications; while Chapter III provides for the establishment of the CPMP. Chapters VI and VII set out general requirements. Chapter III of the Directive has been substantially revised and amended by Directive (EEC) 93/39[5].

---

1. The complete list is : COM(79) 59 of 22 February 1979; COM(80) 149 of 31 March 1980; COM(81) 363 of 13 July 1981; COM(82) 787 of 3 December 1982; COM(84) 437 of 3 December 1984 (in the form of an explanatory memorandum); COM(88) 143 of 22 March 1988; COM(91) 39 of 15 February 1991; and SEC(93) 771.
2. OJ L15 17.1.87 p38. See Appendix 4 post.
3. The name of the CPMP itself is a particularly blatant anachronism : the Committee's activities are not of course now limited to those relating to "proprietary medicinal products" and a more accurate name would now be "Committee for Medicinal Products for Human Use".
4. OJ L142 25.5.89 pp14-15, 16-18; OJ L181 28.6.89 p44; OJ L297 13.10.92 p12.
5. OJ L214 24.8.93 p22. See Chapter 8 post.

5.2   Further requirements in respect of the application for marketing authorisation : Chapter I, articles 1 to 3

Article 1 requires that the "particulars and documents" listed at articles 4(7) and 4(8) of Directive (EEC) 65/65 (that is to say the description of the control methods employed by the manufacturer and the results of tests and clinical trials), should be "drawn up by experts with the necessary technical or professional qualifications" and signed by those experts.

Article 2 sets out the duties of the experts :

(1)   "to perform tasks falling within their respective disciplines (analysis, pharmacology and similar experimental sciences, clinical trials)";

(2)   "to describe objectively the results obtained (qualitatively and quantitatively)" (article 2(a)); and

(3)   "to describe their observations in accordance with Council Directive (EEC) 75/318", in particular :

    (a)   the analyst should state "whether the product is consistent with the declared composition, giving any substantiation of the control methods employed by the manufacturer";

    (b)   the pharmacologist/similar specialist should state "the toxicity of the product and the pharmacological properties observed"; and

    (c)   the clinician should state :

       -   "whether he has been able to ascertain effects on persons treated with the product which correspond to the particulars given by the applicant in accordance with article 4 of Directive (EEC) 65/65";

       -   "whether the patient tolerates the product well";

       -   "the posology the clinician advises";

       and

       -   "any contra-indications and side-effects";

(4)   finally, where published references are used relying on articles 4(8)(a) and (b) of Directive (EEC) 65/65[1], to state the grounds for such use.

The second paragraph of article 2 provides that :

"[d]etailed reports by the experts shall form part of the particulars accompanying the application which the applicant submits to the competent authorities".

Article 3 states in effect that failure to observe the requirements of articles 1 and 2 will be deemed to be non-compliance with the requirements of article 4 of Directive (EEC) 65/65, and therefore for refusal of authorisation under article 5, second paragraph, of that Directive[2].

---

1.   See section 3.4.2 ante.
2.   See section 3.2 ante.

5.3   Guidance to the Member States in examining applications for marketing authorisation : Chapter II, articles 4 to 7

Article 4(a) imposes two *duties* on "the competent authorities of the Member States". They must :

(1)   "verify whether the particulars submitted in support of the application comply with [article 4 of Directive (EEC) 65/65]"; and

(2)   "examine whether the conditions for issuing an authorisation to place proprietary medicinal products on the market (marketing authorisation) are complied with".

These two duties obviously relate respectively to what were called the "formal" and "substantive" criteria in article 5 of Directive (EEC) 65/65[1] : the first duty requires the Member State authorities to confirm that the application is accurate; the second duty requires them to ensure that the product satisfies the substantive criteria of being non-harmful and efficacious. As such, article 4(a) adds nothing of substance to Directive (EEC) 65/65.

Article 4(b) gives the Member State authorities the *power* to :

"submit the[2] medicinal product, its starting materials and, if need be, its intermediate products or other constituent materials for testing by a State laboratory or a laboratory designated for that purpose in order to ensure that the control methods employed by the manufacturer and described in the particulars accompanying the application in accordance with the second subparagraph of point 7 of article 4, second paragraph, of Directive (EEC) 65/65 are satisfactory".

Article 4(c) gives the Member State authorities a further power to demand supplementary information from an applicant in respect of the items listed in the second paragraph of article 4 of Directive (EEC) 65/65. If they do so, the usual time limits[3] are suspended, until either the extra information has been provided or any extra time granted to the applicant to give "oral or written explanation" has expired.

Article 4(b) and (c) are thus somewhat more significant in that they clarify the national authorities' powers to conduct their own investigations and to demand further information. These powers clearly give those authorities a wide discretion in performing their role, to accelerate or retard the authorisation process.

Article 5(a) imposes a further duty on the Member States, to "take all appropriate measures to ensure that their competent authorities" verify that "manufacturers and importers of products coming from third countries" (ie non-EEC countries) :

(1)   can manufacture the products "in compliance with the particulars supplied pursuant to point 4 of article 4, second paragraph, of Directive (EEC) 65/65"; and/or

(2)   can "carry out controls according to the methods described in the particulars accompanying the application in accordance with point 7 of article 4, second paragraph, of [Directive (EEC) 65/65]".

---

1.   See section 3.2 ante.
2.   This is one of the few places in Directive (EEC) 75/319 where the word "proprietary" has been deleted by Directive (EEC) 89/341.
3.   See article 7 of Directive (EEC) 65/65 and section 3.6 ante.

Article 5(b) requires the Member States to permit the authorities to allow manufacturers and importers from third countries :

"in exceptional and justifiable circumstances, to have certain stages of manufacture or certain of the controls referred to in [5(a)] carried out by third parties".

In such cases, the authorities must perform the verifications required by 5(a) in "the establishment designated".

Chapter IV of Directive (EEC) 75/319 specifically deals with authorisation of manufacture and of imports from third countries and introduces a new layer of regulation by requiring that the manufacturer should obtain authorisation as a manufacturer in addition to obtaining authorisation of the product itself. That regime is considered in Chapter 10 below. Article 5 does not add anything to those provisions in respect of the manufacturer but links the authorisation of manufacture to the Member States' obligations in respect of marketing authorisation : the Member States must not only operate each separate authorisation regime; they must also ensure that products can be properly manufactured before granting authorisation for those products to be marketed within the Community.

Articles 6 and 7 concern leaflets "enclosed with the packaging of a proprietary medicinal product". Like articles 13 to 20 of Directive (EEC) 65/65, those provisions are repealed by article 13 of Directive (EEC) 92/27[1].

5.4 The Committee for Proprietary Medicinal Products : Chapter III, articles 8 to 15

Chapter III of Directive (EEC) 75/319 is central to what has been, at least until very recently, one of the most contentious of the issues involved in the Community's efforts to create a single market for pharmaceuticals : how far should a central Community body usurp the national authorities' right to control the authorisation of the marketing of pharmaceutical products on its national markets in the interests of free movement of goods within the Community ? The wording of Chapter III discussed here represents the complete replacement of the original text of articles 8 to 15 of Directive (EEC) 75/319 by article 3 of Council Directive (EEC) 83/570[2]. The radical reform of the Chapter contained in Directive (EEC) 93/39, which again completely replaces Chapter III of Directive (EEC) 75/319, is considered in Chapter 8, where the differences between the old and the new regimes are also discussed. The procedures described below will continue to be operative until 1 January 1995.

Article 8, which sets up the CPMP, makes its purpose quite clear :

"to facilitate the adoption of a common position by the Member States with regard to decisions on the issuing of marketing authorisations and to promote thereby the free movement of proprietary medicinal products" (article 8(1)).

1.　　　OJ L113 30.4.92 p8. See Chapter 15 post.
2.　　　OJ L332 28.11.83 p1. The text of Chapter III of Directive (EEC) 75/319 in force from 1 January 1995 is incorporated in Appendix 3 post, with the rest operative until that date included at the end of Appendix 3.

Again, article 9 states the purpose of its provisions to be :

> "to make it easier to obtain a marketing authorisation in at least two other Member States taking into due consideration an authorisation issued in one Member State in accordance with article 3 of Directive (EEC) 65/65".

Likewise, article 15 provides for the Commission to report to the Council every two years and to submit a proposal within four years :

> "containing appropriate measures leading to the free movement of proprietary medicinal products".

It has thus always been clear that the Community regarded the setting up of the CPMP as no more than a first step, and the Chapter was amended by Council Directive (EEC) 78/420[1] and replaced by Directive (EEC) 83/570 even before the wide-ranging reform proposals included as part of the 1992 Programme for pharmaceuticals emerged for discussion. The current system remains very modest, principally because the CPMP has no power to impose its views on the national authorities, but it represents a *more* significant role for the Community than that included in the original text of Directive (EEC) 75/319[2].

As stated above, article 8 sets up the CPMP :

(1) article 8(1) states that it "shall consist of representatives of the Member States and of the Commission";

(2) article 8(2) defines the CPMP's task :

> "to examine, at the request of a Member State or the Commission and in accordance with articles 9 to 14, questions concerning the application of articles 5, 11 or 20 of Directive (EEC) 65/65";

> (it will be remembered that those latter articles concern respectively authorisation, supervision of authorised products and labelling; authorisation is considered here, but supervision is considered in Chapter 11 below and labelling in Chapter 15)[3];

(3) article 8(3) simply requires the CPMP to draw up its own rules of procedure; the CPMP does not have complete discretion, because articles 9 to 14 of Directive (EEC) 75/319 lay down quite a detailed procedural framework to be observed by the national authorities and by the CPMP itself.

5.4.1   Initiating the multi-State procedure : articles 9 and 10

Article 9 provides the holder of a marketing authorisation in one Member State with the power to re-use the material submitted to that Member State in its application for authorisation in *at least two* other Member States. Where the holder exercises his power to :

---

1. OJ L123 11.5.78 p26.
2. The principal extension of the CPMP's competence resulted from Directive (EEC) 83/570, which reduced the number of additional Member States where a company had to apply to market a product already authorised in one Member State from five to two for the purposes of activating the articles 9, 10 and 14 procedures.
3. A minor anomaly has been present in the legislation since the repeal of article 20 of Directive (EEC) 65/65 by Directive (EEC) 92/27. That will be removed by the coming into force of Directive (EEC) 93/39, which gives the CPMP more general powers: see Chapter 8.

"submit an application to the competent authorities of the Member States concerned together with the information and documents referred to in articles 4, 4a and 4b of Directive (EEC) 65/65",

he falls under a number of obligations. He is required :

(1) to testify to the identity of any subsequent application "with the dossier accepted by the first Member State";

(2) to specify any additions the subsequent application may contain; and

(3) to "certify that all the dossiers filed as part of this procedure are identical" (article 9(1));

Requirement (2) is on its face mysterious, as it appears to undermine requirement (1) and also perhaps requirement (3). In practice, and as further explained by requirement (8) below, the substance of these requirements is to ensure that the original Member State and any subsequent Member States are ultimately all in possession of identical information upon which to base their decisions. If necessary, the original "dossier" must be amended or amplified to take subsequent developments into account.

The holder is further required :

(4) to notify the CPMP of such subsequent applications;

(5) to inform the CPMP as to the Member States concerned;

(6) to send the CPMP a copy of the original authorisation;

(7) to inform the Member State which granted the original authorisation (presumably of the same items as those given to the CPMP);

(8) to notify that Member State of any additions to the original dossier (article 9(2)); and

(9) to notify (it is not stated to whom, but presumably to the CPMP) "the dates on which the dossiers were sent to the Member States concerned" (article 9(3)).

The Member State issuing the initial authorisation may impose a further obligation :

(10) "to provide it with all the particulars and documents necessary to enable it to check the identity of the dossiers filed with the dossier on which it took its decision" (article 9(3)).

Article 9(3) further requires that the CPMP, as soon as it has "noted" that all the Member States concerned are in possession of the dossier :

"shall forthwith inform all the Member States and the applicant of the date on which the last Member State concerned received the dossier".

(It is not wholly clear whether "all the Member States" means all the Member States *concerned* or all the Member States of the Community. In practice, it is not likely to be of significance, since the only interest in the procedure likely to be taken by Member States where no application for marketing authorisation has been made or granted is via their representatives' involvement in the CPMP deliberations themselves, where of course they will be informed with all other representatives of the Member States.)

The most significant requirement of article 9(3) is however imposed on the *Member States* receiving an application modelled on an application in another Member State where authorisation has already been granted. Those Member States are required either to :

> "grant the authorisation valid for their markets within a period of 120 days of the [date on which the last Member State concerned received the dossier], taking into due consideration the authorisation issued [by another Member State]"

or to "put forward a reasoned objection".

The substance of article 9 is therefore that on obtaining an authorisation from one Member State, the holder of that authorisation can compel other Member States (provided that there are at least two) either to grant authorisation themselves on the basis of the material submitted to the original Member State or else to state a reasoned objection, in either case within 120 days. Given that the time limit laid down by article 7 of Directive (EEC) 65/65 for ordinary applications is 120 days in any event, this may not appear a huge advance. The significance of the procedure is :

(1) that the same material can be used simultaneously or successively in different applications; and

(2) that increased transparency is introduced into the decision-making process by the requirement that a Member State must support any decision to adopt an attitude different from that previously taken by another Member State *to exactly the same material* by formulating a reasoned objection.

Article 10 sets out basic procedural requirements to be observed where one or more of the Member States in receipt of a subsequent application do wish to put forward a reasoned objection :

(1) the Member State or States concerned are required to send their reasoned objection or objections both to the CPMP and to the holder of the original authorisation; the reasoned objection must comply with two requirements :

    (a)   it must be "in accordance with article 5 of Directive (EEC) 65/65", that is to say that it must object to the application only on one or more of the three permitted grounds set out in article 5[1];

    (b)   it must be submitted within the time limits set down in article 9(3) (article 10(1));

(2) the matter shall be referred to the CPMP and the procedure referred to in article 14 shall be applied, as to which see below (article 10(2)); and

(3) the holder of the original authorisation is required to send a copy of the dossier submitted to the Member States immediately on receiving the reasoned objection of one of the Member States (article 10(3)).

5.4.2   Other mechanisms, for consultation of the CPMP : articles 11 and 12

Articles 9 and 10 concern the case where one Member State has granted marketing authorisation and the holder of that authorisation wishes to extend that authorisation to other Member States. Article 11 deals with the different situation where a number of applications have been made to various Member States and the

---

1.   See section 3.2 above.

results have not been the same. Where such applications have been made in accordance with Directive (EEC) 65/65 :

"one of the Member States concerned or the Commission may refer the matter to the [CPMP] for application of the procedure referred to in article 14 of this Directive".

(The same applies in relation to suspension or revocation of the authorisation[1].

The third paragraph of article 11 is oddly phrased :

"[where article 11 applies], the person responsible for placing the proprietary medicinal product on the market shall be informed of any decision of the [CPMP] to apply the procedure laid down in article 14".

This appears to imply that the CPMP enjoys a discretion as to whether or not it should apply the article 14 procedure. Nothing else in Chapter III suggests that to be the case and article 14(1) appears to state the contrary. It seems therefore to be no more than a drafting error, the paragraph meaning in effect that the CPMP must notify the applicant in the various Member States whenever either a Member State or the Commission refers a matter to the CPMP under article 11.

Article 12 gives the competent authorities of Member States a general discretion to refer cases to the CPMP :

"before reaching a decision on a request for a marketing authorisation or on the suspension or revocation of an authorisation".

Although the discretion is general, it is limited to : "specific cases where the interests of the Community are involved". The article is vaguely drafted : no guidance is given on what the above expression means; nor on whether the CPMP can reject such a reference if it fails to satisfy this requirement; nor indeed what procedure should be followed if article 12 were to be appropriately relied on by a national authority. Article 14 refers only to articles 9 and 10, so that it may be that the CPMP could rely on article 8(3) and regulate its own procedures in relation to article 12.

In practice, however, article 12 has been of some importance in that it has permitted the involvement of the CPMP in a number of cases where national authorities have taken divergent views in respect of particular applications. Examples are contained in the Commission's Report on the Operation of the CPMP[2].

5.4.3   Assessment reports : article 13

Article 13 is to some extent misplaced in Chapter III. Like article 4 in Chapter II of the Directive, article 13 imposes a duty on the competent authorities of a Member State, in this case to :

"1.   ... draw up an assessment report and comments on the dossier as regards the results of the analytical and toxico-pharmacological tests on, and clinical trials of, any [medicinal products] containing a new active substance which are the subject of a request for a marketing authorisation in the Member States concerned for the first time.

---

1.   See section 11.2 post.
2.   SEC(93) 771.

2.   ...

The competent authorities shall bring the assessment report up to date as soon as it is in possession of information which is of importance for the evaluation to the balance between effectiveness and risk."

Article 13(1) is particularly obscurely drafted : it appears to impose a quite general duty on the Member States to prepare reports, but it also refers to a request for marketing authorisation for a new product in more than one Member State. It is not clear when the duty imposed by the Directive is activated, whether it only arises when a difference of opinion emerges between the Member States or whether it arises whenever more than one Member State is concerned with an application for authorisation. The provision appears in a more generalised form as part of the new article 4b of Directive (EEC) 65/65.

The parts of article 13 relevant to Chapter III are the first and second sub-paragraphs of article 13(2) :

(1)   the first sentence of the first sub-paragraph apparently refers to requirement (7) on the holder of an authorisation in one Member State applying for authorisation in another Member State set out above in relation to article 9, to notify the original Member State of subsequent applications; where the original Member State receives such a notification, it must immediately send its "assessment report accompanied by a summary of the dossier relating to a particular proprietary product" to the other Member States concerned; it is not at all clear why it needs to send a summary of the dossier, given that article 9 of the Directive already requires all Member States concerned to be in possession of identical dossiers; the only purpose would apparently be to permit a cross-check of the application;

(2)   the second sentence of the first sub-paragraph of article 13(2) requires the assessment report to be sent to the CPMP "where a matter is referred to the [CPMP] pursuant to article 10" (see above);

(3)   the second subparagraph of article 13(2) requires that the report :

"shall also be forwarded to the other Member States concerned and to the [CPMP] as soon as a matter is referred to the [CPMP] under the procedure laid down in article 11";

in this case presumably a number of assessment reports will circulate between the Member States that have come to the same or different conclusions about the product (this sub-paragraph has a further odd feature in that its second sentence provides that any assessment report forwarded under this provision "shall remain confidential"; it would be natural to assume that all such reports were confidential, but this provision appears to imply that reports sent to other Member States or to the CPMP in accordance with articles 9 or 10 are not so protected).

5.4.4   Procedure : article 14
Article 14 sets out the outline of the procedure to be followed by the CPMP and the scope of its activities :

(1)   procedurally, the CPMP is required :

(a)   to "consider the matter concerned"; and

(b)   to "issue a reasoned opinion within 60 days of the date on which the matter was referred to it" (article 14(1), first sub-paragraph);

(2) under the article 10 procedure, the holder of the authorisation has the right to "explain himself orally or in writing" before the CPMP issues its opinion and time can be extended in order to make this possible (article 14(1), second sub-paragraph);

(3) under the article 11 procedure, the applicant or holder of an authorisation has no right to be heard, but "may be asked to explain himself orally or in writing"; there is no provision for extension of time in such a case; it is not stated who may ask the applicant or holder to explain himself, but presumably it is the CPMP itself rather than the Commission or the Member States (article 14(1), third sub-paragraph); it is not obvious why the applicant's or holder's rights should be more limited in an article 11 case than an article 10 case[1];

(4) the CPMP is required to inform both the Member States concerned and the "person responsible for placing the product on the market" of "its opinion or of those of its members in the case of divergent opinions"; (article 14(2), second sub-paragraph); nothing in the Directive appears to require any degree of consensus in the opinions of the CPMP members;

(5) the Member States are required to :

"decide what action to take on the Committee's opinion within 60 days of receipt [of that opinion]";

(6) the Member States must immediately inform the CPMP of their decision (article 14(3)).

The impotence of the CPMP is clear from this procedural account : there is no requirement that the CPMP should reach a clear single opinion, nor is there any requirement that the Member States should take any notice at all of the CPMP's view (in theory, there is no requirement even to read the opinion); further, there is no provision for the CPMP to prevent, object to or even comment on the Member States' response to the opinion, however perverse or unyielding.

Substantively, the scope of the CPMP's activities is defined at article 14(2), sub-paragraph 1 :

"[t]he [CPMP]'s opinion shall concern the grounds for the objection provided for in article 10(1) and the grounds on which the marketing authorisation has been refused, suspended or withdrawn in the cases described in article 11."

The CPMP's opinion is limited in scope to commenting either :

(1) on the objections raised by a Member State asked to give an authorisation subsequent to an authorisation issued in another Member State; or

---

1.   The Commission is clearly sensitive to such criticism : its Report on the Operation of the CPMP, SEC(93) 771, states at p40 that the applicant or holder of an authorisation "may generally avail of the opportunity for written oral explanation to the CPMP" under article 11. Article 14 makes no provision for article 12 cases, but the Report states the CPMP's view to be that "when practical, the applicant or the marketing authorisation holder would be offered the opportunity to make a submission, orally or in writing, before the CPMP issues its opinion". There must be doubt as to whether the CPMP's practices would withstand scrutiny by a court.

(2) on the grounds for refusal, suspension or withdrawal of authorisation where opinions differ between Member States.

The CPMP has no power to comment on positive decisions to grant or continue authorisation in either case or to suggest other grounds on which authorisation might be refused, suspended or withdrawn. Again, the scope of the CPMP's activities is plainly limited by comparison to the power of the national authorities, which are of course free to raise novel objections at their discretion, subject only to bringing them within the terms of article 5 of Directive (EEC) 65/65. There is no substantive guidance as to the CPMP's role under article 12.

5.4.5   Review of the multi-State procedure
Article 15 sets out a timetable for review and amendment of the provisions of Chapter 3 :

(1) article 15(1) requires the Commission to report to the Council every 2 years :

> "on the operation of the procedure laid down in this chapter and its effect on the development of intra-Community trade";

(2) article 15(2) requires the Community to submit proposals to the Council containing :

> "appropriate measures leading towards the abolition of any remaining barriers to the free movement of proprietary medicinal products."

within four years of the entry into force of Directive (EEC) 75/319[1];

(3) the Council is required to decide on the Commission proposal within a year.

The fact that the Future System legislation will not come into full effect until 1 January 1998 indicates that this timetable was over-ambitious, although the amending provisions of Directives (EEC) 78/420 and (EEC) 83/570 represented continuing efforts by the Community to promote the effectiveness of the "multi-State" procedure.

5.5   "Miscellaneous provisions" : Chapter VI, articles 30 to 40[2]

Articles 30 to 33 are largely concerned with the revocation or suspension of marketing and manufacturing authorisations and the withdrawal of products from the market and are therefore considered in Chapters 10 and 11, but certain provisions are relevant to marketing authorisations. Article 31 requires, inter alia, that reasons be given for negative decisions under article 5(b) (third party

---

1.   The wording of article 15(2) is clear enough but, given that it was incorporated in Directive (EEC) 75/319 by Directive (EEC) 83/570, it seems likely that the date referred to was intended to be the date of entry into force of Directive (EEC) 83/570, which was in fact 31 October 1985.

2.   As stated at section 5.1 ante, Chapters IV and V, articles 16 to 29, are concerned with the authorisation and supervision of the manufacture and marketing of medicinal products. Those issues are dealt with in Chapters 10 and 11 post. Article 26, first paragraph is widely drafted : "The competent authority of the Member State concerned shall ensure, by means of repeated inspections, that the legal requirements governing medicinal products are complied with." However, the substance of article 26 and of Chapter V generally relates to manufacture and supervision and it is therefore considered in the Chapters dealing with those issues.

manufacture) and article 11(3) (CPMP decision on a matter where two Member States disagree)[1]. Article 33(1) also provides in part that :

> "Each Member State shall take all the appropriate measures to ensure that decisions authorising marketing, refusing ... a marketing authorisation [or] cancelling a decision refusing ... a marketing authorisation ... together with the reasons on which such decisions are based, are brought to the attention of the [CPMP] forthwith".

No reason is given for this provision and there is no requirement that the CPMP should do anything with the information provided to it. It is merely a further step in co-ordinating national procedures by creating a common pool of information concerning national decisions. The new European Agency for the Evaluation of Medicinal Products described in Chapter 7 should increase considerably the scope and importance of such initiatives. Article 33(3) and (4) impose two other requirements : the first on the Member States to bring to the attention of the World Health Organisation any action they have taken pursuant to article 33(1) or 33(2) "which may affect the protection of public health in third countries", and to send a copy to the CPMP; the second on the Commission, to publish a negative list annually of "the medicinal products which are prohibited in the Community". Given that all medicinal products which are not specifically authorised are prohibited by article 3, this second requirement is theoretically unlimited. Common sense dictates that the list is intended to specify only those products for which authorisation has been either refused or revoked by a national competent authority.

Article 34 defines the scope of the Directive, but it does so in an unsatisfactory way and it has also been overtaken by the changes introduced by the "extension" Directives listed at footnote 3 above. Paragraph 1 provides that :

> "[t]his Directive shall apply to medicinal products for human use, within the limits referred to in Directive (EEC) 65/65".

The meaning of "medicinal products" has been discussed in Chapter 2 above. The problem with the provision does not lie in the wording itself but in the inconsistency of that wording with the remainder of the Directive (and of article 34 itself).

The second paragraph of article 34 excludes vaccines, toxins and serums, products based on human blood or blood constituents or radioactive isotopes and homeopathic products from the scope of the Directive[2]. This provision has been to a large extent effectively repealed by Directives (EEC) 89/342, 89/343, 89/381 and 92/73. The paragraph refers to "proprietary medicinal products" but it is again absurd to suppose that (once the limitation of the scope of the Community rules to proprietary medicinal products had been removed in the first paragraph) non-proprietary versions of those products could have been intended to be within the scope of the Community rules while proprietary versions of such products remained excluded under article 34.

---

1. Article 11(3) refers to a "decision of the [CPMP] to apply the procedure laid down in article 14" but the significant decision in practice would be a negative opinion by the CPMP in respect of a product whose quality, safety or efficacy were differently assessed by the national authorities. Article 31 was not amended by Directive (EEC) 93/39, but article 11(3) has ceased to exist in the newly amended article 11.
2. The Annex to the Directive gives examples of "vaccines, toxins and serums" in three categories: "agents used to produce active immunity (such as cholera vaccine, BCG, polio vaccine, smallpox vaccine); agents used to diagnose the state of immunity including in particular tuberculin and tuberculin PPD, toxins for the Schick and Dick Tests, brucellin; agents used to produce passive immunity (such as diphtheria antitoxin, anti-smallpox globulin, antilymphocytic globulin)".

Articles 35 to 37 are incorporated in Directive (EEC) 65/65.

The last significant article, article 39, lays down certain time limits :

(1)   article 39(1) contains a transitional provision for manufacturing authorisations and is considered in Chapter 10 below;

(2)   article 39(2) is an important provision, providing that :

> "Within 15 years of the notification referred to in article 38, the other provisions of this Directive [ie those not concerned with manufacturing authorisations] shall be applied progressively to [medicinal products] placed on the market by virtue of previous provisions";

in effect, this requires the Member State authorities to review all pre-existing marketing authorisations in the light of Directive (EEC) 75/319 before May 1990 to ensure that the procedures applied to those products, both at the time of authorisation and subsequently, conformed to the requirements of the Directive;

(3)   article 39(3) requires the Member States to notify the Commission, within 3 years, of the number of products "covered by" article 39(2) :

> "and, each subsequent year, of the number of these products for which a marketing authorisation referred to in article 3 of Directive (EEC) 65/65 has not yet been issued".

On their own, those provisions make little sense, since the provisions of Directive (EEC) 75/319 concerning marketing authorisation and supervision are to a large extent merely expanding on the terms of Directive (EEC) 65/65, so that they could not be implemented without parallel implementation of the earlier Directive. It is therefore necessary to read article 39(2) and (3) in conjunction with article 24 of Directive (EEC) 65/65. The overall effect of those provisions is that :

(1)   all products marketed under national regimes prior to the introduction of the (EEC) 65/65 regime must be confirmed by the national authorities to comply with the Community regime by May 1990[1];

(2)   the administrative procedures set out in Directive (EEC) 75/319 must also be applied to such products by May 1990[2];

(3)   the Member States must provide the Commission with a list of products which have not yet been brought within the terms of the two Directives, initially within 3 years from the date of notification of the Directive but updated annually thereafter[3].

Given that all the relevant time limits have now expired, those provisions should now be redundant and the Directive be straightforwardly effective to all products within its terms.

---

1.   See article 24 of Directive (EEC) 65/65.
2.   See article 39(2) of Directive (EEC) 75/319.
3.   See article 39(3) of Directive (EEC) 75/319.

Chapter 6 : Directive (EEC) 87/22[1] - High Technology Products and the "Concertation" Procedure

6.1 The path towards centralisation

After the coming into force of Directives (EEC) 75/318[2] and 75/319[3], a number of Directives were passed amending them and extending their scope and also amending or extending Directive (EEC) 65/65[4]. However, the very tentative steps by which the Community sought to introduce common procedures through the CPMP initially proved almost useless in addressing the fundamental aim of free movement of medicinal products within the Community, since the Member States (with the exception of Luxembourg) have invariably refused to accept the authorisation granted by another Member State and have referred the case to the CPMP for its opinion before making its own decision. None of the amendments addressed the central difficulty, that a "decentralised" system where mutual recognition is either the norm or is made compulsory raises the natural fear that each product will be authorised by the least demanding regulatory regime, with the potentially disastrous result that consumer protection and proper control of the drugs market is significantly reduced in at least some, and perhaps all, Member States. On the other hand, any other form of decentralised system has little or no impact on continuing national divisions. There has always been good reason to suppose, therefore, that a "centralised" system of authorisation is the only effective solution, but to achieve a centralised regime the Community had to overcome the national authorities' natural reluctance to surrender responsibility in so sensitive an area.

In the circumstances, Directive (EEC) 87/22 on the approximation of national measures relating to the placing on the market of high-technology medicinal products, particularly those derived from biotechnology represented, like the introduction of the "multi-State" procedure in Directive (EEC) 75/319, a small step towards centralised control. Whereas the "multi-State" procedure introduced a modest consultative machinery of general application, Directive (EEC) 87/22 introduced a somewhat more ambitious procedure, but limited its scope very narrowly, to "High-Technology Medicinal Products" as defined in the Annex to the Directive. The *general* significance of the initiative was as another "trial run" by the Community for a more centralised system. Chapters 7 to 9 set out the solution to the difficulty that has ultimately been agreed, in particular in Regulation (EEC) 2309/93[5] and Directive (EEC) 93/39[6].

---

1. OJ L15 17.1.87 p38. See Appendix 4 post.
2. OJ L147 9.6.75 p1. See Appendix 2 post.
3. OJ L147 9.6.75 p13. See Appendix 3 post.
4. OJ No 22 9.2.65 p369/65. See Appendix 1 post and footnotes to Appendices 1 to 3 for the relevant amendments.
5. OJ L214 24.8.93 p1. See Appendix 5 post.
6. OJ L214 24.8.93 p22. See Appendix 6 post and the amendments to Appendices 1 to 3.

6.2   Industrial policy and guaranteed standards : the recitals

The most important recitals for the purposes of understanding the motivation for Directive (EEC) 87/22, apart from the general motivation just described, are recitals 2, 5 and 6[1]:

> "Whereas high-technology medicinal products requiring lengthy periods of costly research will continue to be developed in Europe only if they benefit from a favourable regulatory environment, particularly identical conditions governing their placing on the market throughout the Community;
>
> ...
>
> Whereas, however, [the procedures introduced by Directive (EEC) 75/319] are not sufficient to open up to high-technology products the large Community-wide single market they require;
>
> Whereas, in this technically advanced sector, the scientific expertise available to each of the national authorities is not always sufficient to resolve problems posed by high-technology products".

Recitals 2 and 5 clearly point to a justification in terms of industrial policy, familiar from other high technology sectors, namely a perceived need to establish economic and regulatory conditions which enable European manufacturers to compete effectively in the global market, particularly against their American and Japanese commercial rivals.

Recital 6 refers to a quite distinct motivation, related to the fear described above, that a system of decentralised authorisations coupled with automatic mutual recognition between Member States would reduce safety standards to the lowest tolerated in any single Member State. Such a fear would become acute where it was believed that particular Member States were not technically capable of assessing certain types of product. Recital 6 itself states that certain individual Member States' authorities may not have the technical expertise to assess such products.

Recital 7 and the terms of the Directive itself provide a tactful way out for such authorities : the substance of what would have happened in practice was likely in any event to have been that one of the technically most sophisticated authorities would have been asked by an applicant for marketing authorisation to assess the product; that assessment would then have been relied on in applications for authorisations in other Member States. The mechanism of Directive (EEC) 87/22 enables that procedure to be co-ordinated at the Community level through a "Community mechanism for concertation, prior to any national decision relating to a high-technology medicinal product, with a view to arriving at uniform decisions throughout the Community". All the Member States have a share in such a process, at least through their representation on the CPMP. This procedure can be compared with the new procedures envisaged in the Future System proposals whereby the European Agency for the Evaluation of Medicinal Products will be established and will take responsibility for Community assessments of high technology products and of products concerning which the Member States cannot reach agreement : see Chapters 7 and 8. The obvious difference between the two systems is that there is

---

1.   Recital 1 stresses the primacy of safeguarding public health, Recitals 3 and 4 refer to Directive (EEC) 75/319 and the equivalent Directive in relation to veterinary products, Directive (EEC) 81/851, while recitals 7, 8 and 9 set out the contents of the Directive in general terms.

no mechanism for any opinion of the CPMP under Directive (EEC) 87/22 to bind any national authority in its subsequent decision.

6.3   The scope of the Directive : articles 1 and 2 and the Annex[1]

Just as Directives (EEC) 75/318 and 75/319 are heavily dependent on Directive (EEC) 65/65, so Directive (EEC) 87/22 is dependent on Directive (EEC) 75/319. Article 1, the principal provision of the Directive, expressly refers back to the CPMP as created by article 8 of Directive (EEC) 75/319 :

> "Before taking a decision on a marketing authorisation or on the withdrawal or, subject to article 4(2),[2] suspension of a marketing authorisation in respect of the medicinal products listed in the Annex, Member States' authorities shall, in accordance with articles 2, 3 and 4, refer the matter for an opinion to the [CPMP]."

The wording of the article is somewhat misleading, since it clearly implies that there is a mandatory requirement on the national authorities to refer all such products to the CPMP, whereas in fact that is not the case for *all* the products listed in the Annex and there are exceptions even where reference is the norm, so that in a sense it is not the case for *any* such products. This is explained below.

The Annex to the Directive has two categories, "List A" and "List B" :

> "A.   Medicinal products developed by means of the following biotechnological processes :
>
> —   recombinant DNA technology,
> —   controlled expression of genes coding for biologically active proteins in prokaryotes and eukaryotes, including transformed mammalian cells,
> —   hybridoma and monoclonal antibody methods.
>
> B.   Other high-technology medicinal products :
>
> —   other biotechnological processes which, in the opinion of the competent authority concerned constitute a significant innovation,
> —   medicinal products administered by means of new delivery systems which, in the opinion of the competent authority concerned, constitute a significant innovation,
> —   medicinal products containing a new substance or an entirely new indication which, in the opinion of the competent authority concerned, is of significant therapeutic interest,
> —   new medicinal products based on radio-isotopes which, in the opinion of the competent authority concerned, are of significant therapeutic interest,

---

1.   Like Directive (EEC) 65/65, but unlike Directives (EEC) 75/318 and 75/319, Directive (EEC) 87/22 is applicable both to products for human use and to veterinary products. In keeping with the general aim of this work to simplify the complexity of the legislation as it appears in the texts themselves, the present exposition of the terms of the Directive ignores all references to veterinary products and to the related Community legislation, in particular Directive (EEC) 81/851 (OJ L317 6.11.81 p1) on the approximation of the laws of the Member States relating to veterinary medicinal products, which, in broad terms, introduced an equivalent Committee, the Committee for Veterinary Medicinal Products ("CVMP"), to the CPMP and equivalent procedures to those introduced by Directive (EEC) 75/319.

2.   See section 6.4 post.

> — medicinal products the manufacture of which employs processes which, in the opinion of the competent authority concerned, demonstrate a significant technical advance such as two-dimensional electrophoresis under micro-gravity."

This classification is important, since the two categories are differently affected by article 2 of the Directive. It is clear from the terms of the Annex that the Member States enjoy a wide discretion in relation to products potentially within the scope of List B : each category on that list is included only in accordance with "the opinion of the competent authority concerned". It would be hard to challenge a national authority which was of the opinion that a product was not sufficiently innovative to be included on List B.

Article 2(1) applies to products in each category and *requires* the competent authorities of a Member State to "bring the matter before" the CPMP as soon as an application for a marketing authorisation is received, but only :

> "at the request of the person responsible for placing the product on the market... Any such request shall be submitted in writing ... at the same time as the application for marketing authorisation and a copy shall be sent to the [CPMP]".

Thus, the applicant for marketing authorisation of such a product can effectively compel a national authority to refer the issue to the CPMP. On the other hand, subject to the subsequent paragraphs, the national authorities cannot apparently refer the matter if the applicant does not make such a request (and the authorities can avoid the need to refer products not on List A by refusal to place them on List B).

Article 2(2) and (3) apply specifically to products in category A. Article 2(2) requires the Member State authorities to refer all applications for marketing authorisations :

> "relating to a medicinal product developed by means of new biotechnological products and referred to in List A in the Annex"

immediately to the CPMP, but article (3) qualifies that requirement. Article 2(2) is stated by article 2(3) not to apply if the applicant certifies with his application that :

> "(i) neither he nor any other natural or legal person with whom he is connected has, during the preceding five years, applied for authorisation to place a product containing the same active principle(s) on the market of another Member State; and
> (ii) neither he nor any other natural or legal person with whom he is connected intends, within the five years following the date of the application, to seek authorisation to place a product containing the same active principle(s) on the market of another Member State."

Where those two conditions are both satisfied, a different procedure is laid down :

(1) "the competent authorities shall notify the [CPMP] of the application and forward to it a summary of product characteristics"

either in accordance with article 4a of Directive (EEC) 65/65[1] or else a similar document (where the product falls outside the scope of Directive (EEC) 65/65); in practice, this is now effectively redundant, as Directive (EEC) 65/65 now covers virtually all medicinal products);

---

1.   See section 3.4.3 ante.

(2) if the original applicant in fact makes further applications to other national authorities, within five years of the original application, for marketing authorisation for "a product containing the same active principle derived from the same route of synthesis", then the original authorities must be informed and the matter referred to the CPMP for its opinion.

In substance, therefore, a product on List A must be referred to the CPMP unless it is certified to be intended for marketing in one Member State only for a period of five years before and after the application, whereas a product on List B only has to be referred to the CPMP at the request of the applicant.

The Directive clearly envisages that the applicant will perceive there to be significant advantages in involving the CPMP at an early stage. It should be noted that there is no requirement that the product is to be marketed in more than one Member State, only the converse, that it is not certified to be marketed in only one Member State. In this respect, Directive (EEC) 87/22 differs markedly from Directive (EEC) 75/319 even as amended, since there has always been a requirement under Directive (EEC) 75/319 that at least two States are concerned, in addition to the original authorising State[1].

Article 2(4) is a further small step towards making CPMP opinions binding on the Member States. It provides that national authorities may not normally withdraw or suspend marketing authorisation for a high-technology product for which the CPMP has issued a favourable opinion without "referring the matter to the [CPMP] for a new opinion". The second sentence of article 4(2) (which would be more appropriately positioned as the second sentence of article 2(4)) qualifies article 2(4) by permitting the Member States to :

"suspend the marketing authorisation in question without waiting for the opinion of the [CPMP] provided that they forthwith inform the [CPMP] thereof, indicating the reasons for the suspension and justifying the urgency of this measure".

The Member States are therefore obliged to take notice of a favourable CPMP opinion if they have granted authorisation for the marketing of a product falling within the scope of the Directive, unlike under the procedure established by Directive (EEC) 75/319[2]. That gives the CPMP some power, but it also serves to highlight the weakness of the CPMP in relation to the original authorisation, where Directive (EEC) 87/22 still does not require the Member States to act in accordance with the CPMP opinion nor even to justify a contrary view[3].

Article 2(5), provides that either the national authorities or the Commission :

"may also consult the [CPMP] on any technical question concerning the proprietary medicinal products referred to in the second paragraph of article 34 of Directive (EEC) 75/319".

Whatever limited importance this special provision may once have had, for those products excluded from the scope of the earlier Directives by article 34(2) of Directive (EEC) 75/319, has vanished since those products were brought within the

---

1. In practice, somewhat ironically, the "multi-State" procedure has generally involved about half the Member States (average 5.20, 1988-1990; 6.32, 1991-1992), whereas the "concertation" procedure has almost always involved all twelve : Commission Report on the Operation of the CPMP in 1991 and 1992, SEC(93) 771 at pp 21 and 35. Those statistics appear to confirm the reasoning set out in the recitals to the Directive : see ante.
2. See section 5.4 ante.
3. See the discussion of article 4(4) post.

scope of the general regime. In theory, since the paragraph has not been amended or repealed, those products apparently still enjoy the special status conferred by article 2(5), but it seems unlikely to be relied on by the Member States in future.

6.4   Procedural requirements : articles 3 and 4

Article 3 lays down the procedural requirements for reference to the CPMP under the Directive.

Article 3(1) makes the representative of the Member State which initiated the procedure "rapporteur" and requires him to "provide all information relevant to the evaluation of the medicinal product". There is no provision for more than one Member State to have initiated the procedure, though article 2 does not exclude the possibility that more than one Member State may be involved; the only guidance from the wording of the Directive comes from the word "initiated" itself but in practice the first Member State to notify the CPMP becomes the "rapporteur". It is therefore in the applicant's interest to time its applications carefully (or, in the case of List B products, to request only one Member State to refer the matter to the CPMP). Article 3(1) also provides for the strict confidentiality of the information disclosed to the CPMP.

Article 3(2), requires the applicant to be informed of the referral to the CPMP and also provides for his right to "provide the [CPMP] with oral or written explanations".

Article 3(3) places the Member State referring the matter under an obligation to ensure that the applicant supplies all members of the CPMP with :

> "an identical summary of the dossier consisting of the summary of the product characteristics together with the reports of the analytical, pharmaco-toxological and clinical experts".

The applicant must also provide a "complete and updated copy of the dossier" submitted to the Member State or States concerned and must certify that all the various copies submitted are identical[1].

Article 3(4) places both the national authorities and the applicant under a duty to provide the CPMP with :

> "[a]ll available evaluation reports and drug-monitoring reports relating to the same medicinal product".

Article 4 specifies relevant time limits :

Article 4(1) refers back to the time limits laid down in article 7 of Directive (EEC) 65/65 and article 4(c) of Directive (EEC) 75/319 (as to which see 3.6 and 5.3 above); the CPMP must issue its opinion at least 30 days before the expiry of such time limits and the Member States must inform the CPMP without delay :

> "of any extension and of the beginning and end of any suspension of the time limits concerned".

No time limits are prescribed for a CPMP opinion which refers to a proposed suspension or withdrawal of authorisation under the procedure laid down by article 2(4) and article 4(2).

---

1.   For a comparison with the requirements of the "multi-State" procedure see section 5.4 ante.

Article 4(2), first sentence, simply provides that :

"the [CPMP] shall fix an appropriate time limit for issuing its reasoned opinion having regard for the requirements for the protection of public health";

the second sentence of article 4(2) was considered at 6.3 above.

Article 4(3), requires the CPMP to notify forthwith :

"its opinion and, where relevant, any dissenting opinions expressed therein, to the Member State concerned"

and to the applicant; and the Member State concerned is required by article 4(4) to reach its decision "on the action it intends to take following the [CPMP]'s opinion" within 30 days of receipt of the opinion and to inform the CPMP of its decision forthwith.

Article 4(4) weakly implies that the Member State's decision should be in some unspecified way linked to the CPMP opinion, but it remains the case :

(1) combining article 4(1) and 4(4), that the national authorities are under the same obligation as before[1] to reach a decision on marketing authorisation within 120 days (unless the time limit is extended for some special reason); and

(2) that they are under no obligation to take any notice of the CPMP's views; that would be particularly apparent where the "Member State concerned" itself expressed one of the dissenting views contained in the CPMP opinion in accordance with article 4(3).

One anomalous feature of articles 2 to 4 is that they generally refer to the "Member State concerned" in the singular. Although in theory the procedure is available for use by a single Member State, and although the "rapporteur" Member State has a special role in the procedure, in practice it is, of course, the procedure is naturally suited to multiple applications to several Member States. The weakness of the CPMP would be starkly exposed were several Member States to take different views of a product and to express those views in the CPMP opinion.

6.5   Miscellaneous provisions : article 5

Article 5 is effectively a "miscellaneous provisions" section :

(1) The first paragraph of article 5 refers to articles 8 and 9 of Directive (EEC) 83/189 relating to the provision of information concerning technical standards[2] and requires the Member States to submit draft technical regulations relating to the production and marketing of "proprietary medicinal products" as defined in article 1 of Directive (EEC) 65/65. It is unclear what effect the amendment of Directive (EEC) 65/65 has had on this requirement; presumably the provision should now relate to "medicinal products" generally[3].

(2) The second paragraph of article 5 provides for the "extension" Directives[4], extending the scope of the Community regime to all pharmaceutical products.

1.   See article 7 of Directive (EEC) 65/65 and compare the position under Directive (EEC) 75/319 discussed at section 5.4 ante.
2.   OJ L109 26.4.83 p8.
3.   See section 3.2 ante.
4.   See Directives (EEC) 89/342 (OJ L142 25.5.89 p14), 89/343 (OJ L142 25.5.89 p16), 89/381 (OJ L181 28.6.89 p44) and 92/73 (OJ L297 13.10.92 p2).

Of those, only Directive (EEC) 92/73, establishing a simplified regulatory regime for homeopathic medicines, is discussed in this work[1].

6.6   Conclusion

Directive (EEC) 87/22 was an important development in the harmonisation process. For the first time, a unitary assessment mechanism was put in place at the Community level, involving the CPMP in assessment of a medicinal product prior to any national authorisation decisions. The CPMP's opinions were of persuasive force only but it emerges clearly from the recitals to Regulation (EEC) 2309/93 that Directive (EEC) 87/22 was an important precursor to the binding rules discussed in Chapters 7 and 8.

---

1.   See Chapter 9 post.

PART III : MARKETING AUTHORISATION - THE FUTURE SYSTEM

Chapter 7 : Regulation (EEC) 2309/93[1] - The "Centralised" Procedure and the European Agency for the Evaluation of Medicinal Products

7.1   The purpose and structure of the Regulation : the recitals

Regulation (EEC) 2309/93 is one of only two pieces of Community legislation relating to the pharmaceutical sector which takes the form of a Regulation rather than a Directive (or a Recommendation)[2]. It is also the only legislation to have been introduced in reliance on article 235 rather than article 100 or 100a of the EC Treaty. Both those unusual features relate to the fact that it is not simply a harmonisation measure but establishes for the first time independent Community procedures for the authorisation of marketing of at least some medicinal products and also establishes a new Community institution, the European Agency for the Evaluation of Medicinal Products ("the Agency")[3].

Recitals 1 to 7 of the Regulation set out the reasons for the establishment of "a centralised Community authorisation procedure". Recitals 1 and 2 refer to the experience of the "concertation" procedure established under Directive (EEC) 87/22[4], described in Chapter 6 ante. That procedure had operated "prior to any national decision relating to a high-technology medicinal product, with a view to arriving at uniform decisions throughout the Community". Recital 1 states that "this route should be followed, particularly to ensure the smooth functioning of the internal market in the pharmaceutical sector". Recital 2 states the need to establish a "centralised" procedure, in the first instance for "technologically advanced products, in particular those derived from biotechnology" but also to be available "to persons responsible for placing on the market medicinal products containing new active substances which are intended for use in human beings or in food-producing animals". The dichotomy established in Directive (EEC) 87/22 is thus preserved, between those products that should and those that can use the new procedure[5].

Recitals 3, 4, 6 and 7 refer to the procedures necessary to make the new system effective and in particular to ensure that the new "centralised" Community authorisations to be granted are based on the criteria laid down by article 5 of

1.   OJ L214 24.8.93 p1. See Appendix 5 post.
2.   Council Regulation (EEC) 1768/92 (OJ L182 2.7.92 p1) concerning the creation of a supplementary protection certificate for medicinal products is the other Regulation in this field: see Appendix 14 hereto and section 1.4.1 ante.
3.   See recital 20. Article 235 provides : "If action by the Community should prove necessary to attain, in the course of the operation of the common market, one of the objectives of the Community and this Treaty has not provided the necessary powers, the Council shall, acting unanimously on a proposal from the Commission and after consulting the European Parliament, take the appropriate measures." One of the principal causes of delay in the enactment of the Future System package was the need for unanimity under article 235. In earlier drafts, the Commission had attempted to put forward the Regulation (or at least the parts other than that setting up the Agency) under the harmonisation provisions of article 100a.
4.   OJ L15 17.1.87 p38. See Appendix 4 post.
5.   Directive (EEC) 87/22 itself is repealed by Directive (EEC) 93/41 (OJ L214 24.8.93 p40) with effect from 1 January 1995 : see section 8.6 post.

Directive (EEC) 65/65[1], of "quality, safety and efficacy". Recital 5 refers to the equivalent provisions for veterinary products.

Recital 3 states "the article 5 criteria" and confirms that those criteria apply "to the exclusion of economic or other considerations"; however, two very general qualifications are placed on this :

> " ... Member States should exceptionally be able to prohibit the use on their territory of medicinal products for human use which infringe objectively defined concepts of public order or public morality".

Those expressions are reminiscent of the wording of article 36 of the Treaty ("public morality, public policy or public security"). The only provision in the newly amended legislation that appears to rely on this recital remains article 6 of Directive (EEC) 65/65, expressly preserved by article 12(1) of the Regulation, but the recital leaves it open that the Member States might prevent the marketing within its territory of a Community authorised product on one of the two stated grounds. It should be noted that the most obviously relevant provision of article 36, "the protection of the health and life of humans, animals or plants", is no longer available to the Member States as a ground for prohibition.

Recitals 4 and 6 refer to Directives (EEC) 65/65, 75/318[2] and 75/319[3] as having "extensively harmonised" the article 5 criteria and state that "the same criteria must be applied to medicinal products which are to be authorised by the Community".

Recital 7 summarises the ambition of the Regulation in establishing the new "centralised" procedure :

> " ... only after a single scientific evaluation of the highest possible standard of the quality, safety or efficacy of technologically advanced medicinal products, to be undertaken within the [Agency], should a marketing authorisation be granted by the Community by a rapid procedure ensuring close co-operation between the Commission and Member States".

The watchwords are thus quality, speed and co-operation and the way they are to be achieved is through the establishment of the Agency.

Recital 8 summarises what is to be the other main task of the Agency, in relation to a new "decentralised" procedure. Like the "centralised" procedure in relation to Directive (EEC) 87/22's "concertation" procedure, the "decentralised" procedure is intended to be the development of Directive (EEC) 75/319's "multi-State" procedure. The new procedure is based on the newly amended Directives 65/65, 75/318 and 75/319, whose effect is summarised :

> " ... in the event of a disagreement between the Member States about the quality, safety or efficacy of a medicinal product which is the subject of the decentralised Community authorisation procedure, the matter should be resolved by a binding Community decision following a scientific evaluation of the issues within a European medicinal product evaluation agency".

Recitals 9 and 10 draw the natural conclusion that it is necessary to provide the Community with "the means to undertake scientific evaluation" for the purposes of the "centralised" procedure and also necessary to provide the Community with "the

---

1.   OJ No 22 9.2.65 p369/65. See Appendix 1 post.
2.   OJ L147 9.6.75 p1. See Appendix 2 post.
3.   OJ L147 9.6.75 p13. See Appendix 3 post.

means to resolve differences between the Member States" over national authorisations. The Agency is to provide such means.

Recitals 11 and 12 provide for the essential duties and procedures of the Agency : "to provide scientific advice of the highest possible quality to the Community institutions and the Member States" in the exercise of their powers of authorisation and supervision of medicinal products (recital 11); and "to ensure close co-operation between the Agency and scientists working within the Member States (recital 12).

Recitals 13 and 14 relate to the role of the CPMP within the Agency : the CPMP is entrusted with "the exclusive responsibility for preparing the opinions of the Agency on all matters relating to medicinal products for human use" (recital 13); recital 14 states that the establishment of the Agency :

> "will make it possible to reinforce the scientific role and independence of [the CPMP], in particular through the establishment of a permanent technical and administrative secretariat".

The expanded role of the CPMP accords with the general approach of the Regulation, to build on the experience of almost thirty years of gradual harmonisation and to retain the involvement of the Member States, while increasingly establishing central Community powers and bodies. The CPMP is of course largely composed of representatives of the national authorities and is thus well suited to the co-operative role assigned to it by the Regulation.

Recitals 15 to 17 relate to supervision and pharmacovigilance and provide that the Commission, "working in close co-operation with the Agency, and after consultation with the Member States" is responsible for the co-ordination of the Member States' various supervisory roles[1]. The Agency is given specific responsibility for pharmacovigilance (recital 17).

Recital 18 is an important indicator that the Future System regime is not intended to be the final step in harmonisation of Community procedures for authorisation. The recital speaks of the "orderly introduction of Community procedures alongside the national procedures of the Member States" and concedes only that "it is appropriate in the first instance to limit the obligation to use the new Community procedure to certain medicinal products". The scope of the procedures are to be reviewed "at the latest six years after the entry into force of this Regulation" (ie by 1 January 2001). It is plainly envisaged that the use of the Community procedures will be expanded at that date.

Recital 19 provides for environmental risk assessments in the specific case of "medicinal products containing or consisting of genetically modified organisms" in accordance with Council Directive (EEC) 90/220[2].

Recital 20 states the need to use the Member States' residual power under article 235 of the EC Treaty, on the ground that the Treaty does not provide any other powers for "the adoption of a uniform system at Community level, as provided for by this Regulation".

Regulation (EEC) 2309/93 is divided into five "Titles" : I Definitions and scope, articles 1 to 4; II Authorisation and supervision of medicinal products for human use, articles 5 to 26; III Authorisation and supervision of veterinary medicinal products, articles 27 to 48; IV The European Agency for the Evaluation of Medicinal

---

1.   See Chapters 11 and 12 post.
2.   OJ L117 8.5.90 p15.

Products, articles 49 to 66; and V General and final provisions, articles 67 to 74. The two principal sections for the purposes of this work are Titles II and IV, respectively setting out the new "centralised" procedure and establishing the Agency. Title III, which introduces similar procedures for veterinary products to those introduced for products for human use by Title II, falls outside the scope of this work.

7.2   Definitions and scope : Title I, articles 1 to 4

Article 1 consists of two paragraphs :

The first paragraph sets out the "objective" of the Regulation :

> "to lay down Community procedures for the authorisation and supervision of medicinal products for human and veterinary use and to establish a European Agency for the Evaluation of Medicinal Products".

The generality of this "objective" is somewhat misleading, since the subsequent provisions of the Regulation make it clear that its scope is, at least for the foreseeable future, strictly limited : many products have already been authorised by the Member State authorities under the existing regimes; and the majority of new applications for authorisation will continue to be dealt with primarily at the national level even under the new regime[1]. It is only in the case of a limited range of sophisticated products, closely related to those previously subjected to the "concertation" procedure under Directive (EEC) 87/22, that the provisions of the Regulation will apply. The paragraph anticipates the future extension of the Agency's field of action.

The second paragraph gives substance to recital 3's reference to the "exclusion of economic or other considerations" as a criterion of assessment of medicinal products and confirms that the Regulation does not affect the national authorities' powers :

> "as regards the price setting of medicinal products or their inclusion in the scope of the national health system of the Member States' authorities or their inclusion in the scope of the social security schemes on the basis of health, economic and social conditions. For example, the Member States may choose from the marketing authorisation those therapeutic indications and pack sizes which will be covered by their social security organisations."

This is clearly an extremely important residual power, permitting the Member States' authorities to refuse to pay for centrally authorised products or to control the price at which such products may be sold on the national market. Given the diversity of approaches adopted by the national authorities, such a power remains a major obstacle to free trade[2]. The final sentence of the paragraph gives the Member States the power specifically to limit the treatments for which a specific product will be financed and to specify the pack sizes for which the social security system will pay. It is clear that the national authorities will retain considerable control even over centrally authorised products.

The first paragraph of article 2 incorporates by reference the "definitions laid down in article 1 of Directive (EEC) 65/65"[3].

---

1.   See Chapter 8 post.
2.   See section 1.4.2 ante.
3.   See Chapter 2 ante.

The second paragraph of article 2 requires the "person responsible for placing products on the market" to be "established in the Community". The concept of "establishment" is not defined in the Regulation but there is a great deal of Community jurisprudence on the term deriving from articles 52 et seq of the EC Treaty concerning "Right of Establishment" (see in particular article 58 in respect of "Companies or Firms"). The aim of this provision is to simplify administration throughout the Community in the face of the increased burden of administration and co-operation between the Member States and the Community implicit in the new system. In effect, the supplier of medicinal products within the Community must have "an address for service" within the Community[1].

Articles 3 and 4 set out the fundamental terms of the Regulation : the centralised Community procedure is made compulsory for a limited range of products and made available for a further wider range at the option of the applicant for authorisation; the application for authorisation is to the European Agency for the Evaluation of Medicinal Products and the Community itself is made responsible for the issue and supervision of marketing authorisations.

Article 3(1) refers to the Annex to the Regulation and states that :

"[n]o medicinal product referred to in Part A of the Annex may be placed on the market within the Community unless a marketing authorisation has been granted by the Community in accordance with the provisions of this Regulation."

The wording of article 3(1) is very similar to that of article 3 of Directive (EEC) 65/65 in respect of national marketing authorisations. It is only in respect of "Part A products" that the provisions of Directive (EEC) 65/65 have been completely superseded by the Regulation. All other products *may* still be authorised under the national procedures.

Part A of the Annex is, in relation to medicines for human use, identically worded to Part A of the Annex to Directive (EEC) 87/22. In relation to veterinary products, the following category of products are included in List A :

"products, including those not derived from biotechnology, intended primarily for use as performance enhancers in order to promote the growth of treated animals or to increase yields from treated animals".

Article 3(2) refers to Part B of the Annex and provides that the person responsible for marketing such a product :

"may request that authorisation to place the medicinal product on the market be granted by the Community in accordance with the provisions of this Regulation".

This wording appears to envisage a direct application by the applicant to the Community authorities without reference to the national authorities, so the applicant would have a clear choice of approach for products in Part B of the Annex : he could either apply to the various national authorities for authorisation; or he could apply directly to the Community authorities, bi-passing the national authorities altogether (the old "concertation" procedure will cease to be available after the repeal of Directive 87/22[2]).

---

1. A national requirement to the same effect was struck down as contrary to articles 30 and 36 of the EC Treaty in Case 247/81 *Commission v Germany* [1984] ECR 1111; clearly different considerations apply where the requirement is Community-wide.
2. See section 8.6 post.

The products for human use in Part B of the Annex to the Regulation are similar to those in Part B to the Annex to Directive (EEC) 87/22 but they include three significant changes : because the new procedure is "centralised", the discretion formerly enjoyed by the Member States' competent authorities to determine whether a product fell within the scope of List B passes to the Agency, which can thus determine whether an applicant enjoys the right granted by article 2(2) to apply for a Community authorisation; new medicinal products "derived from human blood or human plasma" are included as a separate category of product; and the position in relation to products containing a new active substance is clarified :

> "Medicinal products intended for administration to human beings, containing a new active substance which, on the date of entry into force of this regulation, was not authorised by any Member State for use in a medicinal product intended for human use."[1]

This provision appears potentially to widen the scope of the Regulation considerably as against the scope of Directive (EEC) 87/22 : the equivalent provision in List B of the Annex to Directive (EEC) 87/22 is ambiguous, but appears to relate only to products "containing a new substance ... of significant therapeutic interest". In addition, this category and the new category of human blood and plasma products are automatically included in Part B of the Annex to the Regulation whereas List B of the Annex to Directive (EEC) 87/22 was entirely at the discretion of the Member States. The full list of products in Part B is contained in Appendix 5 hereto.

Article 3(3) to (5) provide for amendments to Parts A and B of the Annex to the Regulation : article 3(3) provides for Parts A and B to be revised before entry into force of the Regulation and after consultation of the CPMP. It is hard to see any meaning for such a provision, which required action to be taken before the requirement took legal effect. Article 3(4) is an equivalent provision in relation to veterinary medicinal products, but the most significant provision is article 3(5), which provides that the procedures referred to in paragraphs (3) and (4) are to continue to apply after the entry into force of the Regulation. The procedure laid down in article 3(3) is for the lists in Parts A and B to be re-examined :

> "in the light of scientific and technical progress with a view to making any amendments necessary which will be adopted under the procedure laid down in article 72".

The article 72 procedure is considered at section 7.6 post. It should be noted that there are no criteria laid down for products to be considered suitable for either Part A or Part B of the Annex; given the very significant powers given to the Community authorities in relation to products on those two lists, the re-examination process to be conducted under article 3(5) is therefore potentially of the greatest significance; the Standing Committee on Medicinal Products for Human Use, in co-operation with the Commission and the CPMP, will have the power to propose that any new product should be brought within the scope of the Regulation, either within the scope of Part A, leading to a compulsory Community authorisation procedure under article 3(1), or Part B, where there will be an option, *of the applicant alone*, to choose a Community procedure under article 3(2). It remains to be seen whether those powers will be used.

Article 4 sets out the structure of the new Community authorisation procedure in the most elementary terms :

(1) to obtain the authorisation referred to in article 3 of the Regulation, the person responsible for placing a medicinal product on the market shall submit an application to the Agency (article 4(1));

(2) the Community "shall issue and supervise marketing authorisations for medicinal products for human use in accordance with Title II of this Regulation" (article 4(2)); and

(3) Article 4(3) makes an equivalent provision for veterinary products in relation to Title III of the Regulation.

It should be noted that there is no provision for any involvement of the Member States at any stage of the process, though of course the Member States will in practice be involved in the operation of the Community institutions, both in the Agency - via the CPMP and the Standing Committee and the provision of expert assistance to the Agency - and in the Council, where the Council becomes involved in the authorisation procedure[1].

7.3 The granting of a Community authorisation : Title III, Chapter 1; articles 5 to 14

Chapter 1 of Title III is entitled "Submission and examination of applications - authorisations - renewal of authorisation". The substance of the Chapter is the laying down of procedural rules to be followed within the Agency and by the other Community bodies from the time of receipt of an application under article 3 of the Regulation until the moment of granting or refusal of authorisation. Those rules are very similar to the rules laid down in Directive (EEC) 93/39 amending Directives 65/65, 75/318 and 75/319 and develop out of the old "concertation" procedure.

Article 5 refers back to Directive (EEC) 75/319 and appoints the CPMP to be :

"responsible for formulating the opinion of the Agency on any question concerning the admissibility of the files submitted in accordance with the centralised procedure, the granting, variation, suspension or withdrawal of an authorisation to place a medical product for human use on the market arising in accordance with the provisions of this Title and pharmacovigilance".

The "centralised procedure" is the procedure triggered off by an application within the scope of article 3(1) or (2) and described in this Chapter; the wording is odd in so far as the responsibility for formulating the Agency's opinion on such applications and the other issues cited is granted to a pre-existing body rather than to the Agency itself.

7.3.1 The substance of the authorisation process : articles 6 to 8
Article 6 sets out the various administrative requirements of an application under the Regulation. They are very similar to the requirements under the traditional national regimes as harmonised by Directives (EEC) 65/65, 75/318 and 75/319, as to which see Chapters 3 to 5 ante, and Chapter 8 post for the amended versions.

---

1.   See section 7.6 post for description of the articles 72 and 73 procedures.

Article 6(1) simply refers back to the earlier Directives and requires that the "particulars and documents" referred to in :

(1) articles 4 and 4a of Directive 65/65 (the repeatedly amended general provision in relation to applications)[1];

(2) the Annex to Directive (EEC) 75/318 (the detailed guidelines for applicants to be used in conjunction with Volumes II and III of *The rules governing medicinal products in the European Community*)[2];

(3) article 2 of Directive (EEC) 75/319 (expert reports)[3];

should accompany the application for authorisation.

Article 6(2) refers to medicinal products :

"containing or consisting of genetically modified organisms within the meaning of article 2(1) and (2) of Directive (EEC) 90/220".

Article 2(1) and (2) of Council Directive (EEC) 90/220[4] are, in part, as follows :

"(1) "organism" is any biological entity capable of replication or of transferring genetic material;

(2) "genetically modified organism (GMO)" means an organism in which the genetic material has been altered in a way that does not occur naturally by mating and/or natural recombination".

Article 2(2) is further qualified by reference to the Annexes to Directive (EEC) 90/220, where techniques which do and those which do not constitute "genetic modification" for the purposes of the Directive are set out in categories. Part B of that Directive sets out rules for the granting of written consent by competent authorities in the individual Member States to the release of GMO's into the environment and article 6(4) of the Directive provides that release may only occur once written consent has been obtained from the relevant competent authority. Part C of Directive (EEC) 90/220, articles 10 to 18, relates to the "Placing on the market of products containing GMO's" and articles 11 to 18 set out detailed procedures to be followed by the Member States in assessing products for the purposes of authorisation, in particular the carrying out of an "environmental risk assessment" involving the supply of information to the authority in accordance with Annexes II and III to the Directive. Article 10(1) and (2) provides :

"1. Consent may only be given for the placing on the market of products containing, or consisting of GMO's, provided that :

— written consent has been given to a notification under Part B or if a risk analysis has been carried out based on the elements outlined in that Part;
— the products comply with the relevant Community product legislation;
— the products comply with the requirements of the Part of this Directive, concerning the environmental risk assessment.

---

1. See sections 3.4 ante and 8.2 post.
2. See section 4.3 ante and Appendix 2 hereto.
3. See section 5.2 ante.
4. Directive (EEC) 90/220 (OJ L117 8.5.90 p15) on the deliberate release into the environment of genetically modified organisms.

2.   Articles 11 to 18 shall not apply to any products covered by Community legislation which provides for a specific environmental risk assessment similar to that laid down in this Directive."

Article 6(2) of Regulation (EEC) 2309/93 is closely modelled on the requirements of article 10 of Directive (EEC) 90/220 : in accordance with article 10(1) of the Directive, an application for a marketing authorisation for a product consisting of or containing a GMO must be accompanied by a copy of "any written consent or consents of the competent authorities" under Part B of the Directive and by :

"the complete technical dossier supplying the information requested in Annexes II and III to Directive (EEC) 90/220 and the environmental risk assessment resulting from this information; the results of any investigations performed for the purposes of research or development".

In accordance with article 10(2) of Directive (EEC) 90/220, the detailed rules laid down by articles 11 to 18 of the Directive are declared by article 6(2), second sub-paragraph, of Regulation (EEC) 2309/93 not to apply to "medicinal products for human use containing or consisting of genetically modified organisms".

The overall practical effect is that applications for marketing authorisations for such products must be accompanied by further technical information in addition to that required under article 6(1), as specified in the Regulation and Directive (EEC) 90/220. The reference to "any written consents of the competent authorities" is to article 6(4) of Directive (EEC) 90/220; under Part B of the Directive, it is possible to obtain consents from the national competent authorities on an individual basis, but article 10(1) of the Directive and article 6(2) of the Regulation do not *require* that such consents have been obtained. What is required before a marketing authorisation is granted is *either* a written consent *or* the carrying out of a risk analysis *and* compliance with the "relevant Community product legislation", in the present instance Regulation (EEC) 2309/93.

Article 6(3) merely requires that the application should be accompanied by the fee payable to the Agency for the examination of the application. Although that is a simple provision, its effects are important : the cost of the Agency has been a major issue in the debate over whether or not such an Agency should be set up at all; the fees to be paid by the pharmaceutical industry are a major factor in the assessment of the viability of the Agency[1].

Article 6(4) first sub-paragraph, requires the Agency to ensure that the CPMP gives its opinion within 210 days of receipt of a valid application; the CPMP is thus given the same extended period in which to reach an opinion as that granted to the Member State authorities under article 7(1) of Directive (EEC) 65/65[2]; the two regimes have clearly been designed to run in parallel, with no advantage in terms of speed in pursuing one route rather than the other.

Article 6(4), second paragraph, is related to article 6(2), discussed ante : a CPMP opinion relating to a medicinal product consisting of or containing a genetically modified organism is required to :

"respect the environmental safety requirements laid down by Directive (EEC) 90/220 to ensure that all appropriate measures are taken to avoid adverse effects on human health and the environment which might arise from the deliberate release or placing on the market of genetically modified organisms. During the process of evaluating applications for marketing authorisations for

---

1.   See section 7.5.2 post.
2.   See section 8.2 post.

products containing or consisting of genetically modified organisms, necessary consultations will be held by the rapporteur with the bodies set up [by] the Community in accordance with Directive (EEC) 90/220."

The wording of this paragraph relates to the third indent of article 10(1) of Directive (EEC) 90/220, requiring such products to be authorised for marketing in the Community only if they "comply with the requirements" of Part C of the Directive, and to article 10(2), which disapplies the substantive provisions of Part C where other provision is made for a "specific environmental risk assessment similar to that laid down in this Directive".

Article 6(5) requires the Commission, in consultation with the Agency, the Member States and "interested parties", to draw up detailed guidance on the form in which applications for authorisation are to be presented. The most significant "interested parties" will be potential applicants under the Regulation, the pharmaceutical companies themselves. Notice to Applicants IIA, published in July 1993, before the adoption of the Regulation, expressed the Commission's intention to produce a new Notice in 1995 "to coincide with the entry into force of the "Future System" and to include procedures for centralised and decentralised applications as well as structure and content of the application dossier".

Article 7 is closely modelled on article 4 of Directive (EEC) 75/319 and imposes equivalent duties on the CPMP and grants equivalent powers to the CPMP, in the preparation of its opinion, to those imposed on and granted to the Member State authorities in their examination of applications under Directive (EEC) 65/65 :

(a) Under article 7(a), the CPMP is obliged to verify that the particulars and documents submitted in accordance with article 6 comply with the requirements of Directives (EEC) 65/65, 75/318 and 75/319[1]. It must also examine whether the conditions specified under the Regulation for issuing a marketing authorisation for the product are satisfied; those criteria are set out in article 11 of the Regulation (in combination with article 68), as to which see post. As was stated in section 5.3 ante in relation to article 4(a) of Directive (EEC) 75/319, the assessment procedure falls into two parts : a "formal" examination of the information submitted, to confirm that it is adequate; and a "substantive" examination to ensure that the criteria for authorisation are satisfied.

(b) Article 7(b) gives the CPMP a power equivalent to that enjoyed by the Member State authorities under article 4(b) of Directive (EEC) 75/319 to ask for :

"a State laboratory or a laboratory designated for this purpose to test the medicinal product, its starting materials, and, if need be, its intermediate products or other constituent materials in order to ensure that the control methods employed by the manufacturer and described in the application documents are satisfactory".

The Agency itself will not apparently have the technical competence to perform such tests and will therefore "contract out" the scientific evaluations to the existing national medical agencies[2].

(c) Article 7(c) is equivalent to article 4(c) of Directive (EEC) 75/319 : it permits the CPMP to "request the applicant to supplement the particulars accompanying the application within a specific time limit"; where it does so, the time limit laid down in article 6(4) of the Regulation is suspended until the

---

1.   See Chapters 3 to 5 and 8.
2.   See for further discussion section 7.5 post.

supplementary information is provided; the time limit is likewise suspended "for the time allowed to the applicant to prepare oral or written explanations". That final provision does not make it clear whether the CPMP is *obliged* to grant the applicant such time, or whether the CPMP enjoys a discretion as to the measures necessary; the equivalent provision of Directive (EEC) 75/319 applies only "where appropriate", and it seems that the procedure should be co-operative rather than confrontational, so that there is no need to provide rigid procedural safeguards for the applicant. The CPMP should be required to act reasonably, so that it should not refuse to grant such a hearing where it is reasonably necessary for the proper assessment of the application.

Article 8 corresponds approximately to article 5 of Directive (EEC) 75/319, giving the CPMP the power to confirm, in co-operation with the Member States, that the product subject to the authorisation procedure can be manufactured under satisfactory conditions in the Community or elsewhere. It does not seem that the CPMP is under any obligation to use this power other than its general obligation under article 7(a) to verify the adequacy of the application as submitted. As with article 5 of Directive (EEC) 75/319, the provision is naturally linked to Chapter IV of Directive (EEC) 75/319; that Chapter establishes Community rules for the authorisation of manufacture of pharmaceuticals[1]. Given that the Member State authorities retain control over the authorisation of manufacture under the Future System[2], there is a need for some mechanism for the exchange of information between the national and Community bodies to ensure that the applicant for authorisation is capable of producing the product as authorised.

Article 8(1) places an obligation on the Member States, on receipt of a written request from the CPMP, to :

"forward the information establishing that the manufacturer of a medicinal product or the importer from a third country is able to manufacture the medicinal product concerned and/or carry out the necessary control tests in accordance with the particulars and documents supplied pursuant to article 6".

Presumably, the Member State in question will normally perform that task by confirmation that the applicant has obtained a manufacturing authorisation for the product in accordance with Chapter IV of Directive (EEC) 75/319.

Article 8(2) provides for manufacturing site inspections where considered necessary by the CPMP in order to complete its examination of an application :

"The inspection, which shall be completed within the time limit referred to in article 6, shall be undertaken by pharmaceutical inspectors from the Member State who possess the appropriate qualifications and who may, if need be, be accompanied by a rapporteur or expert appointed by the [CPMP]".

This sentence is vague : it makes it clear that the conduct of a site inspection does not lead to an extension of the time limit of 210 days for the CPMP opinion set out at article 6(4), so that article 7(c) in relation to supplementary information does not apply in such a case; but it does not explain what are the "appropriate qualifications" for a national inspector nor when it is necessary for a rapporteur or an expert to accompany the national expert. The CPMP appears to enjoy a wide discretion to regulate its own procedures.

---

1.   See Chapter 10 post.
2.   See section 10.6 post.

7.3.2 CPMP procedures : article 9

Article 9 relates to the procedure to be adopted by the CPMP when it has reached its opinion. An appeal procedure is established for negative and qualified positive opinions and certain administrative requirements are imposed on the CPMP in the transmission of the final opinion. The procedures to be followed are again very similar to those followed under the new procedures for the resolution of differences between national authorities introduced by Directive (EEC) 93/39[1].

Article 9(1) establishes an appeal procedure to come into effect in four distinct sets of circumstances :

> "— the application does not satisfy the criteria for authorisation set out in this Regulation, or
> — the summary of product characteristics proposed by the applicant in accordance with article 6 should be amended, or
> — the labelling or package leaflet of the product is not in compliance with ... Directive (EEC) 92/27 ... , or
> — the authorisation should be granted subject to the conditions provided for in article 13(2)".

The "criteria" referred to under the first of these categories are contained in article 11 of the Regulation; article 11 is considered post, but the first three categories can be taken together, since they form the three reasons set out in article 11 for the refusal of authorisation under the Regulation. The fourth category, the granting of authorisation subject to conditions, is provided for in article 13(2) of the Regulation, considered post (see also the discussion of article 9(3)(b) post).

Procedurally, the requirements of the Regulation are identical to those of Directive (EEC) 93/39 in relation to the CPMP's opinion on divergent national opinions : the *Agency* is required "forthwith" to inform the applicant of a negative or conditional positive opinion by the CPMP; the *applicant* must notify the Agency of its intention to appeal within fifteen days of receipt of the opinion and must forward its "detailed grounds of appeal" to the Agency within 60 days *of receipt of the CPMP opinion*. The *CPMP* must then decide whether its opinion should be revised within 60 days of receipt of the appeal. Where the appeal procedure is followed, the CPMP must annex the conclusions reached on the appeal to the assessment report prepared for the purposes of article 9(2).

Article 9(2) sets out the procedure to be followed by the Agency once the CPMP's "final opinion" has been "adopted" (there is no guidance on what procedure is to be used to "adopt" the opinion but see article 52(4) of the Regulation and section 7.5.1 post). The Agency is required to forward the opinion to the Commission, the Member States and the applicant within 30 days of its adoption. The opinion must be accompanied by "a report describing the assessment of the product by the [CPMP] and stating the reasons for its conclusions". It is not clear whether "its" refers to the Agency, the CPMP, the CPMP's opinion, the report or the assessment, but the effect is the same. Where there have been supplementary conclusions reached on an appeal, presumably the assessment report should also be supplemented as necessary to give the reasons for those supplementary conclusions.

---

1.   See section 8.4 post.

Article 9(3) requires four documents to be annexed to a *positive* opinion; the fourth document, the "assessment report" is already required to be attached by article 9(2) but the first three documents are distinct :

"(a)   a draft summary of the product characteristics, as referred to in article 4a of Directive (EEC) 65/65;

(b)   details of any conditions or restrictions which should be imposed on the supply or use of the medicinal product concerned, including the conditions under which the medicinal product may be made available to patients, having regard to the criteria laid down in ... Directive (EEC) 92/26 ..., without prejudice to the provisions in article 3(4) of that Directive.

(c)   the draft text of the labelling and package leaflet proposed by the applicant, presented in accordance with ... Directive (EEC) 92/27 ..., without prejudice to the provisions of article 7(2) of that Directive"[1];

Article 4a of Directive (EEC) 65/65 is considered at section 3.4.3 ante, Directives (EEC) 92/26 and (EEC) 92/27 in Chapters 14 and 15. Article 9(3)(b) clearly envisages one possibility to be that the CPMP might recommend that the product should only be supplied to patients under more or less restrictive conditions of prescription[2]; Article 9(3) goes further than the equivalent provision of Directive (EEC) 75/319 as amended, article 13(5), where no guidance is given as to the nature of the conditions that might be deemed appropriate and no reference is made to a draft text of the labelling and packaging leaflet. The difference is the result of the different circumstances surrounding the two opinions : under the "centralised" procedure, the CPMP opinion will lead to a Community authorisation decision; under the "decentralised" procedure, the opinion will lead ultimately to a decision by the Member State authorities which will retain direct responsibility for the details of the authorisation, if granted. In addition, of course, Directives (EEC) 92/26 and 92/27 are directly binding on the Member States to whom they are addressed, but not on the Community institutions. There is therefore no need for a further reference under Directive (EEC) 75/319 as amended.

Article 9(3)(c) refers to article 7(2) of Directive (EEC) 92/27, which permits the "competent authorities" to decide to permit the omission of certain "therapeutic indications" where their inclusion would have serious disadvantages for the patient. In the present context, it appears most natural to regard the "competent authorities" to be the Agency (in practice the CPMP) rather than the Member States although the wording of article 9(3)(c) of the Regulation is far from clear[3].

7.3.3   Binding Community decisions : article 10
Article 10 sets out the procedures to be followed by the Community institutions upon receipt of the CPMP opinion. In summary : the Commission must prepare a draft decision, normally basing itself on the CPMP opinion; the draft decision must be approved by the Standing Committee on Medicinal Products for Human Use - and possibly the Council - in accordance with the procedure set out at article 73 of the Regulation; provision is also made for the Member States to express their views to the Committee and to require the decision to be reviewed.

Article 10(1) requires the Commission to prepare a draft decision within 30 days of receipt of the CPMP opinion, "taking into account Community law" (article 10(1),

---

1.   Article 3(4) of Directive (EEC) 92/26 and article 7(2) of Directive (EEC) 92/27 preserve certain powers of the Member States to waive or restrict the operation of those Directives; they are discussed in Chapters 14 and 15.
2.   See further 14.3 post in relation to Directive (EEC) 92/26.
3.   For the meaning of article 7(2) see section 15.4 post.

first sub-paragraph). This is a very wide requirement, somewhat reminiscent of article 164 of the EC Treaty[1]. It requires the Commission to take into account general principles of good administration as understood by the European Court of Justice in addition to the wording of the Community pharmaceutical legislation, for example, the applicant's right to a fair hearing, the need to observe principles of equality and proportionality and the need to state reasons for Community legislation in accordance with article 190 of EC Treaty. Given that the decision will relate to the Community as a whole, it does not seem that article 30 of the EC Treaty could be relevant[2].

If the Commission's draft decision is positive, the requirements set out at article 9(3) of the Regulation in relation to the CPMP opinion apply also to the draft decision : the draft decision must be accompanied by a summary of product characteristics, details of any proposed conditions or restrictions on supply or use of the product, and the draft text of the proposed labelling and package leaflet (article 10(1), second sub-paragraph).

The third sub-paragraph of article 10(1) provides that :

> "[w]here, exceptionally, the draft decision is not in accordance with the opinion of the Agency, the Commission shall also annex a detailed explanation of the reasons for the differences".

The word "exceptionally" is clearly intended to provide some sort of demarcation between the roles of the Commission and the Agency : the primary role in the assessment of medicinal products lies with the Agency through the CPMP and it will be an exceptional case where the Commission finds it necessary to oppose the Agency's view of the matter. Whether such wording has any effect in practice in constraining the Commission is open to question and it is difficult to see how it could have any binding legal force. Far more significant practically are the requirement that the Commission should state its reasons for any divergence in detail and the procedural requirements in article 10(2) and (3) : see below.

The fourth sub-paragraph of article 10(1) requires the draft decision to be sent to the Member States and the applicant and article 10(2) requires the procedure laid down in article 73 of the Regulation to be followed in adopting a final decision. Article 73 is considered at section 7.6 post, but article 10(2) imposes a number of further procedural requirements guaranteeing the rights of the Member States to express their views.

The procedure is different depending on whether the Commission draft is or is not in accordance with the CPMP opinion. Where the opinion and the draft decision are in agreement, the opinion of the Standing Committee (required under article 73 of the Regulation) is to be obtained in writing (article 10(3), second sub-paragraph, first indent); by implication, therefore, where the opinion and draft decision do not agree, it is necessary to hold a Standing Committee meeting to discuss the matter.

In either case, the Member States have two absolute procedural guarantees and one other guarantee at the discretion of the Commission :

(1) each Member State must be allowed at least 28 days to forward written observations on the draft decision to the Commission (article 10(3), second sub-paragraph, second indent); and

---

1. "The Court of Justice shall ensure that in the interpretation and application of this Treaty the law is observed."
2. The Commission proposal used an even vaguer expression: "taking into account the objectives of Community policies and considering all the relevant information" (COM(90) 283 final-SYN 309 at p68).

(2) each Member State can require the draft decision to be discussed by the Standing Committee, though it must assert its requirement in writing and state its reasons in detail (the Regulation does not say what happens if inadequate reasons are given, nor which body is competent to decide whether they are or are not adequate) (article 10(3), second sub-paragraph, third indent);

(3) "[w]here, in the opinion of the Commission, the written observations of a Member State raise important new questions of a scientific or technical nature which have not been addressed in the opinion delivered by the Agency, the Chairman shall suspend the procedure and refer the application back to the Agency for further consideration" (article 10(3), third sub-paragraph).

The third of these possibilities is clearly the most complex, raising the prospect of disputes between the Commission and individual Member States as to whether the State's observations raise "important new questions of a scientific or technical nature" and whether those questions have been addressed in the CPMP opinion; will it be necessary that the questions should have been *adequately* addressed, and if so, how is the Commission to judge the issue ? Procedurally, the Regulation gives no guidance as to the timetable for the Agency's "further consideration", whether another 210 days could be granted or whether it is entirely at the Commission's discretion.

The fourth sub-paragraph of article 10(3) requires the necessary implementing provisions for the purposes of article 10(3) to be adopted in accordance with the procedure laid down in article 72 of the Regulation[1].

Article 10(4) requires the Agency, upon request, to inform "any person concerned" of the final decision. No guidance as to the meaning of "person concerned" is given, but it must have a wider meaning than the Member States and the applicant. Although the wording of the Regulation does not require anybody other than the applicant ("the party concerned" at article 67 post) to be notified automatically of the final as against the draft decision (the Member States and the applicant must receive the draft decision under article 10(1), discussed ante), the expression "any person concerned" cannot refer only to the Member States, but its precise scope must be uncertain; see further article 12(4), considered post, where the expression used is "interested person".

It should be noted that article 10 gives *no* rights to the applicant to be heard in relation to the draft decision, even if that decision is different from the opinion of the CPMP. The applicant's rights are exhausted by the appeal procedure before the CPMP (the Regulation leaves it unclear whether the applicant has any further rights to express its views to the Agency or the CPMP in the case considered above, where the Commission refers the matter back to the Agency for further consideration after a Member State has raised a significant technical question not previously addressed).

7.3.4 The criteria for authorisation : article 11

Article 11 lays down three types of criterion to be applied in order to determine whether authorisation should be granted. Each corresponds to one of the traditional criteria for national authorisation applied by the Member States under the Directive (EEC) 65/65 regime. Authorisation shall be refused :

(1) "if, after verification of the information and particulars submitted in accordance with article 6, it appears that the quality, the safety or the efficacy of the medicinal product have not been adequately or sufficiently demonstrated by the applicant" (article 11, first paragraph);

---

1.   As to which see section 7.6 post.

(2) "if the particulars and documents provided by the applicant in accordance with article 6 of this Regulation are incorrect"; or

(3) "if the labelling and package leaflets proposed by the applicant are not in accordance with Directive (EEC) 92/27" (article 11, second paragraph).

Criterion (1) clearly corresponds to the threefold basis for refusal set out in the first paragraph of article 5 of Directive 65/65[1]; criterion (2) corresponds to the second paragraph of article 5 of Directive (EEC) 65/65; and criterion (3) corresponds to the requirements of article 10(2) of Directive (EEC) 92/27[2].

The first paragraph of article 11 is stated to be "[w]ithout prejudice to other provisions of Community law". It is not clear what is meant by this provision, which does not correspond to article 5 of Directive (EEC) 65/65 and which appears to contradict article 68 of the Regulation. Article 68 states that authorisation shall not be refused except on the grounds and according to the procedures set out in the Regulation. The only possibility appears to be that the authorisation might be *granted* notwithstanding an applicant's failure adequately or sufficiently to demonstrate the product's quality, safety or efficacy. That could only arise in exceptional circumstances, where general principles of Community law such as proportionality, procedural fairness or equality required that the application should be leniently treated (article 68(2) would still require that the *procedures* laid down by the Regulation should be followed). See also the discussion post of article 13(2) and Part 4G of the Annex to Directive (EEC) 75/318 in relation to authorisation subject to conditions.

7.3.5   Administrative details : articles 12 to 14
Article 12 sets out the effects of the grant of a marketing authorisation under the Regulation and various administrative requirements to be followed by the Community institutions after authorisation or refusal of authorisation.

Article 12(1) is intended to make the effects of an authorisation under the Regulation equivalent to an authorisation under Directive (EEC) 65/65, apart from the fact that it is Community wide rather than national. The first sentence of article 12(1), first sub-paragraph, provides that :

"[w]ithout prejudice to article 6 of Directive (EEC) 65/65, a marketing authorisation which has been granted in accordance with the procedure laid down in this Regulation shall be valid throughout the Community."

Article 6 of Directive (EEC) 65/65, as amended by Directive (EEC) 93/39, preserves the rights of the Member States under the Directive to apply national legislation "prohibiting or restricting the sale, supply or use of medicinal products as contraceptives or abortifacients".[3] The relevance of article 6 of Directive (EEC) 65/65 to Regulation (EEC) 2309/92 is that article 3 of Directive (EEC) 65/65, as amended, provides that *either* a national authorisation under the Directive *or* an authorisation under the Regulation is required for marketing in a Member State. The first sentence of article 12(1) of the Regulation therefore confirms that there is no inconsistency between the Regulation and article 6 of the Directive. The sentence is not satisfactorily drafted, however, since article 6 limits the effect *only of the Directive*; it has no effect on the scope of the Regulation, so that strictly it remains the case under this provision that "a marketing authorisation which has been granted in accordance with the procedure laid down in this Regulation shall be

---

1.   See section 3.2 ante.
2.   See section 15.5 post.
3.   See section 8.2 post.

valid *throughout* the Community" (emphasis added), notwithstanding article 6 of the Directive. It seems that this is simply a drafting error.

The second sentence of article 12(1), first sub-paragraph, grants "the same rights and obligations" in each of the Member States as a national authorisation under Directive 65/65; those rights and obligations are considered in Chapter 3 ante, but also include numerous other obligations under later Directives, described in Chapters 4, 5, 8 and 10 to 16 of this work. The provision is somewhat confusing, in that Chapters 2 and 3 of Title I to the Regulation, considered in Chapters 11 and 12 post, lay down rules for supervision and pharmacovigilance in relation to products authorised under the Regulation; products authorised under Directive (EEC) 65/65 do not fall under that regime, so that it is incorrect to say that all the rights and obligations are "the same" under the two systems. Presumably, the provision means in effect that Directive (EEC) 65/65 and other relevant Directives apply unless otherwise stated in the Regulation.

The second sub-paragraph of article 12(1) requires the authorised product to be entered in the "Community Register of Medicinal Products" and to be given a number which must appear on the packaging of the product.

Article 12(2) states that :

> "[t]he refusal of a Community marketing authorisation shall constitute a prohibition on the placing on the market of the medicinal product concerned throughout the Community".

This provision appears to add nothing in relation to products on List A of the Annex to the Regulation, since they *must* be authorised under the Regulation (article 3(1)). The significance of article 12(2) appears to be limited to products on List B : where the person responsible for marketing a particular medicinal product, on List B, opts for the Community procedure in accordance with article 3(2) of the Regulation, article 12(2) prevents that person subsequently attempting to obtain national authorisations under the "decentralised" procedure; the Community procedure, once initiated, excludes other procedures and binds national authorities.

Article 12(3) requires the "notification of the marketing authorisation" to be published in the Official Journal, quoting in particular the date of authorisation and the number of the product included in the Community Register in accordance with article 12(1), second paragraph. The Regulation does not state when the authorisation comes into effect, so presumably the situation is governed by article 191 of the Treaty of Rome and the authorisation takes effect on the date on which the addressee of the decision, the applicant, is notified of that decision. However, "the date of authorisation" may well refer to the date on which the final decision is taken even if that is earlier than the date on which the applicant receives notification of the decision and thus earlier than the date on which the decision "takes effect".

Article 12(4) provides for the provision of information by the Agency in relation to the work of the CPMP in assessing any product under the Regulation :

> "Upon request from any interested person, the Agency shall make available the assessment report of the medicinal product by the [CPMP] and the reasons for its opinion in favour of granting authorisation, after deletion of any information of a commercially confidential nature."

This is a general provision, but it clearly only applies to *positive* opinions of the CPMP. It is not clear from the wording of the Regulation whether article 12(4) is intended to apply only where authorisation has been granted : that would be the natural assumption, but the provision on its face appears to leave it open that any interested person could request to see the CPMP evaluation report and the reasons given by the CPMP for a positive decision, even if the Commission did not accept the CPMP's reasoning and at any time, including before any final decision had been taken on the product in question. Such an interpretation of the wording of article 12(4) would be potentially highly embarrassing for the Agency, should serious disagreement break out between the Commission and the CPMP over a particular product. "Any interested person" is presumably at least as wide as "any person concerned" in article 10(4) and could include, for example, competing manufacturers and medical researchers.

Article 13 lays down a number of administrative details in relation to authorised products.

Article 13(1) corresponds to article 10(1) of Directive (EEC) 65/65 as amended by Directive (EEC) 93/39 : authorisation is valid for five years; it can be renewed for further five year periods by application at least three months before the authorisation expires; such an application for renewal is to be granted by the Agency only after consideration of "a dossier containing up-to-date information on pharmacovigilance"[1].

Article 13(2) corresponds to article 10(2) of Directive 65/65 as amended and provides for conditions to be imposed on an authorisation. The provisions in the Regulation are not exactly the same as those of the Directive (the terms of the Directive are rather more specific)[2] :

"In exceptional circumstances and following consultation with the applicant, an authorisation may be granted subject to certain specific obligations, to be defined and reviewed annually by the Agency.

Such exceptional decisions may only be adopted for objective and verifiable reasons and must be based on one of the causes mentioned in Part 4G of the Annex to Directive (EEC) 75/318."

Part 4G of the Annex to Directive (EEC) 75/318 provides :

"When, in respect of particular therapeutic indications, the applicant can show that he is unable to provide comprehensive data on the quality, efficacy and safety under normal conditions of use, because :

— the indications for which the product in question is intended are encountered so rarely that the applicant cannot reasonably be expected to provide comprehensive evidence, or
— in the present state of scientific knowledge comprehensive information cannot be provided, or
— it would be contrary to generally accepted principles of medical ethics to collect such information,

marketing authorisation may be granted on the following conditions :

(a) the applicant completed an identified programme of studies within a time period specified by the competent authority, the results of which shall form the basis of a reassessment of the benefit/risk profile,
(b) the medicinal product in question may be supplied on medical prescription only and may in certain cases be administered only under

---

1. See Chapter 12 post in relation to "pharmacovigilance".
2. See section 8.2 post.

strict medical supervision, possibly in a hospital and for a
radiopharmaceutical, by an authorised person,

(c)   the package leaflet and any medical information shall draw the attention
of the medical practitioner to the fact that the particulars available
concerning the medicinal product in question are as yet inadequate in
certain specified respects."

Article 13(3) provides for a further possible restriction :

"Some products may be authorised only for use in hospitals or for prescription
by specialists."

That provision relates back to article 9(3)(b) of the Regulation, where the CPMP is
empowered to recommend conditions of supply as restrictions on authorisation,
and to Directive (EEC) 92/26 where more detailed criteria are laid down in this
area. Directive (EEC) 92/26 is expressly referred to at article 9(3)(b) and is
considered in Chapter 14. It does not appear from the Regulation that the Agency
will be *bound* to adopt the same criteria as the Member States under the Directive
(Directives bind the Member States, not Community bodies like the Agency), but it
is natural to assume that in practice the Agency will operate in accordance with the
newly formulated Community guidelines and article 9(3)(b) does require the CPMP
to take the criteria laid down in Directive (EEC) 92/26 in finalising its opinion and
the documents annexed thereto.

Article 13(4) grants products authorised under the Regulation the benefit of the ten
year period of protection provided for "in point 8 of the second paragraph of article
4 of Directive (EEC) 65/65". That provision is considered in section 3.4.2 ante, but
in summary it prevents the majority of applicants for authorisation of an "essentially
similar" product evading the full technical and administrative requirements of
article 4 of Directive (EEC) 65/65 until the original product has been on the
Community market for at least ten years. After that period the later applicant is not
required to provide all the information normally required under article 4. Other
products may obtain only a six year period of protection.

Article 14 corresponds to article 9 of Directive (EEC) 65/65[1] and states that :

"[t]he granting of authorisation shall not diminish the general civil and criminal
liability in the Member States of the manufacturer or, where applicable, of the
person responsible for placing the medicinal product on the market".

Article 9 of Directive (EEC) 65/65 uses the word "affect" rather than "diminish", but
it is not clear how the granting of authorisation could *increase* the liability of the
manufacturer, so in substance the provisions appear to be the same.

7.4   Supervision and pharmacovigilance : Title III, Chapters 2 and 3; articles 15 to 26

Chapters 2 and 3 of Title III of the Regulation are considered in Chapters 11 and 12
post.

---

1.   As to which see section 3.6 ante and section 8.2 post.

7.5   The European Agency for the Evaluation of Medicinal Products : Title IV, articles 49 to 66

Title IV of Regulation (EEC) 2309/93 contains three Chapters : 1 Tasks of the Agency, articles 49 to 56; 2 Financial Provisions, articles 57 and 58; and 3 General provisions governing the Agency, articles 59 to 66.

7.5.1   The tasks of the Agency : Title IV, Chapter 1; articles 49 to 56

Article 49 establishes the Agency and states its general responsibility (the objectives of the Agency are set out in article 51) :

> "The Agency shall be responsible for co-ordinating the existing scientific resources put at its disposal by the competent authorities of the Member States for the evaluation and supervision of medicinal products".

The wording suggests a weak role for the Agency, dependent on the national competent authorities for its scientific resources and with an ill-defined task of "co-ordinating" those resources. Such wording reflects the intense reluctance of certain Member States to surrender any power over the assessment of medicinal products to an external body and the insistence of the Member States that the Agency should be closely controlled by the national authorities both in terms of its conduct and in terms of cost. It remains uncertain how the Agency will emerge in practice and to what extent it will be able to operate effectively and independently of national interests.

At the time of writing, it is clear that the Agency will be purely administrative in its operation. The current intention is to have a total staff of 300 of whom approximately one half will be administrative personnel. Of the latter, it is inevitable in a Community institution that a high proportion will be involved in the translation of documents between the nine Community languages and/or acting as interpreters.

In December 1992, the workload of the Agency was estimated by "DRT Europe Services" and those figures were annexed by the Commission to a Background Report on the Agency published on 3 December 1993[1]. It was estimated that between 1995 and 1999, the total number of "centralised" applications would fluctuate between 50 and 80 annually, of which between 40 and 64 would be for products for human use. The figures for "decentralised" arbitrations were much higher, fluctuating between 200 and 720, of which between 160 and 576 would be products for human use. The most notable feature is that the estimate forecasts that the introduction of the article 7a procedure for compulsory decentralised arbitrations after 1 January 1998 will more than double the workload of the Agency, from 256 decentralised arbitrations in 1997 to 576 in 1998[2].

Article 50(1) sets out the composition of the Agency :

> "(a)   the [CPMP], which shall be responsible for preparing the opinion of the Agency on any question relating to the evaluation of medicinal products for human use;
>
> (b)   the Committee for Veterinary Products [with equivalent responsibilities for veterinary medicinal products];
>
> (c)   a Secretariat, which shall provide technical and administrative support for the two Committees and ensure appropriate co-ordination between them;

---

1.   ISEC/B33/93.
2.   The procedures are described in section 7.3 ante and section 8.4 post.

(d)   an Executive Director, who shall exercise the responsibilities set out in article 55;

(e)   a Management Board, which shall exercise the responsibilities set out in articles 56 and 57."

The composition and functions of the CPMP (and the CVMP) are set out in articles 5 to 7 of the Regulation (and the role of the CPMP has already been described in relation to product authorisation); the functions of the Executive Director and the Management Board are described in articles 55 and 56; the role of the Secretariat is not expressly stated beyond the brief outline at (c) above, but its responsibilities as a technical bureaucracy are clearly indicated in the detailed statement of the objectives and tasks of the Agency set out in article 51 of the Regulation.

Article 50(1) and (2), sets out two specific powers of the CPMP and the CVMP : to establish working parties and expert groups; and to "seek guidance on important questions of a general scientific or ethical nature". The first possibility is a continuation of the developing practice of the CPMP to delegate specific tasks to such subordinate groups as a necessary reflection of its increasing workload. In its latest report to the Council on the work of the CPMP, the Commission describes the present situation as follows :

"The CPMP supports its scientific activities with expertise from the competent authorities of the Member States. Given this large pool of resource, a number of structures have been set up.

—   Working parties : A working party gathers experts from all 12 Member States, and generally treats questions relating to the manufacture, demonstration of safety and efficacy of medicinal products and/or administrative procedures. Although there is a tendency for the same expert to follow developments within the working party, the attendance at any given meeting will be determined by the content of the agenda. Working parties generally meet twice a year, although additional drafting group meetings, for specific topics, may also be called.

—   Ad hoc groups : Experience has shown that flexible structures which can respond to specific needs and which can regroup expertise either of differing disciplines or specialist interests, are required. Thus ad hoc groups are formed in order to deal with clearly identified tasks/questions. The number of meetings of an ad hoc group will depend on the time scale given for the resolution of the problem and the complexity of the issue."[1]

The reference to the CPMP seeking guidance on general scientific or ethical questions is less easy to understand. There is no explanation of the type of guidance or the source of the guidance that is envisaged. In the absence of such explanation, it appears that the CPMP is granted a very general power to commission special studies or to consult national or international experts on problems which arise.

Article 51 falls into two parts : a statement of the objectives of the Agency; and a statement of the "tasks" to be undertaken by the Agency in pursuance of those objectives. The objectives of the Agency are as follows :

---

1.   SEC (93) 771 at pp11-12. The current list of working parties is: Quality; Safety; Efficacy; Operations; Biotechnology/Pharmacy; and Pharmacovigilance. The current list of "ad hoc groups" is: Blood Products; Radiopharmaceuticals; Hypnotics; Herbal Remedies, and Over the Counter (OTC's). The activities of the various groups is described at pp13-16 of the Commission Report.

"In order to promote the protection of human and animal health and of consumers of medicinal products throughout the Community, and in order to promote the completion of the internal market through the adoption of uniform regulatory decisions based on scientific criteria concerning the placing on the market and use of medicinal products, the objectives of the Agency shall be to provide the Member States and the institutions of the Community with the best possible scientific advice on any question relating to the evaluation of the quality, the safety, and the efficacy of medicinal products for human or veterinary use, which is referred to it in accordance with the provisions of Community legislation relating to medicinal products."

The twofold purpose of the Agency - to protect public health and to promote the achievement of the single market - is closely modelled on the recitals to the original pharmaceutical Directive (EEC) 65/65[1]; as is the case with the new article 8 of Directive (EEC) 75/319[2], the final achievement of a single market is much more explicit than it had been in the 1965 (or the 1975) Directive. The objectives of the Agency in seeking to achieve that purpose are likewise derived from the original provisions of Directive (EEC) 65/65 in the threefold criteria of assessment of medicinal products[3]; the objective of providing "the best possible scientific advice" will only be fulfilled if the new Agency can be guaranteed to be given the resources necessary to provide the best advice *available in the Community*, rather the best advice available *given the limited resources allotted to it by the Member States*. It is clearly crucial to the credibility of the Agency as a source of final authority on the very difficult scientific and ethical problems likely to arise in the future that its findings should be generally accepted as at least as good and preferably better than those available from any national authority. The wording of article 49 does not dispel all possible doubts as to the Member States' will to create such a body.

In order to achieve the objectives laid down, article 51 also assigns ten specific tasks to the Agency :

"(a)   the co-ordination of the scientific evaluation of the quality, safety and efficacy of medicinal products which are subject to Community marketing authorisation procedures;

(b)   the transmission of assessment reports, summaries of product characteristics, labels and package leaflets or inserts for these medicinal products;

(c)   the co-ordination of the supervision, under practical conditions of use, of medicinal products which have been authorised within the Community and the provision of advice on the measures necessary to ensure the safe and effective use of these products, in particular by evaluating and making available through a database information on adverse reactions to the medicinal products in question (pharmacovigilance);

(d)   advising on the maximum limits for residues of veterinary medicinal products which may be accepted in foodstuffs of animal origin in accordance with Regulation (EEC) 2377/90.

(e)   co-ordinating the verification of compliance with the principles of good manufacturing practice, good laboratory practice and good clinical practice;

---

1.   See section 3.1 ante.
2.   Considered at section 8.4 post.
3.   See article 5 of Directive (EEC) 65/65 and section 3.2 ante.

(f)   upon request, providing technical and scientific support for steps to improve co-operation between the Community, its Member States, international organisations and third countries on scientific and technical issues relating to the evaluation of medicinal products;

(g)   recording the status of marketing authorisations for medicinal products granted in accordance with Community procedures;

(h)   providing technical assistance for the maintenance of a database on medicinal products which is available for public use;

(i)   assisting the Community and Member States in the provision of information to health care professionals and the general public about medicinal products which have been evaluated within the Agency;

(j)   where necessary, advising companies on the conduct of the various tests and trials necessary to demonstrate the quality, safety and efficacy of medicinal products."

That list clearly envisages a considerable administrative burden being accepted by the Agency, which again raises the question of the level of resources to be provided by the Community and the industry for its operation. The references to "Community procedures" are not explained but they must include not only the "centralised" procedures introduced by Regulation (EEC) 2309/93 but also the "decentralised" procedures introduced by Directive (EEC) 93/39. The most notable omission from the list is any reference to the conduct of technical scientific work by the Agency itself. That omission confirms that the Agency will have only a modest supportive role in the assessment of new products and will remain highly dependent on the technical resources of the Member States. That is confirmed by the description of the role of the CPMP at articles 52 to 54.

Articles 52 to 54 make quite detailed provision for the composition and functions of the CPMP and CVMP. As elsewhere in the Community pharmaceutical legislation, the structure is confusing : it remains the case that the CPMP is established by article 8 of Directive (EEC) 75/319 as amended, but other detailed provisions in relation to the CPMP are contained in the Regulation, a distinct piece of legislation.

Article 52 sets out the composition and general function of the CPMP[1]. Article 52(1), provides that the CPMP is to consist of two members nominated by each Member State and chosen "by reason of their role and experience in the evaluation of medicinal products for human ... use", who represent the national competent authorities. The Executive Director of the Agency or his representative and Commission representatives are entitled to attend all CPMP meetings and also meetings of working parties and expert groups. Members of the CPMP "may arrange to be accompanied by experts".

By article 52(2), the members of the CPMP have the task of ensuring "appropriate co-ordination between the tasks of the Agency and the work of competent national authorities, including the consultative bodies concerned with the marketing authorisation" (in the United Kingdom, the relevant body is the Medicines Commission established pursuant to Section 2 of the Medicines Act 1968; alternatively a committee established pursuant to Section 4 of the Act to deal with a specific product). The CPMP members' co-ordinating role is additional to their principal task of "providing objective scientific opinions".

---

1.   The CVMP is also provided for, in identical terms.

Crucially, article 52(3) provides that the work of the CPMP is dependent on the national authorities :

"The members of the [CPMP] and the experts responsible for evaluating medicinal products shall rely on the scientific assessment and resources available to the national marketing authorisation bodies. Each Member State shall monitor the scientific level of the evaluation carried out and supervise the activities of members of the [CPMP] and the experts it nominates, but shall refrain from giving them any instruction which is incompatible with the tasks incumbent on them."

The technical work in relation to the assessment of products under the new procedures will remain in the hands of the Member States, subject only to the rather vague prohibitions placed on the Member States' interference in that work. Under the "concertation" procedure, there were very clear trends as to the Member States which in practice carried out the initial assessments as "rapporteurs" : the United Kingdom was by far the most common State chosen as rapporteur, followed by France, the Netherlands, Denmark, Germany and Italy. Greece, Luxembourg, Spain and Portugal have never been rapporteurs[1]. There seems good reason to suppose that similar trends will emerge under the new regime[2].

Article 52(4) provides the outline of a procedure in reaching CPMP opinions : the CPMP must "use its best endeavours to reach a scientific consensus"; if that is impossible, then the opinion "shall consist of the position of the majority of members and may, at the request of those concerned, include the divergent positions with their grounds". Articles 5 to 14, setting out the "centralised" procedures, did not suggest the possibility of dissenting opinions forming part of a CPMP opinion. Clearly, the possibility of such dissenting opinions greatly increases the chance that the Commission might disagree with the majority opinion and therefore activate the procedure under article 10(1), third sub-paragraph. The existence of dissenting opinions under the Future System will not have the same debilitating effect as under the old "multi-State" and "concertation" procedures, because the new procedures have a mechanism for resolving the differences of opinion and reaching a binding decision. The old opinions could simply be ignored by Member States which did not agree with them.

Article 53 provides for the appointment of rapporteurs and experts to assist the CPMP. Article 53(1) provides that the CPMP shall appoint one of its members to be "rapporteur" where it is "required to evaluate a medicinal product". The rapporteur's task is "the co-ordination of the evaluation" and the appointment must take into consideration "any proposal from the applicant for the choice of rapporteur". The CPMP has the option to appoint a second member as "co-rapporteur" and is required to ensure that "all its members undertake the role of rapporteur or co-rapporteur". It is as yet uncertain to what extent the applicant's proposal will be taken into account in the choice of rapporteur. If it is normally treated as decisive then it is likely that in practice only a limited number of members of the CPMP will be appointed rapporteurs, in accordance with the wishes of applicants, and the other members will generally take part as co-rapporteurs (compare the Commission statistics in relation to Directive (EEC) 87/22 referred to previously).

Article 53(2) simply requires the Member States to supply the Agency with a list of "experts with proven experience in the assessment of medicinal products" who could serve on working parties and expert groups, with an indication of their

---

1. See figure 13 on page 36 of the Commission's latest Report on the Operation of the CPMP, SEC (93) 771.
2. Whether the location of the Agency in London will consolidate the United Kingdom's status as an authority favoured by applicants for authorisation of high technology products remains to be seen.

qualifications and specific areas of expertise, and to keep the list updated. Article 53(3), provides for written contracts between such rapporteurs and experts and the Agency, or where appropriate between the Agency and his employer. Payment is to be on a fixed scale established by the Management Board. Article 53(4) gives the Agency a general power, on a proposal from the CPMP, to use rapporteurs or experts "for the discharge of other specific responsibilities of the Agency". There are a number of technical or administrative functions for which such expertise might be useful. The involvement of the CPMP suggests that under this provision at least the task to be performed will be broadly scientific.

Article 54(1) requires the membership of the CPMP to be made public, and that the professional qualifications of each member should be specified when he is appointed. Article 54(2) relates to an important issue in pharmaceutical regulation, the great difficulty in separating the regulator from the regulated. The paragraph provides :

> "Members of the Management Board, Committee members, rapporteurs and experts shall not have financial or other interests in the pharmaceutical industry which could affect their impartiality. All indirect interests which could relate to this industry shall be entered in a register held by the Agency which the public may consult."

There is obviously a wide area for disagreement as to what might be an interest which could affect a regulator's partiality. Article 54(2) is a minimum first step to provide some degree of openness in the regulatory process[1].

Article 55 provides for the Executive Director of the Agency. He is to be appointed by the Management Board for a renewable term of five years on a proposal from the Commission and is the legal representative of the Agency. His responsibilities are set out at article 55(2) : day to day administration; provision of technical support for the CPMP, its working parties and expert groups; ensuring time limits laid down in Community legislation for the adoption of opinions by the Agency are respected; co-ordination between the CPMP and the CVMP; preparation of the accounts and the execution of the budget; and staff matters. Article 55(3) requires him to present four documents for approval to the Management Board each year, distinguishing the activities concerning veterinary products and those for human use : a draft report covering the activities of the Agency, in particular statistics concerning applications, duration of evaluations, and the products authorised, rejected or withdrawn; a draft programme of work for the next year; draft annual accounts for the previous year; and a draft budget for the next year. Article 55(4) requires the Executive Director's approval for all expenditure by the Agency.

Article 56 provides for the Management Board, which is to consist of two representatives from each Member State, two from the Commission and two appointed by the European Parliament, each pair comprising one member having responsibility for veterinary products and one for products for human use. Each representative may arrange to be replaced by an alternative and shall serve for a renewable term of three years. The Board is to elect a Chairman for three years and to adopt its rules of procedure, subject to the requirement that its decisions require a two-thirds majority. The Executive Director is to provide the Secretariat of the Board. Before 31 January each year, the Board is required to adopt the general report on the activities of the Agency for the previous year and its programme of work for the coming year and to forward them to the Member States, the Commission, the Council and the European Parliament.

---

1.   See Hancher *Regulating for Competition* (1990) Clarendon Press for a detailed discussion of these issues.

7.5.2   Financial provisions for the Agency : Title IV, Chapter 2; articles 57 and 58

Chapter 2 of Title IV, articles 57 and 58, sets out the financial provisions in relation to the Agency. Those provisions for the Agency remain a major source of uncertainty in attempting to predict how the Agency will work in practice (and finance will of course be a major factor in limiting the technical facilities and personnel available to the Agency).

Article 57 sets out, in eleven paragraphs, the essential procedures to be followed by the Executive Director and the Management Board in managing the finances of the Agency. Article 57(1) is of general significance :

"The revenues of the Agency shall consist of a contribution from the Community, and the fees paid by undertakings for obtaining and maintaining a Community marketing authorisation and for other services provided by the Agency."

It has not been finally resolved what proportion of the Agency's costs is to be borne out of central expenditure and what proportion by the pharmaceutical industry but the current intention is that fees should be set at a level that will, at least in the long term, make the Agency self-financing[1].

Article 57(2) states the scope of the Agency's expenditure : "the staff, administrative, infrastructure and operational expenses and expenses resulting from contracts entered into with third parties". No special provision is made for capital costs or the costs of setting up the Agency.

Article 57(3) to (6) deal with the mechanics of the budget : the Director is required to produce a preliminary draft budget for the Board by 15 February each year in relation to the next financial year's[2] anticipated activities; revenue and expenditure are required to balance and the Board must approve the draft and send it to the Commission for inclusion in the Community draft budget in accordance with article 203 of the EC Treaty; the final budget must be adopted before the beginning of each financial year, "adjusting it where necessary to the Community subsidy and the Agency's other resources"; the Director is responsible for implementation of the Budget. The difficulties in the operation of those provisions in practice will naturally arise in anticipation of the level of work and of Community subsidy each year and their relationship to the appropriate level of fees charged to industry by the Agency.

Article 57(8) to (11) concern supervision of the budget : the general task of monitoring the budget is the task of a financial controller appointed by the Board; in addition, the Director is required to send accounts for the preceding financial year to the Commission, the Board and the Court of Auditors[3] by 31 March each year; the Court of Auditors is required to examine the accounts in accordance with article 188c of the EC Treaty; the Board must "give a discharge to the Director in respect of implementation of the budget" (that expression is not explained but it presumably implies approval of the Director's conduct). Article 57(11) provides :

---

1.   See further article 58 post.
2.   The Community's financial year corresponds to the calendar year: article 203(1) of the EC Treaty.
3.   The Court of Auditors is established by Part Five, Title I, Chapter 1, Section 5 of the EC Treaty, articles 188a to 188c. The Court has general responsibility for financial supervision of the Community institutions and is required under article 188c to produce a financial report after the end of each financial year based on an audit of the accounts of the institutions.

"After the Court of Auditors has delivered its opinion, the Management Board shall adopt the internal financial provisions specifying, in particular, the detailed rules for establishing and implementing the Agency's budget."

Article 188c(4) of the EC Treaty provides for opinions to be delivered by the Court of Auditors "at the request of one of the institutions of the Community". It is not clear that there has been any such request or that any is provided for in article 57 of the Regulation. Article 57(11) appears to envisage a "one-off" action by the Board to adopt detailed budgetary rules in the light of guidance from the Court. It would of course be open to either the Commission or the Director, as the legal representative of the Agency, to seek such guidance under article 188c(4).

Article 58 is an important practical provision :

"The structure and amount of the fees referred to in article 57(1) shall be established by the Council acting under the conditions provided for by the Treaty on a proposal from the Commission, following consultation of organisations representing the interests of the pharmaceutical industry at Community level."

The Commission is thus required to consult with industry representatives with a view to reaching an agreed attitude to fee levels and proposing such a scheme to the Council for approval. The Commission submitted a draft scheme in February 1993 in which specific figures for an initial budget were proposed and a draft proposal for a Council Regulation on fees payable to the Agency was issued on 2 December 1993.

The draft proposal[1] is prefaced by an explanatory note (also reflected in the recitals to the draft Regulation) expressing the general intention that : the Agency should as far as possible be self-financing; that the level of fees should "neither lay an undue burden on the applicants nor endanger the achievement of the Agency's primary task of providing scientific advice of the highest possible quality in relation to the authorisation and supervision of medicinal products"; and that the Agency's finances should reflect its expenses as a supranational body obliged to incur, in particular, translation costs not generally incurred by national authorities. The guiding principle as to the level of fees is stated to be that it should be "more or less equivalent to but in no case substantially higher than the total of fees charged by the 12 Member States" on the basis that the Community procedures will replace separate applications in each Member State.

On that basis, article 2 of the draft Regulation proposes the following fee structure : (1) full Community authorisation : 200,000 ECU; (2) abridged application pursuant to article 4(8)(a) of Directive 65/65[2] : 100,000 ECU; (3) extension of authorisation to a new strength or form of an authorised product : 40,000 ECU; (4) Minor variation (article 15(4) of Regulation (EEC) 2309/93) : 5,000 ECU; (5) Major variation : 40,000 ECU; (6) Five-yearly renewal : 40,000 ECU; (7) Post-authorisation inspection within the European Community : 10,000 ECU[3]. Article 3 provides for an "arbitration fee" for resolution of disputes between Member States under the new "decentralised" procedure established by Directive (EEC) 93/39 and described in Chapter 8. The flat fee for such procedures is set at 40,000 ECU. No separate provision is made for charges in respect of amendments made pursuant to article 15 of Directive (EEC) 75/319 as amended. It is possible that the rates would

---

1. Draft Proposal for a Council Regulation on Fees Payable to the European Medicines Evaluation Agency; the rest is based on the 2 December 1993 draft III/5680/93-REV2.
2. See section 3.4.2 ante.
3. Inspection fees outside the Community are to be supplemented by a travel fee "on the basis of effective cost".

be the same as those specified at article 2(4) and (5) in respect of centrally authorised products.

Article 3 also provides that all Member States other than the authority responsible for initial authorisation are to reduce their fees by one half to reflect the reduced workload of those national authorities where the Community procedure is adopted.

Articles 4 and 5 set out an equivalent fee structure (at approximately one half of the level) for veterinary products and article 6 provides for the possibility of "waivers and fee reductions" in special cases, in particular where a product is designed to treat "only a limited number of patients of a particular disease (so-called orphan drugs)". Article 9 provides that where an application previously governed by the "concertation" procedure under Directive (EEC) 87/22 is converted into a "centralised" application, by article 2 of Directive (EEC) 93/41[1], the applicable fee will be the "arbitration fee" specified at article 3 of the draft Regulation rather than the full fee.

The draft Regulation is currently undergoing a process of consultation with the pharmaceutical industry but it must clearly be in place before 1 January 1995 when the Agency comes into operation. The precise legal basis for the adoption of the Regulation is left unclear by article 58 of Regulation (EEC) 2309/93 and the possibility of further difficulties of the kind described at section 7.1 cannot be excluded. Different national authorities have traditionally had quite different attitudes to the charging of fees for authorisation and the national industries' responses to the prospect of substantial Community fees reflect their national traditions.

7.5.3   General provisions governing the Agency : Title IV, Chapter 3; articles 59 to 66

Chapter 3 of Title IV consists of a range of diverse provisions. Article 59 grants the Agency legal personality, full legal rights in the Member States including the rights to acquire and dispose of land and other property and to institute legal proceedings. Article 60 governs the contractual and non-contractual liability of the Agency and the personal liability of the Agency. The provisions are substantially the same as article 215 of the EC Treaty, with the addition that the European Court of Justice is given jurisdiction to rule on any arbitration clause contained in a contract concluded by the Agency. Article 61 applies the Protocol on the Privileges and Immunities of the European Communities to the Agency.[2] Article 62 applies the Staff Regulations of Officials of the European Communities and the Conditions of Employment of Other Servants of those Communities to the staff of the Agency, gives the Agency the powers of the "appointing authority" under those Regulations and Conditions, and requires the Board to adopt necessary implementing provisions. Article 63 imposes continuing obligations of professional secrecy on the members of the Board, the CPMP and of the staff of the Agency. Articles 64 and 65 give the Commission and the Board powers to make certain contacts on behalf of the Agency : the Commission may, in agreement with the Board and the CPMP, invite international observers "with interests in the harmonisation of regulations" to participate in the work of the Agency; and the Board, in agreement with the Commission, is required to develop contacts between the Agency and representatives of the pharmaceutical industry, consumers and patients and the health professions.

---

1.   See section 8.6 post.
2.   That Protocol was annexed to the Treaty establishing a Single Council and a Single Commission of the European Communities of 8 April 1965.

Article 66 states simply that the Agency shall take up its responsibilities on 1 January 1995. Now that the issue of the location has been resolved, no legal impediment remains to that starting date. Many practical issues remain unresolved.

7.6   General and final provisions : Title IV, articles 67 to 74

Article 67 sets out two essential administrative requirements that go naturally together with the provisions of articles 12 to 14 of the Regulation : all decisions to "grant, refuse, vary, suspend, withdraw or revoke a marketing authorisation" under the Regulation must "state in detail the reasons on which they are based"; and the decisions must be notified to the party concerned. Those requirements correspond to article 12 of Directive (EEC) 65/65[1] in relation to negative decisions (though that provision requires that the party concerned be informed of any remedies available to him and of the time limits applicable to such remedies), and, more generally, to the general Community requirements set out in articles 190 and 191 of the EEC Treaty, though the requirement to state reasons is strengthened in Directive (EEC) 65/65 and the Regulation to require that reasons be given "in detail". The omission of any reference to available remedies does not of course exclude the possibility of judicial review of a Community decision under article 173 of the EC Treaty or of failure to reach a decision under article 175.

Article 68 states that the Community bodies must apply *only* the grounds (in practice the substantive criteria are those set out in article 11) and the procedures contained in the Regulation. Article 68(1) provides that an authorisation :

"shall not be refused, varied, suspended, withdrawn or revoked except on the grounds set out in this Regulation";

Article 68(2) provides that the authorisation :

"shall not be granted, refused, varied, suspended, withdrawn or revoked except in accordance with the procedures set out in this Regulation".

The substantive criteria therefore relate to refusals of authorisation only, as with article 21 of Directive (EEC) 65/65[2]. The Regulation's procedural requirements apply to all applications, whether or not they result in an authorisation. The justification of that difference is that the Community legislation does not require a positive evaluation of a product before it is authorised beyond that implied by the imposition of the three negative criteria of quality, safety and efficacy. In particular, there is no positive criterion of cost effectiveness. That is a matter for the consumer, whether the individual purchaser or the State security system.

Article 69 requires the Member States to "determine the penalties to be applied for the infringement of the provisions of this Regulation". The penalties must be "sufficient to promote compliance" with the Regulation. The Member States are required to inform the Commission forthwith of "any infringement proceedings"; the Council Minutes attached to the Commission Proposal of 10 June 1992 states that this refers only to the institution of formal legal proceedings, not to investigations of alleged infringements. The penalties established by the Member States are qualified, since they are to be :

"[w]ithout prejudice to article 68, and without prejudice to the Protocol on the Privileges and Immunities of the European Communities".

---

1.   Considered at section 3.6 ante.
2.   As to which see section 3.2 ante.

The effect of this qualification is that the Member States are prevented from derogating from the criteria or the procedures for authorisation set out in the Regulation or from the rights and privileges of the Community institutions and their employees accorded to them under the Protocol[1].

Article 70 is concerned with veterinary products and is therefore not considered here.

Article 71 requires the Commission, within six years of the entry into force of the Regulation, to publish :

"a general report on the experience acquired as a result of the operation of the procedures laid down in this Regulation, in Chapter III of Directive (EEC) 75/319 and in Chapter IV of Directive (EEC) 81/851".

In relation to the Regulation and Directive (EEC) 75/319, those procedures are the new "centralised" and "decentralised" procedures involving the CPMP and the Agency and leading to binding Community decisions on marketing authorisations. The procedures under Directive (EEC) 81/851 involving the CVMP and veterinary medicines are similar. The provision corresponds to the old obligation included in article 15 of Directive (EEC) 75/319[2] and corresponds to recital 18 of the Regulation[3].

Articles 72 and 73 were introduced at a late stage in the negotiations, by the Common Position reached on 26 October 1992. Previous drafts had simply referred to the procedures set out in article 2c of Directive (EEC) 75/318 where implementing measures were required under the Regulation[4] (article 2c remains unamended in Directive (EEC) 75/318 and the procedure laid down therein is still applicable for amendments to the Annex to that Directive under article 2a). The two new articles lay down the procedures to be followed in accordance with Council Decision (EEC) 87/373[5] laying down procedures for the exercise of implementing powers conferred on the Commission. The procedures are of great political significance because of the relative roles of the Council and the Commission in adopting or amending proposed secondary legislation.

Article 72 corresponds to variant (a) of procedure III set out in Directive (EEC) 87/373 and is in substance identical to article 2c of Directive (EEC) 75/318; article 73 corresponds to variant (b) of procedure III. The only, and crucial, difference between the two procedures is in the final paragraph of each. If the Commission and the Standing Committee on Medicinal Products for Human Use (which is the Committee established by Directive (EEC) 75/318) agree on the measures to be adopted, then the Commission simply adopts those measures. It is only if the measures proposed by the Commission do not attract the support of a qualified majority of the members of the Committee (in accordance with article 148 of the EC Treaty) that the Council is involved, the Commission then submitting to the Council a proposal for the measures to be taken, on which the Council must act, again by qualified majority. Article 72 provides that :

---

1.   A reservation by Germany entered on the 10 June 1992 draft, that the Commission should waive its staff's immunity in accordance with article 18(2) of the Protocol in the case of infringements of their secrecy obligation regarding statistical data, has not apparently been accepted.
2.   As to which see section 5.4 ante.
3.   See also the new article 15c of Directive (EEC) 75/319 discussed at section 8.4 post.
4.   See section 4.2 ante.
5.   OJ L197 18.7.87 p33.

"If on the expiry of a period of three months from the date of referral to the Council, the Council has not acted, the proposed measures shall be adopted by the Commission."

Article 73 by contrast provides that :

"If on the expiry of a period of three months from the date of referral to the Council, the Council has not acted, the proposed measures shall be adopted by the Commission, save where the Council has decided against the said measures by a simple majority."

Article 73 gives the Council the last word, though the wording of article 73 is somewhat contradictory in that it envisages that the Council may at the same time not act within three months and decide against the measures by a simple majority. The substance of the difference between the two measures is that under article 72 the Council needs a qualified majority either accepting or rejecting the Commission proposal for the Council to be able to block that proposal; whereas under article 73 the Council can block the Commission proposal by a simple majority of the Member States.

The article 72 procedure is to be used for :

— amendment of the Annexes to the Regulation (article 3);

— adoption of procedures for the Commission to refer the CPMP's opinion back for reconsideration (article 10(3));

— adoption of arrangements for variations to marketing authorisations (article 15(4)); and

— amendment to Title II, Chapter 3 on pharmacovigilance in the light of scientific and technical progress (article 26).

The article 73 procedure is reserved for :

— the decision to authorise itself (article 10(2)), where the article 73 procedure is adjusted in accordance with article 10(3) to increase the powers of the Member States to intervene in the consultative procedure before the Standing Committee[1]; and

— decisions to suspend or withdraw authorisations (article 18(3) referring to article 10; in urgent cases, the Committee is required to reach an opinion within fifteen days of a proposal from the Commission)[2].

The effect is that the Member States retain a power to block market authorisations and suspensions by simple majority.

Article 74, the final article, states :

"This Regulation shall enter into force on the day following the decision taken by the competent authorities on the headquarters of the Agency.

Subject to the first subparagraph Titles I, II, III, and V shall enter into force on 1 January 1995."

---

1.   See section 7.4 ante.

2.   See sections 11.5 and 12.3 post for more detailed discussion of article 18.

London was selected as the location for the headquarters of the Agency on 29 October 1993. The difficult practical and legal questions that might have arisen if the seat of the Agency had still not been decided on 1 January 1995 do not therefore need to be considered. It should however be noted that the current rules under Directives (EEC) 65/65, 75/318, 75/319 and 87/22, set out in Chapters 3 to 6 ante, continue to apply until 1 January 1995.

One difficulty does remain, however, because two distinct dates, 30 October 1993 and 1 January 1995, are identified by article 74. The period of six years from the date of entry into force of the Regulation, identified by article 71 above, must run from one or other of those dates. In context, it appears that the later date must be meant, when the procedures introduced by the Regulation become operative (see also article 15c(2) of Directive (EEC) 75/319 as amended).

Chapter 8 : Directives (EEC) 93/39[1] and 93/41[2] - The "Decentralised" Procedure and the End of the "Multi-State" and "Concertation" Procedures

8.1 The purpose and scope of the new regime : the recitals to Directive (EEC) 93/39

The recitals to Directive (EEC) 93/39 amending Directives (EEC) 65/65, 75/318 and 75/319[3] in respect of medicinal products and the Directive itself, are clearly complementary to Regulation (EEC) 2309/93[4] described in Chapter 7, in particular to recitals 8 and 9 of the Regulation expressly referring to the new "decentralised" procedure and to the sections of the Regulation establishing the Agency and laying down the functions of the CPMP.

Recitals 1 and 2 of the Directive, which was adopted on 14 June 1993, are both somewhat anachronistic : recital 1 states the need to "adopt measures with the aim of progressively establishing the internal market over a period expiring on 31 December 1992"; while recital 2 refers back to article 15(2) of Directive (EEC) 75/319, which had required the Commission to submit a proposal to the Council "containing appropriate measures leading to towards the abolition of any remaining barriers to the free movement of proprietary medicinal products". The reference to "proprietary" medicinal products is itself anachronistic[5] and Recital 2 omits to mention that the Commission's obligation under article 15(2) of Directive (EEC) 75/319 was to make a proposal *within four years*, ie by 1979[6]!

Recital 3 is equivalent to recitals 3 and 4 of Regulation (EEC) 2309/93, restating the exclusive nature of the criteria of quality, safety and efficacy for the purposes of marketing authorisation "in the interest of public health and of the consumer of medicinal products", and referring to the harmonisation already achieved by Directives (EEC) 65/65, 75/318 and 75/319. Recital 3 of Regulation (EEC) 2309/93 expressly excluded "economic or other considerations" but that is not repeated in the Directive, which does however include the provision that :

> "Member States should exceptionally be able to prohibit the use on their territory of medicinal products which infringe objectively defined concepts of public order or public morality".

That is the same wording as recital 3 of the Regulation[7].

---

1. OJ L214 24.8.93 p22. See Appendix 6 post.
2. OJ L214 24.8.93 p40. See Appendix 7 post.
3. OJ No 22 9.2.65 p369/65, see Appendix 1 post; OJ L147 9.6.75 pp1-12, 13-22, see Appendices 2 and 3 post. The text of Directive (EEC) 93/39 consists entirely of a-mendments to the earlier Directives and is therefore not reproduced at Appendix 6.
4. OJ L214 24.8.93 p1.
5. See section 3.2 ante.
6. The old article 15(2) is itself a strange provision : it was incorporated into Directive (EEC) 75/319 by Directive (EEC) 83/570, but its terms appear to refer back to 1975. It may well have been intended to refer to 1985 : see section 5.4 ante.
7. See section 7.1 ante.

Recital 4 states the purpose of the Directive for all medicinal products intended to be marketed in the Community other than those subject to the "centralised" procedure established by Regulation (EEC) 2309/93 :

"an authorisation to place a medicinal product on the market in one Member State ought in principle to be recognised by the competent authorities of the other Member States unless there are serious grounds for supposing that the authorisation of the medicinal product concerned may present a risk to public health".

Where the Member States disagree, the CPMP should undertake :

"a scientific evaluation of the matter ... leading to a single decision on the area of disagreement binding on the Member States concerned; ... this decision should be adopted by a rapid procedure ensuring close co-operation between the Commission and the Member States".

As with the "centralised" procedure, the essential requirements are scientific quality, speed and co-operation between the Community institutions and the Member States.

Recital 5 provides specifically for the preparation and exchange of assessment reports between the Member States to avoid duplication of effort; also for the suspension of authorisation procedures in one Member State pending results in another. The detailed amendments to Directives (EEC) 75/319 provide not only for voluntary suspension of national procedures after 1994 but for compulsory suspension after 1997[1].

Articles 6 and 7 relate to improved procedures for the supervision of products imported from third countries in the light of the internal market; and to improved information exchange between the Member States in relation to supervision of authorised products and pharmacovigilance. Those issues are considered in Chapters 11 and 12.

8.2   Amendments to Directive (EEC) 65/65; article 1 of Directive (EEC) 93/39

Article 1 consists of nine paragraphs and makes specific amendments to Directive (EEC) 65/65. Reference should be made to Chapter 3 for discussion of the text in force until 1 January 1995.

Article 1(1) replaces article 3 of Directive (EEC) 65/65 and introduces two new and potentially highly significant elements. The new article 3 is in two paragraphs and the first paragraph provides :

"No medicinal product may be placed on the market of a Member State unless a marketing authorisation has been issued by the competent authorities of that Member State in accordance with this Directive or an authorisation has been granted in accordance with Regulation (EEC) 2309/93 ..."

Authorisation is no longer limited to the competent authorities of the Member States in accordance with Directive (EEC) 65/65; it is now possible for a marketing authorisation, valid throughout the Community and thus in each individual Member State, to be obtained by a different route : the "centralised" Community procedure set out in Regulation (EEC) 2309/93[2].

---

1.   See section 8.4 post.
2.   See Chapter 7 ante.

The new second paragraph to article 3 of Directive (EEC) 65/65 provides :

"The provisions of this Directive shall not affect the powers of the Member States' authorities either as regards the setting of prices for medicinal products or their inclusion in the scope of national health insurance schemes, on the basis of health, economic and social conditions."

This provision appears to have two purposes : it confirms that the Directive does not *extend* the powers of Member States to take price into account when establishing price controls for medicinal products; it also confirms that the Directive does not *restrict* those powers, so that a Member State can set prices for drugs and refuse to include drugs within the scope of reimbursement schemes even if those drugs have been authorised for marketing either by themselves or by the Community. The most significant effect in practice is likely to be to permit Member States to refuse to pay for products that have been authorised either through the "centralised" authorisation procedure or after a Community decision pursuant to the "decentralised" procedure. The final words, "on the basis of health, economic and social conditions", leave the Member States a wide margin of appreciation within which to argue that a refusal to finance a product was justified[1]. It is not, however, easy to see how a decision not to finance an authorised product, which was therefore certified to be safe, effective and of suitable quality, could be justified on the basis of health alone. The argument would be that public health is best protected by the Member States establishing priorities and refusing to pay for non-cost-effective treatments.

Article 1(2) adds a further sub-paragraph to article 4 of Directive (EEC) 65/65, between the existing first and second sub-paragraphs, which provides that the "person responsible for placing products on the market" must be established in the European Community and that, in relation to products already authorised on the date of entry into force of the Directive, this new requirement is to be applied progressively by the Member States to those products as and when each product's authorisation comes up for its five-yearly renewal (see article 10 of Directive (EEC) 65/65). The requirement introduced by article 1(2) will thus gradually come to apply to all authorised medicinal products, and that should help to simplify administration throughout the Community in the face of the increased burden of administration and co-operation between the Member States and the Community implicit in the new system : see also the equivalent provision, article 2, of Regulation (EEC) 2309/93.

Article 1(3) replaces points 6 and 11 of the second paragraph of article 4 of Directive (EEC) 65/65, clarifying the administrative requirements of article 4[2].

Point 6 of article 4 is simply extended by the introduction of four specific elements to be included : precautionary measures to be taken for (i) the storage of the product, (ii) its administration to patients and (iii) disposal of waste products, and also (iv) any potential environmental risks posed by the product. The "precautionary" measures are very similar to elements (5) and (6) of the summary of product particulars to be provided pursuant to article 4, point 9 and article 4a of Directive (EEC) 65/65[3].

Point 11 of article 4 is substantially extended. The old version simply required that any authorisation obtained from another Member State or third country should be

---

1.   For the Court of Justice's attitude to this issue, see Case 301/82 *Clin-Midy and Others v Belgium* [1984] ECR 251 and the discussion of articles 3, 5 and 21 of Directive (EEC) 65/65 at section 3.2 ante.
2.   See section 3.4 ante.
3.   See section 3.4 ante.

included with the application for authorisation in a Member State. That provision left it unclear what exactly was required, whether the mere fact of authorisation or the full details of the application and authorisation. The new version explicitly requires four documents to be provided :

(1) copies of other national authorisations (not only within the Community), together with a list of those Member States where an application within the scope of Directive (EEC) 65/65 is currently under examination;

(2) copies of the summary of product characteristics, either the summary submitted to other national authorities pursuant to article 4a or the summary approved pursuant to article 4b (the Directive does not express a preference but it would seem preferable to submit the approved version where available);

(3) copies of the proposed or approved package leaflet under article 6 or article 10 of Directive (EEC) 92/27[1]; and

(4) details of any refusals of authorisation in any Member State or third country, together with the reasons for such a refusal.

Point 11, as amended, now further requires that this information "shall be updated on a regular basis".

Article 1(4) replaces article 4b of Directive (EEC) 65/65. The old version of article 4b simply required the competent authority of a Member State to provide the applicant with an accurate summary of the product as approved. The new version requires in addition that the authorising authority :

(1) send a copy of the decision reached and the summary as approved to the European Agency for the Evaluation of Medicinal Products[2];

(2) draw up an assessment report and comments in relation to the analytical and pharmacological tests and clinical trials carried out on the product and to update it whenever important new information emerges in respect of the quality, safety or efficacy of the product.

Article 1(5) replaces article 6 of Directive (EEC) 65/65 in the following terms :

"This Directive shall not affect the application of national legislation prohibiting or restricting the sale, supply or use of medicinal products as contraceptives or abortifacients. The Member States shall communicate the national legislation to the Commission."

The significant change is the introduction of "abortifacients" as a category of products distinct from contraceptives but, like contraceptives, given special treatment by the Directive. The new article 6 also requires the Member States to notify the Commission of national legislation falling within the terms of the article. Article 6 is referred to by article 12 of Regulation (EEC) 2309/93[3].

Article 1(6) amends and extends article 7 of Directive (EEC) 65/65, while article 1(7) introduces a new article 7a :

The new article 7(1) of Directive (EEC) 65/65 extends the period within which Member States are required to complete their authorisation procedure to 210 days,

---

1.   See Chapter 15 post.
2.   See section 7.5 ante.
3.   See section 7.3.4 ante.

thus recognising the practical realities of the process[1]. The period starts from the date of submission of "a valid application". The concept of a "valid" application is defined by the requirements of Directive (EEC) 65/65 and the Annex to Directive (EEC) 75/318 as elucidated by Commission notices and by CPMP guidelines[2].

The new article 7(2) of Directive (EEC) 65/65 introduces a new procedure to be operated from 1 January 1995. This new procedure applies to applications to more than one Member State where the first State ("A")'s examination of the application is still in progress when the second State ("B")'s examination begins. It provides that in such a situation, B may suspend detailed examination of the application pending the outcome of A's investigation. In practice, B will be made aware of A's investigation by the applicant including details of other applications in accordance with point 11 of article 4 as amended : see above. A will be required by the new article 4b to prepare an "assessment report" and B can await receipt of A's report before itself examining the application. B is required to notify A of its conduct and A is required to send B a copy of its report as soon as it has completed its examination and reached a decision. Within ninety days of receipt of A's decision, B must either : "recognise the decision ... and the summary of product characteristics" as approved by A; or refer the matter to the CPMP under the new procedures introduced by the amended articles 10 to 14 of Directive (EEC) 75/319[3]. Article 7 as amended limits this second option to cases where B :

> "considers that there are grounds for supposing that the authorisation of the medicinal product concerned may present a risk to public health".

A footnote indicates that the expression "risk to public health" refers to the quality, safety and efficacy of the product, ie to all three of the criteria set out at article 5 of Directive (EEC) 65/65, though on its face it appears to relate to only one of those criteria, the harmfulness of the product.

The new article 7(2) is not particularly clearly drafted in that the conduct of B after its decision to suspend or not to suspend is not expressly made conditional on a positive decision to suspend, but in practice that must be the intention. Until 1998, B retains the option to ignore A's assessment under this procedure.

The new article 7a of Directive (EEC) 65/65, to come into effect from 1 January 1998, simplifies the procedure described above and finally introduces a close approximation to a system of compulsory mutual recognition between the national authorities. The difference between 7a and 7(2) as amended above is that in the latter case B *must* request A to send its assessment report as soon as it is made aware of A's investigation. The procedure on receipt of the report is identical in either case. article 7a does not say whether B must or may suspend its own examination of the product pending receipt of A's report. One might have expected that B would be required to suspend its own investigation, but the principal feature of the post-1997 procedure is that B will be required to activate the procedure, which will in turn oblige A to prepare an assessment report for B's use and receipt of A's report will oblige B either to recognise A's decision within 90 days or to refer the matter to the CPMP for a binding Community decision. It will therefore no longer be possible for two divergent national procedures to be completed without a binding Community resolution of the divergence.

Article 1(8) replaces article 9a of Directive (EEC) 65/65, making minor alterations and adding a reference to point 4 of article 4 ("method of preparation") and obliging

---

1.   See section 3.6 ante.
2.   See Chapters 3 and 4 ante.
3.   See section 8.4 below.

the person responsible for putting the product on the market to update its control methods in preparation and manufacture of the product.

Article 1(9) replaces article 10 of Directive (EEC) 65/65 : the new article 10(1) of Directive (EEC) 65/65 amends the old wording slightly and adds a requirement that renewal of a marketing authorisation in future requires examination of an updated dossier on the product :

> "containing in particular details of the data on pharmacovigilance and other information relevant to the monitoring of the medicinal product".

The new article 10(2) of Directive (EEC) 65/65 introduces an important qualification, permitting certain conditions to be imposed on an authorisation in "exceptional circumstances", in particular to carry out "further studies" following authorisation and to notify any adverse reactions to the product. This is intended to be an "exceptional" course of conduct, which may only be adopted for "objective and verifiable reasons" and must be based on one of the causes referred to "in Part 4(G) of the Annex to Directive (EEC) 75/318". That provision is similar to article 13(2) of Regulation (EEC) 2309/93[1].

8.3 Amendments to Directive (EEC) 75/318; article 2 of Directive (EEC) 93/39

Article 2 of Directive (EEC) 93/39 makes only one small change to Directive (EEC) 75/318. "The Committee on the Adaptation to Technical Progress of the Directives on the Removal of Technical Barriers to Trade in the Medicinal Products Sector", established by article 2b of Directive (EEC) 75/318, as introduced by Directive (EEC) 87/19, is given the catchier title of "the Standing Committee on Medicinal Products for Human Use". That Committee has important tasks not only under Directive (EEC) 75/318 but also now under Regulation (EEC) 2309/93 and Directive (EEC) 75/319[2].

8.4 Amendments to Directive (EEC) 75/319 : the new "decentralised" procedure; article 3 of Directive (EEC) 93/39

Article 3(1) of Directive (EEC) 93/39, as Directive (EEC) 83/570 had done previously, completely replaces Part Three of Directive (EEC) 75/319, the section of that Directive governing the operation of the Committee for Proprietary Medicinal Products, the "CPMP". This section therefore describes the whole section afresh, though there are obvious similarities with the description of the old system at section 5.4. The description follows the article numbering of Directive (EEC) 75/319.

The new article 8(1) of Directive (EEC) 75/319 sets up the CPMP, though its purpose has been altered slightly from the previous version. The new version states that the CPMP is set up :

> "[i]n order to facilitate the adoption of common decisions by Member States on the authorisation of medicinal products for human use on the basis of the scientific criteria of quality, safety and efficacy, and to achieve thereby the free movement of medicinal products within the Community".

---

1.   See section 7.3.3 ante.
2.   See section 7.6 ante and section 8.4 post.

The previous version had spoken of the adoption of "a common position" by the Member States and of "promoting" rather than "achieving" the free movement of pharmaceuticals within the Community. The new version clearly (if optimistically) envisages the final *achievement* of the elusive goal of a single market for pharmaceuticals.

A second difference is that the CPMP is now stated to form part of "the European Agency for the Evaluation of Medicinal Products established by Regulation (EEC) 2309/93[1].

Article 8(2) of Directive (EEC) 75/319 requires the CPMP, "[i]n addition to the other responsibilities conferred upon it by Community law" (as to which see articles 52 to 54 of Regulation (EEC) 2309/93), to :

> "examine any question relating to the granting, variation suspension or withdrawal of marketing authorisation for a medicinal product which is submitted to it in accordance with this Directive".

The CPMP is thus given a very wide and general remit under the Directive (the old article 8(2) was much more specific).

The old article 8(3), which authorised the CPMP to draw up its own rules of procedure, has been deleted. The new legislation contains no provision for the procedures to be adopted by the CPMP, although the provisions of Title III of Regulation (EEC) 2309/93 and of Chapter III of Directive (EEC) 75/319 as amended lay down quite detailed procedural rules and articles 52 to 54 of the Regulation make specific provision for the composition and functions of the CPMP. Earlier drafts of the Directive had included the old article 8(3) with proposals that the CPMP rules should be subject to the approval of the Council and the Commission.

8.4.1 Activating the "decentralised" procedure : articles 9 and 10

Article 9 sets out the procedure to be followed by the holder of a marketing authorisation issued in accordance with article 3 of Directive (EEC) 65/65 in order to "obtain the recognition in one or more of the Member States" of that authorisation. There is thus no longer any requirement that at least two further States should be involved and the new version introduces the concept of "recognition" explicitly where the previous version had merely spoken of "making it easier to obtain" authorisation in another Member State and of "due consideration" being given to an authorisation granted in another Member State.

The obligations on the holder of the market authorisation are very similar to those under the earlier regime :

(1) to submit applications to the national authorities concerned together with the information required under articles 4, 4a and 4b of Directive (EEC) 65/65; the new version says "shall" where the earlier said "may", but there is no real difference; the holder is under no obligation to seek recognition rather than applying in each Member State individually;

(2) to testify that the "dossier" is identical to that accepted by the first Member State; this is identical to the earlier version; or

(3) to identify any additions or amendments it may contain; the new wording clarifies but does not change the substance of the earlier version;

---

1.   See Chapter 7 ante.

(4) where (3) applies, to certify that the summary presented in accordance with article 4a in the current application is identical to that accepted by the first Member State in accordance with article 4b of Directive (EEC) 65/65; this is a new obligation; the Directive does not leave open the possibility that there might be good reason for the summary to have changed between the authorisation and the application for recognition;

(5) to certify that all the dossiers filed at this stage to the various national authorities concerned are identical; this is identical to the earlier requirement (article 9(1)).

The overall effect of these provisions is that the original national authority and all subsequent authorities must be certified all to be in receipt of the same application with the same summary of product characteristics.

The applicant is further required :

(6) to notify the CPMP of the application; this is identical to the earlier requirement;

(7) to inform the CPMP of the Member States concerned and of the dates of submission of the applications; this is in substance identical to the old regime;

(8) to send the CPMP a copy of the authorisation granted by the first Member State; this is identical to the earlier requirement;

(9) to send the CPMP copies of any other authorisations granted by other Member States and to indicate whether any other application is currently under consideration in any Member State; this is a new requirement, referring to the procedures introduced by the new article 7(2) and article 7a of Directive (EEC) 65/65 : see above (article 9(2));

(10) until 1 January 1998[1], to inform in advance the Member State granting the original authorisation, upon which the other applications for recognition are based, of the application in accordance with Directive (EEC) 75/319; this is a more precise version of a requirement under the old regime;

(11) to notify that Member State of any additions to the dossier; this is identical to the old regime;

(12) where that Member State so requires, to provide all the particulars and documents necessary to enable it to check that the dossiers filed are identical to the dossier on which it took its decision; this is identical to the old regime;

(13) to request that Member State to prepare an assessment report in respect of the medicinal product concerned or to update an existing report if that is necessary; this is a new requirement, clarifying a separate provision under article 13 of the old version, whereby the obligation was a general one placed on the Member State authorities; that article has been broken up and now appears in articles 4 and 7 of Directive (EEC) 65/65 and in the present article (article 9(3)).

---

1.   On 1 January 1998, the procedure set out in article 7a of Directive (EEC) 65/65 will come into effect. There will then be an automatic requirement that a Member State asked to grant an authorisation subsequent to that granted by another Member State must ask for an assessment report from that other Member State and then either recognise the earlier decision or refer the matter to the CPMP : see ante. It will then be superfluous for the applicant to make a request to the other Member State.

Article 9(3) and (4) place certain obligations on the Member States concerned in the new procedures. The Member State granting the original authorisation is required :

(1) to prepare or update the assessment report, as requested by the holder of the authorisation under (13) above, within 90 days of receipt of the request (the Member State may presumably refuse to do so if the applicant does not agree to make the necessary changes to update the dossier);

(2) to forward the assessment report to the Member States concerned by the application for recognition at the same time as the application (article 9(3));

Article 9(4) is subject to article 10(1) considered below, which introduces the machinery of consultation between Member States and the CPMP. Subject to that provision, the Member States in receipt of an application in accordance with article 9(1) to (3) are required :

(1) to recognise the original marketing authorisation within 90 days of receipt of the application and the report; and

(2) to inform the Member State granting the original application, the other Member States concerned by the application, the CPMP and the person responsible for marketing.

Those obligations imposed on the Member States are new, although they in part simply draw together a number of disparate elements in the old system. Under the old regime, the Member States had 120 days from notification by the CPMP of the last application for recognition in which to state "reasoned objections"; under the new system, a Member State has only 90 days and time runs from receipt of the application and assessment report.

Article 10 sets out a procedure to be followed in the event that :

"a Member State considers that there are grounds for supposing that the authorisation of the medicinal product concerned may present a risk to public health".

As in the equivalent provisions of Directive (EEC) 65/65 as amended (articles 7(2) and 7a) the expression "risk to public health" is not limited to its literal meaning but includes all three of the criteria set out at article 5 of Directive (EEC) 65/65 : quality, safety and efficacy. The previous wording of article 9 was clearer on this issue, expressly referring to article 5 of Directive (EEC) 65/65. The effect of the change seems to be to give as restrictive a tone as possible to the wording of article 10 without in fact changing the meaning of the article.

Article 10(1) requires a Member State harbouring such concerns :

(1) to inform the applicant, the Member State which granted the initial authorisation, any other Member State concerned by the application and the CPMP;

(2) to state the basis for its concerns in detail; and

(3) to indicate what action may be necessary to correct any defect in the application.

This provision is similar to the previous procedure whereby a Member State had either to grant authorisation or state "reasoned objections."

Article 10(2) places obligations on all of the "Member States concerned" :

(1) to use their best endeavours to reach agreement on the action to be taken in respect of the application;

(2) to provide the applicant with the opportunity to make his point of view known orally or in writing; but

(3) to refer the matter to the CPMP for application of the procedure laid down in article 13 of the Directive if they cannot reach agreement within the period laid down by article 9(4).

The overall effect of paragraphs 9(4), 10(1) and 10(2) is therefore that there is a period of ninety days for each Member State, from the date on which it receives an application for recognition and the relevant assessment report, to reach a preliminary view as to whether recognition should be granted; to notify all parties of any concerns; and to enter into discussions with other Member States concerned (with input from the applicant) as to the appropriate action to take. The effect will be that there will be different time periods for the various Member States concerned, depending on the date of receipt of the application and report. The decisive time limit in practice will be ninety days from the first date of receipt of both the application and the report by a Member State expressing concern. Other Member States expressing concern will in effect be bound by that date, even if they were the first Member State to express concern. Likewise, even those Member States that have already granted recognition will be bound to refer the matter to the CPMP if agreement cannot be reached. It will therefore be advisable as far as possible to present reports and applications simultaneously to all the Member States concerned.

Article 10(3) requires the Member States concerned to provide the CPMP with a detailed statement of the matters on which they have been unable to reach agreement and the reasons for their disagreement and to provide a copy of this information to the applicant.

The Member States are required to provide this information to the CPMP within "the time limit referred to in [article 10(2)]". That appears to refer to the ninety day period discussed above rather than to the very short time ("forthwith") granted to the Member States to refer the matter to the CPMP on expiry of the period for discussion. It seems illogical for the Member States to spend time preparing a detailed statement of their irreconcilable differences during the period in which they are supposed to be attempting to reconcile those differences. It would be more natural to allow a period after the 90 days in which such a statement can be prepared, but the decision was taken that disputes should be referred to the CPMP for resolution as quickly as possible[1]. Of course, in some cases it will be clear at an early stage that there is a strong difference of opinion and in such cases it will be possible to refer the matter to the CPMP and prepare a statement within the 90 day period. No time limit is specified for provision of the information to the applicant.

Article 10(4) provides that the applicant shall forthwith send the CPMP a copy of its application and the assessment report on being informed of referral of the matter to the CPMP. Since there is no time limit for the applicant to be informed there can be no firm date by which the CPMP must receive copies of the application and assessment report. This provision corresponds to article 10(3) under the old regime.

---

1. See page 3 of the Council's Reasons for the Common Position in respect of the Directive.

8.4.2   Other mechanisms for consultation of the CPMP : articles 11 and 12
Article 11 is very similar in substance under the old regime and the new. Directive (EEC) 93/39 revises and simplifies the wording, but the purpose remains to enable those concerned to ask the CPMP to resolve differences between Member States where "divergent decisions" have been adopted in relation to authorisation, suspension of authorisation or withdrawal from the market of a product. The only differences of substance are :

(1)   the "person responsible for placing the product on the market" is given the right to refer matters to the CPMP; previously that right was restricted to the Member States themselves and the Commission;

(2)   the question referred must be "clearly identif[ied]"; and

(3)   the Member States and the person responsible for marketing must send the CPMP "all available information relating to the matter in question".

Article 12 expands and clarifies article 12 under the old regime. The new article 12 has the same basic defect as the old article, referring to "specific cases where the interests of the Community are involved" without any explanation of what that expression means. Procedurally however it is much more satisfactory : article 13 is general in scope so that article 12 references are governed by the same general procedures as article 10 and article 11 references. As with article 11, the scope of the new article 12 has been expanded to permit references to the CPMP by the Member States, the Commission and by "the applicant or holder of the marketing authorisation". The wording of the article does not strictly make sense, since each party is given the right to refer matters to the CPMP :

> "before reaching a decision on a request for a marketing authorisation or on the suspension or withdrawal of an authorisation, or on any other variation to the terms of a marketing authorisation which appears necessary, in particular to take account of the information collected in accordance with Chapter Va".

Of course, applicants or holders of authorisations are in no position to take decisions and the Commission's right to take decisions does not come into effect until 1 January 1995 and will remain limited. It appears that the text must mean that each of the parties concerned has the right to refer an important issue of principle to the CPMP before the relevant decision *is taken* by whichever body is responsible, normally a Member State authority. The same general requirements are clearly to identify the question in issue and to send all available information to the CPMP apply under article 12 as under article 11.

8.4.3   The CPMP's procedures : article 13
Article 13 lays down the framework for the CPMP's procedures. It therefore corresponds to article 14 of the old Chapter III; the old article 13 has been replaced by various provisions in article 9 and also by amendments to article 4 and 4b of Directive (EEC) 65/65[1].

Article 13(1) lays down the deadlines for the CPMP to "issue a reasoned opinion" on the matters referred to it under articles 10, 11 and 12 (also under articles 7(2) and 7a of Directive (EEC) 65/65) :

(1)   the normal deadline is 90 days from the date on which the matter is referred to the CPMP; this is extended from 60 days under the old regime; the effect of article 9(4) and article 13(1) in combination is therefore to preserve an overall time limit of 180 days but to shorten the period for consideration by the

---

1.   See ante.

Member States and to lengthen the period for consideration by the CPMP, each by 30 days;

(2) the period of 90 days can be extended by a further 90 days in cases referred to the CPMP under articles 11 and 12; that is a new provision;

(3) in urgent cases the CPMP may agree to a *shorter* deadline on a proposal from the chairman of the CPMP; this is also a new provision, compensating to some degree for the general extension of time.

Article 13(2) introduces a new system of "rapporteurs". The CPMP is given the power to appoint one of its members to act as rapporteur; also to appoint "individual experts to advise it on specific questions" who are to be given defined tasks to be completed within a specified time limit. The system of rapporteurs and experts coheres with the new system introduced for "centralised" authorisations under article 53 of Regulation (EEC) 2309/93[1]. To a large extent, article 13(2) simply recognises the way in which the CPMP has developed in practice under the old "multi-State" and "concertation" procedures described in Chapters 5 and 6[2].

Article 13(3) lays down certain minimum procedural guarantees of good administration :

(1) In cases under articles 10 and 11, the CPMP must give the person responsible for marketing the product in issue an opportunity to present "oral or written explanations"; this provision ends the anomaly of article 14(1) of the old Chapter III under which there were different rules for article 10 and for article 11 cases[3];

(2) Article 12 cases are brought within the scope of the new article 13, but the CPMP has the power (not the duty) to allow the person responsible for marketing the product to explain himself orally or in writing;[4]

(3) the CPMP is given a new general power to invite any other person to provide relevant information;

(4) the CPMP is permitted to suspend the time limits laid down in article 13(1) "to allow the person responsible for marketing to prepare explanations"; this corresponds to the provisions of article 14(1) of the previous version of Chapter III.

Article 13(4) deals with the procedure to be followed by the European Agency for the Evaluation of Medicinal Products where the CPMP is of the opinion that :

"— the application does not satisfy the criteria for authorisation, or
— the summary of product characteristics proposed by the applicant in accordance with article 4a of Directive (EEC) 65/65 should be amended, or
— the authorisation should be granted subject to conditions, with regard to conditions considered essential for the safe and effective use of the medicinal product including pharmacovigilance, or

---

1.   See section 7.5.1 ante.
2.   See the Commission's latest Report on the Operation of the CPMP, SEC(93) 771, Chapters II to IV.
3.   See section 5.4 ante.
4.   According to the Commission's Report on the Operation of the CPMP, SEC(93) 771 at p40, the CPMP considers that in article 12 cases : "when practical, the applicant or the marketing authorisation holder would be offered the opportunity to make a submission, orally or in writing, before the CPMP issues its opinion".

— an existing marketing authorisation should be suspended, varied or withdrawn".

With reference to the first possibility, the criteria for authorisation are laid down in article 5 of Directive (EEC) 65/65 and those criteria should clearly also be applied by the CPMP where it is asked to give its opinion[1]. The second possibility is a specific instance of the requirement in article 5 of Directive (EEC) 65/65 that the particulars and documents submitted by an applicant should comply with article 4 of Directive (EEC) 65/65. The third possibility corresponds to the newly amended article 10 of Directive (EEC) 65/65. Issues relating to suspension of authorisation and pharmacovigilance, the fourth possibility, are considered in Chapters 11 and 12.

The procedure to be followed by the Agency under article 13(4) is "forthwith" to inform the person responsible for marketing of the CPMP opinion. That person has fifteen days from receipt of the CPMP opinion to notify the Agency in writing of its intention to appeal. Where he does notify the Agency of his intention to appeal, he must forward detailed grounds for appeal to the Agency within 60 days *of receipt of the CPMP opinion* (ie he does not have a further 60 days after filing the appeal). The CPMP must decide whether its opinion should be revised within 60 days of receipt of the grounds of appeal. The conclusions reached on appeal must be annexed to the assessment report prepared for the purposes of article 13(5) below.

Article 13(5) sets out the procedure to be followed by the Agency after the CPMP has reached a final opinion, either an initially positive opinion without right of appeal or an initially negative opinion possibly reconsidered on appeal. The Agency must send the final opinion of the CPMP within 30 days of its adoption to the Member States, the Commission and to the person responsible for placing the product on the market. That opinion must be accompanied by an assessment report on the product giving the reasons for the conclusions reached.

A further requirement is laid down where the opinion of the CPMP is positive : the Agency must annex to the opinion :

"(a) a draft summary of the product characteristics, as referred to in article 4a of Directive (EEC) 65/65;

(b) any conditions affecting the authorisation within the meaning of paragraph 4."[2]

Under (a), the CPMP effectively takes the place of the Member State and provides a summary of the product characteristics as approved, but the Member States retain their formal position, as the final approval of the summary of product characteristics remains a matter for the Member States, under article 4b of Directive (EEC) 65/65, when a marketing authorisation is finally issued in accordance with article 3 of that Directive. Clause (b) refers to the third possibility under article 13(4) discussed

---

1. Article 13(4) corresponds to article 9(1) of Regulation (EEC) 2309/93 in relation to Community "centralised" authorisations, but criteria are also set out in article 11 of that Regulation. Articles 9(1) and 11 of the Regulation refer also to defects in the labelling or package insert under article 10 of Directive (EEC) 92/27. It is not clear whether the first indent of article 13(4) of the Directive states that to be one of the "criteria" for authorisation under Directive (EEC) 75/319 as amended. Consistency would require it to do so.

2. The equivalent provision in Regulation (EEC) 2309/93 (article 9(3)) refers specifically to Directive (EEC) 92/26 on the classification for supply of medicinal products for human use and Directive (EEC) 92/27 on labelling and packaging leaflets. Directive (EEC) 75/319 leaves those issues to the national authorities, as to which see Chapters 14 and 15.

above, that authorisation should in the CPMP's view be granted only subject to conditions.

8.4.4   Binding Community decisions : article 14

Article 14 lays down the procedure to be adopted by the Commission in reaching a final decision subsequent to the opinion of the CPMP on behalf of the Agency.

Article 14(1), (2) and (3) are procedurally identical to the provisions of article 10(1), (2) and (3) of Regulation (EEC) 2309/93, considered at section 7.3 above. The only difference between the two derives from the difference between article 13(5) of the Directive and article 9(3) of the Regulation : under the Directive, if the Commission's draft decision envisages the granting of authorisation, it must annex the documents described at article 13(5)(a) and (b), a summary of the product characteristics and any conditions to be imposed on the authorisation; under article 10(1) of the Regulation, the Commission must annex the documents referred to at article 9(3)(a), (b) and (c)[1] of the Regulation, which include the draft text of the packaging leaflet in addition to the documents required under the Directive. Under the Directive, the supervision of the packaging and labelling of the product is left to the national authorities; compare the discussion of article 13(4) above.

The only other differences is that article 10(2) of the Regulation refers to a procedure contained in article 73 thereof whereas article 14(2) refers to article 37b of the Directive; and article 10(3) refers to article 72 of the Regulation whereas article 14(2) refers to article 37a of the Directive. In practice, the wording of the provisions referred to is in substance identical and is discussed at section 7.6.

Article 14(4) deals with the effects of a final decision under the Directive. The decision is to be addressed to the Member States concerned by the matter, presumably those where authorisation has either been granted or applied for, and to the person responsible for placing the product on the market. The Member States must act to comply with the decision within 30 days of notification of the decision, either by granting authorisation, withdrawing authorisation or by varying the terms of an authorisation "as necessary to comply with the decision". That last possibility most obviously applies where the Community decision requires conditions to be imposed on the authorisation. Each Member State must inform the Commission and the CPMP of what action it has taken to comply with the decision.

Article 14(5) concerns a completely different and general point, stating that "cases provided for in article 9(2) of ... Directive (EEC) 92/73 ... on homeopathic medicinal products" shall not be dealt with under the procedures set out in articles 8 to 14 of Directive (EEC) 93/39. Directive (EEC) 92/73 establishes special procedures for such products and is considered in Chapter 9.

8.4.5   Variations and review of the "decentralised" procedure : articles 15 to 15c

Articles 15, 15a and 15b set out procedures for the variation of marketing authorisations granted by the Community procedures under the Directive; article 15c sets out a machinery for the review of the operation of the procedures introduced by the Directive.

Article 15 consists of five unnumbered paragraphs. Article 15, paragraph (1), requires the person responsible for marketing a medicinal product to submit any application to vary an authorisation granted under the Directive to all the Member

---

1.   Article 9(3)(d) further specifically requires that the assessment report should be annexed to a positive opinion. That appears to be redundant as it is already required by article 9(2) of the Regulation and the first para of article 13(5) of the Directive.

States which have granted authorisation to the product. Article 15, paragraph (2), requires the Commission, in consultation with the Agency, to adopt "appropriate arrangements for the examination of variations to the terms of a marketing authorisation". Article 15, paragraph (3), requires that the arrangements put in place by the Commission and the Agency must include a "notification system or administration procedures for minor variations" and must "define precisely the concept of "a minor variation"". The implication of this provision is clearly that minor variations as defined should be dealt with by a simple administrative procedure without substantial involvement of the Community machinery. Article 15, paragraph (4) provides for the Commission's use of the procedure established under article 37a of the Directive, considered below. Draft guidelines have been produced by the Commission but they cannot be finalised until the Agency comes into operation in 1995[1].

Article 15 paragraph (5), is the most significant provision, requiring that the procedure established under articles 13 and 14 of the Directive (the procedures for the formulation of the CPMP's opinion and the draft and final decisions) :

> "shall apply by analogy to variations made to marketing authorisations for products subject to the Commission's arbitration."

At least two things are unclear about this provision : first, it is not wholly clear how close the "analogy" between the original authorisation process and the amendment authorisation is required to be, for example whether a full CPMP opinion and draft decision are required, complete with the annexes provided for in articles 13 and 14, or whether it is simply necessary that the same timetable should be observed with the same procedural rights for the applicant and the Member States; article 15(5) makes no provision for implementing regulations to be passed by the Commission. Secondly, the expression "products subject to the Commission's arbitration" is of uncertain scope. It does not have any technical meaning but presumably means no more that those products to which article 15(1) applies.

Article 15a gives the Member States two further roles in the supervision of products on the market.

Article 15a(1) requires each Member State to refer a matter to the CPMP "forthwith" for the application of the article 13 and article 14 procedures where it :

> "considers that the variation of the terms of a marketing authorisation which has been granted in accordance with the provisions of this Chapter or its suspension or withdrawal is necessary for the protection of public health".

The scope of article 15a, limited to authorisations "granted in accordance with the provisions of this Chapter", might be thought to extend to all cases where more than one Member State was involved, whether or not there was a difference of view under article 10(1). However, where article 9(4) operates, the subsequent Member States "recognise the marketing authorisation granted by the first Member State" so no authorisation is "granted" under article 9(4). It thus appears that article 15a only applies where the full Community procedure is followed.

Article 15a(2) is stated to be without prejudice to the Member State's general right, under article 12 of the Directive, to refer matters to the CPMP for its opinion, and grants the Member States a strictly limited right to "suspend the marketing and the use of the medicinal product concerned on its territory". "The medicinal product concerned" refers back to article 15a(1), and the Member State's right of suspension

---

1. See section 11.5 post for equivalent provisions in respect of Community authorised products.

is limited to "exceptional cases, where urgent action is essential to protect public health". Where the Member State exercises this exceptional right, it is required to inform the Commission and the other Member States "no later than the following working day of the reasons for its action". The Member State's obligations to inform the Community institutions and each other of developments on the national pharmaceutical market is considered further in Chapter 12 post. The provisions of article 15a are analogous to article 18 of Regulation (EEC) 2309/93, where the Member States are granted rights (by article 18(4)) to suspend products authorised by the Community itself, in exceptional cases[1].

Article 15b provides :

"Articles 15 and 15a shall apply by analogy to medicinal products authorised by Member States following an opinion of the [CPMP] given in accordance with article 4 of Directive (EEC) 87/22 before 1 January 1995."

Article 4 of Directive (EEC) 87/22 is considered at section 6.4 : it provides for the timetable for the non-binding opinions of the CPMP to be reached and communicated to the Member States. Directive (EEC) 87/22 is to be repealed with effect from 1 January 1995. The significance of the provision is that it confirms that the variation and suspension procedures set out at articles 15 and 15a are only applicable to products whose original authorisation involved the giving of an opinion by the CPMP under Directive (EEC) 87/22 or Directive (EEC) 93/39. That implies that products which have never been the subject of a CPMP opinion (those which were authorised by the Member States under the ordinary procedures set out in Directive (EEC) 65/65) or which have been subject to a CPMP opinion under one of the old versions of Chapter III of Directive (EEC) 75/319 (the non-binding "multi-State" procedure described at section 5.4) can be varied by the Member States without any necessary consultation with the Community bodies.

Article 15c replaces the old article 15 and imposes obligations on the Agency, the Commission and the Council to consider the operation of the new regime : Article 15c(1) requires the Agency to publish an annual report on the procedures laid down in the new Chapter III of Directive (EEC) 75/319 and to forward it to the European Parliament and the Council for information; article 15c(2), first sub-paragraph requires the Commission to publish a "detailed review" of the operation of the procedures laid down in Chapter III and to propose any amendments necessary to improve those procedures; the Commission is required to produce its proposal by 1 January 2001[2] and the Council is required to act on the proposal within one year of its submission.

The remainder of article 3 of Directive 93/39 is concerned with : a minor amendment to article 22 of Directive (EEC) 75/319, part of Chapter IV on manufacturing authorisation; and a new section, articles 29a to 29h, entitled "Pharmacovigilance". Those changes are considered in Chapters 10 and 12 post.

8.5   Implementation of Directive (EEC) 93/39 : article 4

Article 4 consists of four paragraphs, here referred to as 4(1) to (4). Article 4(1) requires the Member States to take all appropriate measures to comply with the Directive, with the exception of article 1(7), before 1 January 1995. Article 1(7) contains the new article 7a to Directive (EEC) 65/65 introducing a form of

---

1.   See section 11.5 post.
2.   Six years from the date laid down in article 4(1) of Directive (EEC) 93/39, 1 January 1995, the date on which most of the provisions of the Directive must be given effect by the Member States.

compulsory mutual recognition by one Member State of marketing authorisations granted by another Member State[1]. Article 4(2) provides that the Member States must take all appropriate measures to comply with article 1(7) by 1 January 1998. Both 4(1) and (2) require the Member States to inform the Commission of the measures taken to comply with the Directive and article 4(4) requires the Member States to communicate to the Commission the text of the provisions of national law which they adopt in the field governed by the Directive. Article 4(3) simply requires a reference to be made to the Directive in the national implementing provisions in accordance with national practice.

8.6   The repeal of Directive (EEC) 87/22 : Directive (EEC) 93/41

Council Directive (EEC) 93/41[2] is a short Directive repealing Directive (EEC) 87/22. That Directive, described in Chapter 6, was an important development in the process of harmonisation in that it introduced a small degree of compulsion and a significant degree of centralisation into the regulatory process for at least some medicinal products. Regulation (EEC) 2309/93 is to a large extent modelled on Directive (EEC) 87/22 both in its scope and its procedures. However, the new "centralised" and "decentralised" approaches to marketing authorisation are intended to replace not augment the "multi-State" and "concertation" procedures and the new machinery of the Agency and the binding authorisation at the Community level require that the "centralised" procedure be introduced by legislation which goes beyond the amendment of the Directive (EEC) 87/22.

Recital 1 simply states that the provisions of Directive (EEC) 87/22 have been superseded by the provisions of Regulation (EEC) 2309/93[3]. Recital 2 states that provision has been made in Directive (EEC) 93/39 for the continued management of marketing authorisations granted by the Member States following an opinion of the CPMP under Directive (EEC) 87/22. The recital refers to article 15b of Directive (EEC) 93/39[4]. Recital 3 contains an equivalent provision in relation to veterinary products and Directive (EEC) 93/40. Recital 4 simply provides for the repeal of Directive (EEC) 87/22 and Recital 5 requires that transitional provisions should be made.

The text of the Directive consists of four short articles. Article 1 repeals Directive (EEC) 87/22 with effect from 1 January 1995. Article 2 provides that applications for marketing authorisations which have been referred to the CPMP (or CVMP) before 1 January 1995 in accordance with article 2 of Directive (EEC) 87/22 and in respect of which the Committee concerned has not given an opinion by 1 January 1995 shall be considered in accordance with Regulation (EEC) 2309/93. The effect of that provision will be that a referral from a national authority for a CPMP opinion under Directive (EEC) 87/22 which remains outstanding as at 1 January 1995 will be transformed into an application for a Community authorisation under the new "centralised" procedure set out in the Regulation. Because of the close affinity between the products contained in the Annex to Directive (EEC) 87/22 and Regulation (EEC) 2309/93, there should be no substantive difficulty in effecting that transition. In relation to procedural difficulties, no provision is made for the time limits to be observed by the CPMP in relation to applications covered by article 2, in particular whether the CPMP must give its opinion on the product within 210

---

1.   See section 8.2 ante.
2.   OJ L214 24.8.93 p40. See Appendix 7 post.
3.   The recital also refers to the replacement of Council Directive (EEC) 83/189 (OJ L109 26.4.83 p8) by Council Directive (EEC) 88/182 (OJ L81 26.3.88 p75). Those Directives relate to the provision of information in the field of technical standards and regulations and the earlier Directive was referred to in article 5 of Directive (EEC) 87/22 : see section 6.5 ante.
4.   See section 8.4.5 ante.

days of receipt of the referral in accordance with article 6(4) of the Regulation or whether time starts to run on the date of receipt of a valid application by one of the Member States[1].

Articles 3 and 4 are implementing provisions requiring the Member States to take all appropriate measures to comply with the Directive with effect from 1 January 1995 and to inform the Commission of those measures in accordance with the standard national and Community procedures.

---

1.   See sections 6.4 and 7.3 ante for the procedures under the "concertation" and "centralised" procedures.

Chapter 9 : Directive (EEC) 92/73[1] - An "Authorisation" Regime for Homeopathic Medicinal Products

9.1   The purpose of the Directive : the recitals

The exclusion of certain categories of medicinal products from the scope of the established regimes for market authorisation by article 34 of Directive (EEC) 75/319[2]. Since 1990, the only category of products still completely outside the scope of the general rules was homeopathic medicines which naturally raise special considerations requiring special treatment by the legislator. Widely divergent attitudes exist between individuals and between Member States as to the desirability of encouraging homeopathic remedies as against the "allopathic" remedies upon which Western medicine has traditionally relied. In addition, the types of test that have been developed under the Community Directives to confirm the quality, safety and efficacy of pharmaceuticals are not satisfactory for products whose identifiable active ingredients are much less powerful and whose clinical performance under controlled conditions is less impressive than mainstream Western medicines.

As a result, the Community has now established a modified and simplified system for the authorisation of homeopathic products designed to facilitate trade and to impose a level of regulation appropriate to the products in question. The recitals to Directive (EEC) 92/73 set out the reasoning behind the Directive.

Recitals 1 to 3 state the general principles underlying the Directive. Recital 1 states that legal, regulatory and administrative differences between the Member States :

> "may hinder trade in homeopathic medicinal products within the Community and lead to discrimination and distortion of competition between manufacturers of these products".

Recital 2 is similar to the wording of recital 1 of Directive (EEC) 65/65[3] :

> "the essential aim of any rules governing the production, distribution and use of medicinal products must be to safeguard public health."

The only significant difference is that reference is made to "use" of medicinal products, in the light of the new Community rules on wholesale distribution, classification, labelling and advertising of medicinal products[4].

Recital 3 stresses the need for consumer choice, subject to proper protection of public health :

> "despite considerable differences in the status of alternative medicines in the Member States, patients should be allowed access to the medicinal products of

---

1.   OJ L297 13.10.92 p8. See Appendix 8 post.
2.   OJ L147 9.6.75 p13. See Appendix 3 post and section 5.5 ante.
3.   OJ No 22 9.2.65 369/65. See Appendix 1 post.
4.   See Chapters 13 to 16 post.

their choice, provided all precautions are taken to ensure the quality and safety of the said products."

As elsewhere in the Directive, only two of the three criteria set down in article 5 of Directive (EEC) 65/65 are mentioned : the criterion of "therapeutic efficacy" is notably absent[1].

Recitals 4 to 7 of the Directive make four general statements about homeopathic medicinal products. Recital 4 states that :

"the anthroposophic medicinal products described in an official pharmacopoeia and prepared by a homeopathic method are to be treated, as regards registration and marketing authorisation, in the same way as homeopathic medicinal products."

Recital 4 does not precisely correspond to anything in the text of the Directive and no definition is offered of "anthroposophic"; the term refers to systems of treatment, particularly well-established in Germany, depending on "holistic" assessment of the needs of the patient rather than merely combating specific adverse symptoms, as is the case with conventional Western medicines[2].

Recital 5 states that the provisions of Directives (EEC) 65/65 and 73/319 are "not always appropriate" for homeopathic products; recital 6 asserts that "homeopathic medicine is officially recognised in certain Member States but is only tolerated in other Member States"; and recital 7 claims that even if not always officially recognised, such products "are nevertheless prescribed and used in all Member States".

Recitals 8 to 11 summarise the central provisions of the Directive and the aims they are intended to achieve. Recital 8 states a twofold aim :

"to provide users of these medicinal products with a very clear indication of their homeopathic character and with sufficient guarantees of their quality and safety".

The contrast with standard medicinal products is very clear : instead of the requirement of "therapeutic efficacy", homeopathic products are merely required to be labelled as such, with the apparent implication that a consumer who buys such a product must be warned that there may be no "therapeutic efficacy" in the scientifically accepted sense; likewise, the reference to "sufficient guarantees" indicates that a lower standard of testing will be acceptable for homeopathic medicines than for standard pharmaceutical products.

Recital 9 states that rules on manufacture, control and inspection of homeopathic products *must* be harmonised :

"to permit the circulation throughout the Community of medicinal products which are safe and of good quality."

---

1.   See section 3.2 ante for the criteria.
2.   Anthroposophic medicines are not otherwise considered in EC pharmaceutical legislation. If they fulfil the criteria laid down in articles 1 and 2 of Directive (EEC) 65/65 (as to which see Chapter 2 and section 3.2 ante) there seems to be no reason to exclude them from the scope of the general rules unless they are also homeopathic medicines as described in recital 4. In practice, it appears likely that many such products will be on the margins of the Community definitions of "medicinal product".

That recital, reflected in article 4 of the Directive, indicates that there must be no compromise in manufacturing standards for homeopathic as against other types of medicinal products. The compromise of standards relates only to initial authorisation.

Recitals 10 and 11 contrast "traditional homeopathic medicinal products which are placed on the market without therapeutic indications in a pharmaceutical form and dosage which do not present a risk for the patient" with other products which are "placed on the market with therapeutic indications or in a form which may present risks which must be balanced against the desired therapeutic effect". In the case of the former :

> "having regard to the particular characteristics of these medicinal products, such as the very low level of active principles they contain and the difficulty of applying to them the conventional statistical methods relating to clinical trials, it is desirable to provide a special, simplified registration procedure" (recital 10).

In the case of the latter, the usual rules governing marketing authorisation should apply, but subject to the qualification that :

> "those Member States which have a homeopathic tradition should be able to apply particular rules for the evaluation of the results of tests and trials intended to establish the safety and efficacy of these medicinal products provided that they notify them to the Commission" (recital 11).

It is only in relation to the latter products that the Community criteria for authorisation all apply and even in their case, individual Member States can disapply the Community rules, subject to supervision by the Commission, in relation to safety and efficacy so that in practice only the rules laid down by Directive (EEC) 65/65 and the related legislation (in particular the Annex to Directive (EEC) 75/318[1]) in relation to quality apply with full force[2].

9.2   The scope of the Directive : Chapter 1; articles 1 and 2

Article 1(1) defines "homeopathic medicinal product" to mean :

> "any medicinal product prepared from products, substances or compositions called homeopathic stocks in accordance with a homeopathic manufacturing procedure described by the *European Pharmacopoeia* or, in absence thereof, by the pharmacopoeias currently used officially in the Member States."

The component terms of that definition are not further defined; in particular, no references are made to Directive (EEC) 65/65 or to the definitions of "medicinal product" or "substance" in article 1(2) and (3). The definition of substance at article 1(3) discussed at section 2.4.1 is clearly wide enough to include homeopathic products, but the definitions of "medicinal product" discussed in detail in Chapter 2 do not naturally apply to such products. Given the lack of stress on therapeutic efficacy in the legislation, it must be doubtful whether homeopathic medicines could be said either to be clearly "presented for the treatment or prevention of disease" or to be "endowed" with properties which make them suitable for administration either to make medical diagnoses or to "restore, correct or modify

---

1.   OJ L147 9.6.75 p1. See Appendix 2 post.
2.   The derogation permitted to the Member States has one natural consequence : the new procedures introduced by Directive (EEC) 93/39 for mutual recognition of national authorisations and binding Community resolution of national differences of opinion, has no application in relation to homeopathic products : see article 14(5) of Directive (EEC) 93/39 and section 8.4 ante.

physiological functions"[1]. If such products (as a class) come within the Directive (EEC) 65/65 definition at all it appears that they must do so as products which are "presented" as possessing properties for "restoring, correcting or modifying physiological functions". It would be highly undesirable to be forced to conclude that the term "medicinal product" in Directive (EEC) 92/73 had a different meaning from the complex definition contained in Directive (EEC) 65/65 so that it seems necessary to construe it in that way. If that is correct then there will be a large group of products which will be on the borderline between "homeopathic medicinal products" and foodstuffs or cosmetics[2].

"Homeopathic stocks" is given no clear meaning. In the absence of any definition or criterion for identifying such products, there appears to be further room for disagreement as to the scope of the definition of "homeopathic medicinal product."

Article 1(2) provides that a homeopathic medicinal product "may also contain a number of principles". Again no definition is offered of the term "principle". Elsewhere in the Community legislation, the term denotes active chemical substances but in the context of the legislation it is unclear whether it is intended to indicate substances whose action is *not* homeopathic. If that is the case, there will be further room for disagreement as to the classification of specific products.

Article 2(1) defines the scope of the Directive, which is stated to apply to "homeopathic products for human use"[3]. The exceptions set out in article 1(4) and (5) and article 2(4) of Directive (EEC) 65/65, products prepared in accordance with magistral and officinal formulas and products individually prepared by a health care professional for supervised use by his patients, are repeated in article 2(1)[4].

Article 2(2) lays down the first substantive requirement of the Directive :

> "The medicinal products referred to in [article 2(1)] shall be identified by a reference on their labels, in clear and legible form, to their homeopathic nature."

The purpose of that requirement is similar to the "presentation" definition under Directive (EEC) 65/65[5]. Consumers must be protected not only from products which may harm them but also from purchasing products under a misapprehension as to the nature of the products.

9.3   Manufacture, control and inspection : Chapter 2, articles 3 to 5

Articles 3 to 5 concern the application of the rules laid down in Chapters IV and V of Directive (EEC) 75/319 in relation to manufacture and supervision of medicinal products generally in the special case of homeopathic medicines. Those rules are discussed in Chapters 10 and 11 of this work. It should only be noted here that, although the general rules laid down by Chapters IV and V, and also articles 30 to 33, of Directive (EEC) 75/319 continue to apply, the criterion of "therapeutic efficacy" is disapplied in this area as elsewhere in relation to homeopathic products : see article 4, second paragraph, and article 5.

---

1.   See section 2.3 ante for the structure of article 1(2) of Directive (EEC) 65/65.
2.   The facts of Case C-369/88 *Delattre* [1991] ECR I-1487 and Case C-219/91 *Ter Voort* [1992] ECR I-5485, described in summary at section 2.1 ante, provide good examples of the types of difficulty that will inevitably arise, although those cases did not strictly relate to homeopathic remedies.
3.   Directive (EEC) 92/74 applies to homeopathic veterinary products.
4.   See section 3.3 ante for discussion of Directive (EEC) 65/65.
5.   See section 2.4 ante.

9.4   Placing the product on the market : Chapter 3, articles 6 to 9

Article 6 sets out the general principles applicable to the grant of marketing authorisations for homeopathic medicinal products. Article 6(1) provides :

"Member States shall ensure that homeopathic medicinal products manufactured and placed on the market within the Community are registered or authorised in accordance with articles 7, 8 and 9. Each Member State shall take due account of registrations and authorisations previously granted by another Member State."

That short provision is equivalent to article 3 of Directive (EEC) 65/65, requiring market authorisation for all products placed on the market within a Member State, and to the apparatus of the "centralised" and "decentralised" procedures introduced by Regulation (EEC) 2309/93[1] and Directive (EEC) 93/39[2]. The general requirement of authorisation is qualified by the simplified "registration" procedure introduced by article 7 of the Directive. The second sentence of article 6(1) is little more than a pious hope that the Member States will "take due account" of one another's practices in relation to homeopathic products. It is hard to see how such a provision could be relied on by a supplier in possession of a valid authorisation in one Member State who was refused authorisation in another Member State (the third sentence of article 6(2) is more specific in relation to products covered by articles 7 and 8 of the Directive).

Article 6(2) is directed at those Member States which treat homeopathic medicines in the same way as other medicinal products and makes two provisions. First, Member States are permitted to "refrain from establishing a special, simplified registration procedure" for the products referred to in article 7, subject to a requirement of informing the Commission accordingly. Secondly, those Member States who do not set up a simplified regime are nonetheless required, by 31 December 1995 at the latest, to allow the use in their territory of "homeopathic medicinal products registered in other Member States in accordance with articles 7 and 8". That is the most far-reaching provision of the Directive, compelling Member States which do not permit homeopathic products to be marketed without full authorisation to permit at least some such products to be marketed on their territory even when those products have not been subjected to any standardised Community procedure. The significance of the procedure is limited by the strict rules for the products within the scope of article 7.

Article 6(3) applies the general rules on advertising of medicinal products laid down in Directive (EEC) 92/28[3] to the homeopathic medicines identified in articles 7(1) and 6(2). Article 7(1) is clear enough (see below) but article 6(2) refers to two classes of products : "products referred to in article 7" and "products registered by other Member States in accordance with articles 7 and 8". The effect of article 6(3) appears to be to make all products within the scope of article 7(1) subject to Directive (EEC) 92/28 but only those products which are within the scope of article 8 and registered with at least one Member State so subject.

Three specific rules are laid down in relation to those products : article 2(1) of Directive (EEC) 92/28, which requires the Member States to prohibit the advertising of a medicinal product which has not been granted a marketing authorisation "in accordance with Community law", does not apply[4]; only the information specified

---

1.   OJ L214 24.8.93 p1. See Appendix 5 post.
2.   OJ L214 24.8.93 p22. See Appendix 6 post.
3.   OJ L113 30.4.92 p13, see Appendix 13 post. See further Chapter 16 post.
4.   Homeopathic medicinal products are not "authorised" under articles 7 and 8, so the application of article 2(1) of Directive (EEC) 92/28 would have prevented all advertising of products within the scope of article 7(1).

in article 7(2) of Directive (EEC) 92/73 may be used; and each Member State is permitted to prohibit any advertising of such products within its territory. The overall effect is that advertising of the specified products may be prohibited on a national basis but where such advertising is permitted it must conform to Directive (EEC) 92/28 (subject to the qualification just mentioned) and it must also conform to article 7(2) of Directive (EEC) 92/73.

No provisions are made for the advertising of the products referred to in article 9, which suggests that Directive (EEC) 92/28 should apply to those products. If that is correct then it confirms that the expression "medicinal product" in article 1(1) of the Directive has the same meaning as in article 1(2) of Directive (EEC) 65/65 : article 1(1) of Directive (EEC) 92/28 specifically relies on the concept of "medicinal product" as used in Directive (EEC) 65/65 in defining the scope of the Community rules on the advertising of medicinal products[1].

Article 7 lays down the essential requirements for a "special, simplified registration procedure". Article 7(1) specifies the conditions which must be satisfied by the products to which it may be applied :

"— they are administered orally or externally;
— no specific therapeutic indication appears on the labelling of the medicinal product or in any information relating thereto,
— there is a sufficient degree of dilution to guarantee the safety of the medicinal product; in particular, the medicinal product may not contain either more than one part per 10 000 of the mother tincture or more than 1/100th of the smallest dose used in allopathy with regard to active principles whose presence in an allopathic medicinal product results in the obligation to submit a doctor's prescription."

The first criterion is relatively straightforward and appears to exclude at least suppositories and products introduced directly into the bloodstream[2]. The second criterion may be difficult to apply in practice, for example in relation to products which reduce insomnia or flatulence or aid digestion, and it raises the problem again of whether such products are in fact "medicinal products" at all within the scope of Directive (EEC) 65/65[3]. That problem is equally clearly raised by the third criterion which lays down specific levels of dilution required to "guarantee the safety of the medicinal product". The levels of permitted concentration are so low that it is doubtful whether is satisfies the "functional" criterion discussed at section 2.5 above and it is equally doubtful whether the "presentation" criterion discussed at section 2.4 is satisfied by a product which is expressly prohibited from claiming any specific therapeutic indication.

There is a further more technical problem in relation to the second specific test of concentration, that the product should not contain more than one per cent of the smallest dose used in standard medicine which would result in the need for a doctor's prescription. That test clearly assumes that the classification of medicinal products as "prescription only" is based on the level of active ingredient in those products but that does not conform to the Community's own requirements under Directive (EEC) 92/26[4]. The Community's criteria laid down in article 3(1) of Directive (EEC) 92/26 do not mention the level of concentration of active

---

1. The general problems raised by the Rational Use Directives discussed in Chapters 13 to 15 are considered below in relation to article 9.
2. That requirement was challenged in Case C-437/92 (renumbered T-463/93) *Guna Srl v Council* but the challenge (based on the exclusion of injectable products from article 7) was declared inadmissible : OJ C38 12.2.93 p17 and OJ C328 4.12.93 p5.
3. See Chapter 2 ante.
4. OJ L113 30.4.92 p5. See Appendix 11 post.

ingredients as a permissible criterion for making a product "prescription only" and article 2(1) and article 7 of that Directive have required the Member States to adopt the Community rules since 1 January 1993[1].

Article 7(1) further requires a Member State registering such a product to "determine the classification for the dispensing of the medicinal product" at the time of registration. Given the characteristics of the product, it is hard to see how the product could possibly be classified as a "prescription only" product pursuant to article 2(1) and article 3(1) of Directive (EEC) 92/26. The only issue which could possibly arise would therefore be the type of issue that is familiar in France in relation to the "pharmacists' monopoly"[2].

Article 7(2) lays down as the principal requirement for "registration" that "the labelling and, where appropriate, the package insert" for products within the scope of article 7(1) should comply with a number of detailed requirements in addition to the requirement laid down in article 2(2) and repeated at article 7(2) that the products should be clearly marked "homeopathic medicinal product." The products are required to :

"bear the following, and no other, information :

— the scientific name of the stock or stocks followed by the degree of dilution, making use of the symbols of the pharmacopoeia used in accordance with article 1(1),
— name and address of the person responsible for placing the product on the market and, where appropriate, of the manufacturer,
— method of administration and, if necessary, route,
— expiry date, in clear terms (month, year),
— pharmaceutical form,
— contents of sales presentation,
— special storage precautions, if any,
— a special warning if necessary for the medicinal product,
— manufacturer's batch number,
— registration number,
— "homeopathic medicinal product without approved therapeutic indications",
— a warning advising the user to consult a doctor if the symptoms persist during the use of the medicinal product."

Of those requirements, all except the last three correspond to requirements set out at article 2(1) of Directive (EEC) 92/27 (in some cases in more detail) for the outer packaging of medicinal products within the scope of Directive (EEC) 65/65. Directive (EEC) 92/27 is discussed in Chapter 15. The last three requirements clearly only apply to article 7(1) homeopathic products because of :

— the replacement of the "authorisation" requirement by the "registration" requirement;

— the presentation of the products as medicinal products but "without approved therapeutic indications"; and

---

1. The expression "mother tincture" is not defined. The expression is apparently used in homeopathic medicine to denote the original preparation of an alcoholic solution of the original homeopathic product, in practice the highest possible concentration of the product.
2. See Chapter 2 above in relation to Case C-369/88 *Delattre* [1991] ECR I-1487 and Case C-60/89 *Monteil and Sammani* [1991] ECR I-1547.

— the need to ensure that consumers who do not in fact obtain any benefit from treatment with products which have not been shown to have therapeutic efficacy under controlled conditions obtain professional medical treatment within a reasonable time.

Article 7(3) permits the Member States additionally to require :

"the use of certain types of labelling in order to show :

— the price of the medicinal product,
— the conditions for refunds by social security bodies."

That provision expressly preserves the Member States' control over pricing and reimbursement.

Article 7(4) provides :

"The criteria and rules of procedure provided for in articles 5 to 12 of Directive (EEC) 65/65 shall apply by analogy to the special, simplified registration procedure for homeopathic medicinal products, with the exception of the proof of therapeutic efficacy."

Articles 5 to 12 of Directive (EEC) 65/65 are discussed in Chapters 3 and 11 of this work, and the amendments made by Directive (EEC) 93/39 are discussed at section 8.2. The effect of the "analogy" must be that[1] :

— registration will only be permitted where the product is of proven quality and safety and where it is proved to fall within article 7(1) [article 5];

— "contraceptive and abortifacient products" (if such exist) may be refused registration [article 6];

— decisions on registration must be taken within 210 days [article 7];

— adequate controls must be demonstrated and updated [articles 8 and 9a];

— civil liability is unaffected [article 9];

— registration is valid for five years and renewable on three months notice before expiry [article 10];

— registration shall be suspended or withdrawn where the safety or quality of the product is shown to be lacking or where any information submitted at the time of the original registration is shown to have been incorrect [article 11];

— reasons must be given for refusals to register and decisions to register or revoke registration must be published in the appropriate national official publication [article 12].

Article 8 provides for a further relaxation of the rules relating to applications for registration for medicinal products falling within the scope of article 7(1). Such applications "may cover a series of medicinal products derived from the same homeopathic stock or stocks". The purpose of article 8 is to avoid the need for multiple applications for authorisations for a number of products with the same active ingredients where those active ingredients are of the minimal nature specified in article 7(1). To demonstrate "the pharmaceutical quality and the batch-

---

1.   The relevant articles of Directive (EEC) 65/65 are indicated in square brackets.

to-batch homogeneity of the products concerned", the applicant must produce a number of relevant documents :

> "— scientific name or other name given in a pharmacopoeia of the homeopathic stock or stocks, together with a statement of the various routes of administration, pharmaceutical forms and degree of dilution to be registered,
> — dossier describing how the homeopathic stock or stocks is/are obtained and controlled, and justifying its/their homeopathic nature, on the basis of an adequate bibliography,
> — manufacturing and control file for each pharmaceutical form and a description of the method of dilution and potentisation,
> — manufacturing authorisation for the medicinal product concerned,
> — copies of any registrations or authorisations obtained for the same medicinal product in other Member States,
> — one or more specimens or mock-ups of the sales presentation of the medicinal products to be registered,
> — data concerning the stability of the medicinal product."

Those requirements are intended to provide the national competent authority with adequate material to ascertain the chemical composition of the various products and to satisfy themselves that each such product will be safe in use and has been manufactured to the requisite standard.

Article 9 applies to all homeopathic medicinal products which fail to satisfy the requirements of article 7(1), ie they are either not administered orally or externally, or they are marketed as appropriate for a specific therapeutic indication, or their active principles are too concentrated to satisfy the third limb of article 7(1). For those products, article 9(1) provides that they :

> "shall be authorised and labelled in accordance with articles 4 to 21 of Directive (EEC) 65/65 including the provisions concerning proof of therapeutic effect and articles 1 to 7 of Directive (EEC) 75/319."

Those provisions have been discussed at length in Chapters 3 and 5 above. They are the provisions establishing the standard harmonised procedures for the grant or refusal of marketing authorisation by individual Member States. The difficulties in the interpretation of article 9(1) derive from the Rational Use package of Directives discussed in Chapters 13 to 16. The primary difficulty is that article 9(1) clearly intends to apply the Community rules in relation to labelling of medicinal products but does not refer to Directive (EEC) 92/27 but rather to articles 13 to 20 of Directive (EEC) 65/65 and articles 6 and 7 of Directive (EEC) 75/319, all of which were repealed and their provisions replaced by Directive (EEC) 92/27. It seems that article 9(1) must be an old draft that was never changed to reflect the coming into effect of the Rational Use package.

Secondly, there is a more general problem that each of the Rational Use Directives (EEC) 92/25, 92/27 and 92/28 provides at article 1(1) that it covers medicinal products for human use to which Chapters II to V of Directive (EEC) 65/65 apply[1]. It

---

1. The fourth Directive, (EEC) 92/26, relates to "medicinal products", as defined in article 1 of Directive (EEC) 65/65, for human use : see article 1 thereof. Subject to the obvious difficulties in bringing article 7(1) products within the scope of the Community definition of medicinal products, it seems clear that the products covered by Directive (EEC) 92/73 are "medicinal products for human use" and should therefore all be covered by Directive (EEC) 92/26. The difficulty in practice is that the Member States' obligations under article 2 of that Directive arise on the grant of a "marketing authorisation" and article 7(1) of Directive (EEC) 92/73 provides for the Member States to "determine the classification for the dispensing of

is reasonably clear that the products within the scope of article 7(1) of Directive (EEC) 92/73 are not intended to be covered by that provision (only certain provisions from Chapter II of Directive (EEC) 65/65 are stated to apply "by analogy" : see article 7(4)); it is less clear what the position is for article 9(1) products. Chapters II to V run from articles 3 to 25 of Directive 65/65, so that articles 3 and 22 to 25 do not apply to article 9(1) homeopathic products. On the other hand, articles 22 to 25 are now redundant provisions and article 6(1) of Directive (EEC) 92/73, requiring the Member States to ensure, inter alia, that article 9(1) products are authorised if they are placed on the market within that Member State, is closely analogous to the requirements of article 3 of Directive (EEC) 65/65. On balance, therefore, it seems clear that article 9(1) products *are* now intended to be covered by Directives (EEC) 92/25, 92/26 and 92/28[1].

Article 9(2) provides :

> "A Member State may introduce or retain in its territory specific rules for the pharmacological and toxicological tests and clinical trials of homeopathic medicinal products other than those referred to in article 7(1) in accordance with the principles and characteristics of homeopathy as practised in that Member State.
>
> In this case, the Member State concerned shall notify the Commission of the specific rules in force."

The effect of that provision is to permit the Member States in part to disapply the requirements of article 9(1), and thus to preserve, subject only to the general supervision of the Commission, an individual Member State's existing rules, if any, for the testing of those homeopathic medicinal products which would otherwise be made subject to the full requirements of Directives (EEC) 65/65 and 75/319. The corollary of that concession to the Member States with a tradition of homeopathic medicine is a further concession to the other Member States, that they are not required to recognise authorisations granted in other Member States in accordance with special tests or trials, with the result that the aim of market integration will not be achieved for such products authorised in such ways. Article 6(1) of the Directive only requires the Member States to permit the marketing on their respective territories of "registered" products within the scope of articles 7 and 8, and article 14(5) of Directive (EEC) 75/319 (as amended by Directive (EEC) 93/39) specifically excludes "cases provided for in article 9(2)" of Directive (EEC) 92/73 from the scope of the new "decentralised" procedure for ensuring mutual recognition of national marketing authorisations[2].

---

the medicinal product" at the time of registration, suggesting that Directive (EEC) 92/26 does not apply to article 7(1) products. It is quite unclear what criteria are intended to be applied by the Member States in fulfilling its obligations under article 7(1), in particular whether it is required to take note of the provisions of Directive (EEC) 92/26. There is nothing to suggest that article 9(1) products, which are subject to authorisation, are not within the scope of Directive (EEC) 92/26.

1.   If that is correct then article 34, para 2, of Directive (EEC) 75/319, disapplying Chapters II to V of Directive (EEC) 65/65 and the provisions of Directive (EEC) 75/319 inter alia to homeopathic medicinal products, is itself disapplied to article 9(1) homeopathic products. The application of Chapters IV and V of Directive (EEC) 75/319 to medicinal products for human use (relating to manufacture and supervision of such products) is considered in Chapters 10 and 11 below (and the position in relation to article 7(1) products in relation to "registration" was considered ante).

2.   Given that article 9(1) of the Directive specifically refers to articles 4 to 21 of Directive (EEC) 65/65 it might be thought that the new procedures introduced as articles 7 and 7a of Directive (EEC) 65/65, for suspension of the authorisation procedure in the light of a parallel procedure in another Member State, would apply to article 9(1) products seeking authorisation in accordance with article 9(2)

It should be noted that it is only "cases provided for in article 9(2)", *not* products identified by article 9(1), that are covered by article 14(5) of Directive (EEC) 75/319. The new procedures for mutual recognition introduced into Directives (EEC) 65/65 and 75/319 by Directive (EEC) 93/39 should apply in the same way to article 9(1) products authorised in accordance with the standard Community requirements as to other medicinal products. That fact will provide some incentive for manufacturers and suppliers, if they wish to market particular products in more than one Member State, to obtain full authorisation in a Member State where such procedures are applied to article 9(1) products.

9.5   Final provisions : Chapter IV, articles 10 and 11

Articles 10 and 11 are the implementing provisions. Article 10(1) requires the Member States to take the measures necessary to comply with the Directive by 31 December 1993 and article 10(2) requires that applications "for registration or for marketing authorisation for medicinal products covered by this Directive" after 31 December 1993 comply with the Directive. Article 10(3) requires the Commission to present a report to the European Parliament and the Council concerning the operation of the Directive by 31 December 1995. The relatively short timescale for a Commission report indicates that the legislation is not cast in stone.

---

procedures. That is not correct: the new articles 7 and 7a procedures specifically refer to the new "procedures set out in articles 10 to 14 of Directive (EEC) 71/319" and it is those new procedures which are disapplied to cases covered by article 9(2) of Directive (EEC) 92/73 by article 14(5) of Directive (EEC) 75/319. It would therefore be impossible for a Member State to obtain a binding ruling from the European Agency for the Evaluation of Medicinal Products in such a case.

PART IV : CONTINUING SUPERVISION OF AUTHORISED PRODUCTS

Chapter 10 : The Authorisation Of The Manufacture Of Medicinal Products

10.1 The authorisation requirement : Chapter IV of Directive (EEC) 75/319[1], articles 16 to 20

The Community rules on the authorisation of manufacture of medicinal products were laid down for the first time in *Chapter IV* of Directive (EEC) 75/319 entitled "Manufacture and imports coming from third countries", and have remained largely unaltered since 1975[2]. They clearly complement the rules on the substance of the authorisation process set out in the Annex to Directive (EEC) 75/318[3] and also the provisions on supervision of authorised products described in Chapter 11[4]. Although the overall regime has not altered, more detailed rules have been laid down in respect of "Good Manufacturing Practice" by Commission Directive (EEC) 91/356[5] and by the Commission's *Guide to good manufacturing practice for medicinal products*[6].

Article 16 sets out the fundamental requirement of authorisation and defines its scope. The Member States are required to take "all appropriate measures to ensure that the manufacture of medicinal products is subject to the holding of an authorisation". Authorisation is required not only for medicinal products manufactured within the Community for supply within the Community, but also for products manufactured within the Community but "intended for export" (article 16(1)) and for "imports coming from third countries" (article 16(3)). Chapter IV and article 29 (relating to the suspension or revocation of authorisation) are said to have "corresponding application to such imports as they have to manufacture" and the remaining provisions of Chapter IV and article 29 contain specific provisions in relation to imports.

Article 16(2) defines the scope of the authorisation requirement. It is obvious that manufacture of a major industrial product comprises a range of distinct activities and article 16(2) is widely drafted :

> "The authorisation referred to in [article 16(1)] shall be required for both total and partial manufacture, and for the various processes of dividing up, packaging or presentation.

---

1. OJ L147 9.6.75 p13. See Appendix 3 post.
2. One significant exception is article 16(1), the fundamental provision of the Chapter, which has been expanded to cover all medicinal products, not just proprietary medicinal products, and also to apply to products intended for export from the Community. Those changes were made by Directive (EEC) 89/341 (OJ L142 25.5.89 p11).
3. OJ L147 9.6.75 p1. See Appendix 1 post.
4. See also article 5 of Directive (EEC) 75/319, which imposes a requirement on the national competent authorities to confirm that a manufacturer or importer is capable of manufacturing the product in conformity with the requirements of article 4 of Directive (EEC) 65/65: see section 5.3 ante.
5. OJ L193 17.7.91 p30. Appendix 9 post.
6. Those Community instruments were adopted after the introduction of a new article 19a into Directive (EEC) 75/319 requiring such a Directive and such guidelines to be prepared: see post.

However, such authorisation shall not be required for preparation, dividing up, changes in packaging or presentation where these processes are carried out, solely for retail supply, by pharmacists in dispensing pharmacies or by persons legally authorised in the Member States to carry out such processes."

The distinction between "total" and "partial" manufacture indicates that manufacture from intermediate products as well as from raw materials is within the scope of the Directive. The more difficult issue in practice may be how far back up the production chain it is necessary to go, for example when organic products are used as raw materials in a pharmaceutical preparation. Some assistance can be derived from the Commission's *Guide to good manufacturing practice* which has a glossary of terms, including the following :

"Bulk product : any product which has completed all processing stages up to, but not including, final packaging.

Finished product : a medicinal product which has undergone all stages of production, including packaging in its final container.

Intermediate product : partly processed material which must undergo further manufacturing steps before it becomes a bulk product.

Manufacture : all operations of purchase of materials and products, production, quality control, release, storage, distribution of medicinal products and the related controls.

Packaging : all operations, including filling and labelling, which a bulk product has to undergo in order to become a finished product. Note : sterile filling would not normally be regarded as part of packaging, the bulk product being the filled, but not finally packaged, primary containers.

Packaging material : any material employed in the packaging of a medicinal product, excluding any outer packaging used for transportation or shipment. Packaging materials are referred to as primary or secondary according to whether or not they are intended to be in direct contact with the product.

Starting material : any substance used in the production of a medicinal product, but excluding packaging materials."[1]

It appears from the Guide and as a matter of common sense that the object of the Community authorisation procedure is to approve a broadly unitary process that starts when the materials for the creation of the product are assembled at the site of manufacture and ends when the finished product has been divided up and packaged in the form in which it will be presented to the consumer, pharmacist or medical practitioner[2]. The Guide requires that guarantees of quality should be in place at the time when the starting materials for the process of manufacture are purchased[3]. The distribution and marketing process are now governed by the Rational Use Directives discussed in Chapters 13 to 16 post, in particular Directive (EEC) 92/25[4] in relation to wholesale distribution. In that respect at least, the

---

1. *Guide to good manufacturing practice* at pp9-13.
2. Different considerations apply to imported products, where the activity regulated by the Directive is quality control rather than manufacture itself: see article 17(1). For products manufactured within the Community, quality control is an essential element in manufacture rather than an end in itself: see in particular Chapter 6 of the Guide at pp53-58.
3. See *Guide to good manufacturing practice*, paras 5.25 to 5.34 at pp47-48.
4. OJ L113 30.4.92 p1. Appendix 10 post.

"definition" of manufacture given in the Guide's glossary is misleading and too broad.

The qualification in the second sub-paragraph of article 16(2), exempting processes performed by pharmacists or equivalent authorised personnel for the purposes of retail supply, is equivalent to the exclusions contained in article 1(2) and 2(3) of Directive (EEC) 65/65[1] in relation to marketing authorisations for individual preparations. The Community regimes are intended to apply to industrial or semi-industrial processes leading to mass production of uniform products, rather than to the performance of their professional duties by doctors or pharmacists in treatment of individual patients or customers. In such cases, the regulation of manufacture would apply to the materials from which the individually prescribed medicines were made [2].

Articles 17 to 20 set out four distinct elements of the authorisation process : article 17 sets out the requirements to be met by an applicant for authorisation; article 18 gives guidance to the national competent authority in assessing such an application; article 19 imposes certain obligations on the successful applicant, the holder of a manufacturing authorisation; and article 20 sets out the procedures to be followed in granting or varying the initial authorisation.

The requirements of article 17 are that the applicant gives two fundamental pieces of information and that he has the necessary material and human resources to perform the manufacturing process satisfactorily. He must specify (with supporting particulars) :

(1) "the medicinal products and pharmaceutical forms which are to be manufactured or imported"; and

(2) the place where those products are to be manufactured and/or controlled (article 17(a)).

He must also "have at his disposal" :

(3) "suitable and sufficient premises, technical equipment and control facilities" for the manufacture or import of the specified products (article 17(b)); and

(4) "the services of at least one qualified person within the meaning of article 21" (article 17(c)).

The requirement of adequate facilities is made relative to article 5(a) of Directive (EEC) 75/319[3], which itself refers back to the details of manufacturing methods and controls required under article 4(4) and (7) respectively, of Directive (EEC) 65/65. Article 5(a) requires the national competent authorities to verify that the manufacturer or importer is capable of manufacturing and/or carrying out controls on the product in accordance with the particulars supplied for the purposes of marketing authorisation; the applicant for *manufacturing* authorisation must demonstrate that his manufacturing and/or control facilities comply with the requirements of the relevant national authority.

The requirements of articles 21 to 25 in respect of qualified personnel are discussed at section 10.2 below.

---

1.   OJ No22 9.2.65 p369/65.
2.   See the discussion of Case 35/85 *Tissier* [1986] ECR 1207 at section 2.5.4 ante.
3.   Discussed at section 5.3 ante.

No explanation is given of the expression "have at his disposal"; the expression does not appear to be limited to property owned or leased by the applicant or personnel permanently employed by the applicant, though those would be the normal cases. In the case of the "qualified person", article 17(c) is subject to article 21, which makes it clear that the requirement is to have the services of such a person "permanently and continuously" at the manufacturer's disposal. By contrast, article 5(b) of the Directive permits, "in exceptional and justifiable circumstances", certain stages of manufacture or certain of the controls to be carried out by third parties. Such "contracting out" is provided for at article 12 of Directive (EEC) 91/356 and in Chapter 7 of the Commission's Guide and is also permitted by article 22(1) of Directive (EEC) 75/319.

Article 18 makes three simple points in respect of the national authority : article 18(1) requires the competent authority to verify the accuracy of the particulars provided under article 17 "by means of an inquiry carried out by its agents" before granting a manufacturing authorisation to an applicant; article 18(2) permits the national authority to grant an authorisation "conditional on the carrying out of certain obligations imposed either when authorisation is granted or at a later date"; and article 18(3) makes it clear that a manufacturing authorisation is specific to the premises and the products specified in the application under article 17. The last point is clearly highly significant : a manufacturer requires a separate authorisation in respect of each product that he manufactures and in respect of each manufacturing site that he operates.

Article 19 imposes six continuing minimum obligations on a holder of a manufacturing authorisation. Those obligations are :

"(a)   to have at his disposal the services of staff who comply with the legal requirements existing in the Member State concerned both as regards manufacture and controls;

(b)   to dispose of the authorised [medicinal products] only in accordance with the legislation of the Member States concerned;

(c)   to give prior notice to the competent authority of any changes he may wish to make to any of the particulars supplied pursuant to article 17; the competent authority shall in any event be immediately informed if the qualified person referred to in article 21 is replaced unexpectedly;

(d)   to allow the agents of the competent authority of the Member State concerned access to his premises at any time;

(e)   to enable the qualified person referred to in article 21 to carry out his duties, for example by placing at his disposal all the necessary facilities;

(f)   to comply with the principles and guidelines of good manufacturing practice for medicinal products as laid down by Community law."

Those obligations are largely self-explanatory. The references in article 19(a) and (b) to rules laid down by the Member States reveals the extent to which manufacturing authorisation even more than marketing authorisation is a partial harmonisation measure : Member States retain their own rules in these and related areas and the manufacturer must comply not only with Community but also with national rules. The use of the term "disposal" in article 19(b) seems wide enough to include both disposal of waste products and distribution of finished products. Directives (EEC) 75/319 and 91/356 do not otherwise provide for disposal of waste products.

Article 19(f) was introduced by article 3 of Directive (EEC) 89/341[1] and is linked to the new article 19a also introduced by that Directive. Article 19a relates to the "principles and guidelines" referred to in article 19(f), requiring that a Directive laying down such principles and guidelines should be adopted in accordance with

---

1.   OJ L142 25.5.89 p11.

the procedures laid down by article 2c of Directive (EEC) 75/318[1]. That Directive was adopted as Directive (EEC) 91/356[2]. Article 19a also states that the Commission will publish detailed guidelines in line with the principles laid down by the Directive which will be "revised as necessary to take account of technical and scientific progress". Those detailed guidelines appear as Volume IV of the Commission publication "The Rules Governing Medicinal Products in the European Community".

Article 20 lays down time limits for the grant or variation of manufacturing authorisation. Article 20(1) requires the Member States to take all appropriate measures to ensure that the procedure for the granting of initial authorisation does not exceed ninety days from the date of receipt of an application for authorisation. Article 20(2) applies where the applicant notifies the national competent authority that he wishes to change any of the particulars provided to the authority in accordance with article 17(a) or (b) (specification of the products to be manufactured and the place of manufacture, and availability of suitable premises and equipment : see ante). In such a case, the authority's procedure in considering the request must not exceed thirty days. Article 20(3) permits the Member States to require from the applicant "further information concerning the particulars pursuant to article 17 and concerning the qualified person referred to in article 21". Where such further information is required, the time limits set out in article 21(1) and (2) are to be suspended until the information has been provided.

10.2   The need for qualified personnel : Chapter IV of Directive (EEC) 75/319[3], articles 21 to 25

Articles 21 to 25 of Directive (EEC) 75/319 lay down, in considerable detail, the qualifications and experience which must be possessed by at least one person "at the disposal" of the holder of a manufacturing authorisation. Article 21 imposes the general obligation to have such a person; article 22 states the duties of that person; article 23 states the minimum qualifications to be held by the person; article 24 is a transitional measure derogating from article 23 in the case of persons already carrying out the duties specified in article 22; and article 25 provides for national administrative measures to ensure compliance with the Community rules.

Article 21(1) requires the Member States to ensure that the holder of a manufacturing authorisation :

> "has permanently and continuously at his disposal the services of at least one qualified person, in accordance with the conditions laid down in article 23, responsible in particular for carrying out the duties specified in article 22".

Article 21(2) permits the holder himself to assume the responsibility for compliance with article 22 if he fulfils the conditions laid down by article 23. Article 21 thus sets out the structure of the Community rules for "qualified persons".

Article 22 requires the Member States to ensure that the "qualified person" is responsible for two important tasks to ensure the quality of the products manufactured by the holder of the manufacturing authorisation. Those responsibilities are stated to be "without prejudice to his relationship with the holder of the manufacturing authorisation"; that appears to mean that they are to be statutory rather than contractual duties. The responsibilities are to be performed "in the context of the procedures referred to in article 25"; those are described post.

---

1.   See section 4.2 ante.
2.   See section 10.5 post.
3.   OJ L147 9.6.75 p13. See Appendix 3 post.

The "qualified person" is responsible for securing :

"(a) in the case of [medicinal products] manufactured within the Member States concerned that each batch[1] of [medicinal products] has been manufactured and checked in compliance with the laws in force in that Member State and in accordance with the requirements of the marketing authorisation;

(b) in the case of [medicinal products] coming from third countries, that each production batch has undergone in the importing country a full qualitative analysis, a quantitative analysis of at least all the active constituents and all the other tests or checks necessary to ensure the quality of [medicinal products] in accordance with the requirements of the marketing authorisation".

Under sub-paragraph (a), the procedures and criteria to be applied will no doubt vary between the States but each will be based on the common requirements of Directives (EEC) 65/65, 75/318 and 75/319 (and now Regulation (EEC) 2309/93[2]). Sub-paragraph (b) gives the "qualified person" a more difficult and discretionary task in assessing whether all the tests or checks "necessary" have been performed.

Article 22(1) contains two further sub-paragraphs : the second sub-paragraph exempts batches of products which have undergone the controls laid down by (a) or (b) in one Member State from undergoing similar controls in another State "if they are imported into another Member State, accompanied by the control reports signed by the qualified person". Article 22(1), third sub-paragraph, relates to imported products and provides for arrangements to be made between individual Member States and third countries exporting products to the Community whereby the third country ensures that the controls are performed prior to export. In such cases, the Member States may exempt the "qualified person" from his duties under (b). In addition, where the imports are already in their retail packaging, the Member States may allow exceptions to the requirements laid down in article 17[3] : see ante. That further exception does not appear to relate to the "qualified person" in particular but would permit the Member States to authorise a manufacturer of such products which had no manufacturing or control facilities and did not employ any "qualified person" within that State[4].

Article 22(2) requires the "qualified person" to certify in "a register or equivalent document provided for that purpose that each production batch satisfies the provisions of [article 22]". The register must be kept up to date and must be available to the "agents of the competent authority" for five years or such longer period as the Member State in question may specify. The requirement applies "[i]n all cases and particularly where the medicinal products are released for sale".

---

1. In the Annex to Directive (EEC) 75/318, Part 2, para E(1) it is provided that : "[f]or the control of the finished product, a batch of a finished product comprises all the units of a pharmaceutical form which are made from the same initial quantity of material and have undergone the same series of manufacturing and/or sterilisation operations or, in the case of a continuous production process, all the units manufactured in a given period of time".
2. OJ L214 24.8.93 p1. Appendix 5 post.
3. See section 10.1 ante.
4. Article 22(1), third sub-paragraph, was amended by article 3(2) of Directive (EEC) 93/39 (OJ L214 24.8.93 p22) with effect from 1 January 1995. From that date, the Community will replace Member States in respect of the "appropriate arrangements" with third countries. Those arrangements are to ensure that the imported products are manufactured to a standard at least as high as that required in the Community and that the controls required by article 22(1)(b) have been carried out. The exception in respect of packaged products no longer applies from 1 January 1995.

Article 22 of Directive (EEC) 75/319 was the other provision of the Community rules on authorisation of medicinal products effectively disapplied, by the ruling of the European Court of Justice in Case 104/75 *De Peijper*[1], in respect of parallel importers[2]. Parallel importers cannot expect any voluntary co-operation from the manufacturers of pharmaceutical products, their whole purpose being to undercut the prices of such manufacturers. They are therefore normally unable to produce the necessary batch control reports provided for in article 22. The Court in *De Peijper* considered that in the special case of a parallel importer, where the product for which authorisation was sought was identical or virtually identical to a product already authorised, it was contrary to article 30 and beyond the scope of article 36 of the EC Treaty for a Member State to require batch control reports to be produced. The Court considered that the national authorities could adopt "a more active policy" in such cases, either (i) compelling the original manufacturer to produce the requisite information, or (ii) taking steps to obtain such information from another Member State, or (iii) adopting a presumption of conformity, or (iv) accepting proof other than the documents to which, *ex hypothesi*, the parallel importer has no access[3]. The Court's approach was followed and made more specific by the Commission Communication on parallel imports of proprietary medicinal products for which marketing authorisations have already been granted[4].

Article 23 lays down minimum conditions of qualification of the "qualified person". Article 23(a) sets out the minimum academic qualifications in some detail. The basic requirement is for a "diploma, certificate or other evidence of formal qualifications" awarded by a university or equivalent institution as evidence of completion of a four year course of theoretical and practical study in either pharmacy, medicine, veterinary medicine, chemistry, pharmaceutical chemistry and technology, or biology. Variations are allowed : (i) where a three and a half year course is followed by a further period of one year's theoretical and practical training including six months training in a public pharmacy followed by a university level examination; and (ii) where a Member State recognises a three year course offered by one university or other institution as equivalent to a four year course offered elsewhere within that State. Article 23(a) further specifies the core subjects to be covered in the course[5]. Where the formal evidence of qualification does not satisfy the requirements of article 23 (ie if the course is too short or fails to cover all the subjects specified) "the competent authority of the Member State shall ensure that the person concerned provides evidence of adequate knowledge of the subjects involved".

Article 23(b) relates to practical experience and requires a "qualified person" to have spent at least two years in one or more undertakings authorised to manufacture medicinal products :

---

1.   Case 104/75 De Peijper [1976] ECR 613.

2.   See section 1.4.3 ante. *De Peijper* also affected the interpretation of article 5 of Directive (EEC) 65/65: see section 3.2 ante.

3.   Case 104/75 *De Peijper* [1976] ECR 613, paras 23 to 29 of the judgment at pp637-638.

4.   OJ C115 6.5.82 p5. See Appendix 16 post.

5.   Applied physics; General and inorganic chemistry; Organic chemistry; Analytical chemistry; Pharmaceutical chemistry, including analysis of medicinal products; General and applied biochemistry (medical); Physiology; Microbiology; Pharmacology; Pharmaceutical technology; Toxicology; Pharmacognosy (medical aspects) (study of the composition and effects of the active principles of natural substances of plant and animal origin). Those studies are required to be "so balanced as to enable the person concerned to fulfil the obligations specified in article 22", as to which see ante.

"in the activities of qualitative analysis of medicinal products, of quantitative analysis of active substances and of the testing and checking necessary to ensure the quality of medicinal products".

Article 23 permits a "trade-off" between academic study and practical experience : where the person has studied for five years, his practical requirement drops by one year to a minimum of one year; where six years, it drops by a year and a half, to a minimum of six months.

Article 24 contains transitional provisions in relation to those persons already performing the task of a "qualified person" at the date of coming into force of the Directive without fulfilling the requirements of article 23. Given that the Directive came into force in 1976, the provision is no longer of any practical significance, though there will still be persons who benefited from the provision at that time who continue to perform the duties of a "qualified person".

Article 25 imposes an obligation on the Member States to ensure that "qualified persons" perform their duties "either by means of appropriate administrative measures or by making such persons subject to a code of conduct". The Member States are further empowered temporarily to suspend a "qualified person" where administrative or disciplinary procedures are commenced against him for failure to fulfil his obligations.

10.3   Supervision of manufacture : Chapter V of Directive (EEC) 75/319

Chapter V of Directive (EEC) 75/319 is considered in Chapter 11 in so far as it relates to continuing supervision of authorised products. However, much of Chapter V concerns supervision of manufacture rather than of the product itself.

Article 26 provides for repeated inspections by the Member State authorities to ensure compliance with "the legal requirements governing medicinal products". The second paragraph of article 26 requires a report to be written after each such inspection by the officials representing the national competent authorities on "whether the manufacturer complies with the principles and guidelines of good manufacturing practice laid down by Community law". The contents of the report must be communicated to the manufacturer who has been inspected. The provisions in respect of reports and the reference to Community guidelines were added by Directive (EEC) 89/341.

The third paragraph of article 26 gives three specific powers to the officials of the national competent authorities required to carry out the inspections. They may :

"(a)   inspect manufacturing or commercial establishments and any laboratories entrusted by the holder of the authorisation referred to in article 16 with the task of carrying out checks pursuant to article 5(b);
(b)   take samples;
(c)   examine any documents relating to the object of the inspection, subject to the provisions in force in the Member States at the time of notification of this Directive and which place restrictions of these powers with regard to the descriptions of the method of preparation."

The reference to article 5(b) is to third parties entrusted by the manufacturer or importer with certain aspects of the manufacture and/or control of a product. Sub-paragraph (c) preserves national rules on the confidentiality of business secrets relating to the description of the method of preparation of a medicinal product. No such secrecy is permitted at the stage of obtaining marketing authorisation where the method of preparation is a fundamental part of the material to be submitted[1].

Articles 27 and 28 are general provisions governing control procedures and the withdrawal of a product from the market, and are considered in Chapter 11. Article 28a, added by Directive (EEC) 89/341, requires the Member States to certify at the request of the manufacturer, exporter or the authorities of an importing third country, that a manufacturer is in possession of a manufacturing authorisation in accordance with article 16(1). The purpose of such a certification would be to satisfy the equivalent requirements of third countries in respect of pharmaceuticals imported into those countries. The issue of such certification is made subject to three conditions : the Member States must "have regard to the prevailing administrative arrangements of the World Health Organisation" (article 28a(1)); they must supply the summary of product characteristics as approved in accordance with article 4(b) of Directive (EEC) 65/65 where the product is intended for export and has received marketing authorisation in the State in question (article 28a(2)); and the *manufacturer* must provide "the authorities responsible for establishing the certificate" with a declaration explaining why no marketing authorisation is available where the manufacturer does not have such an authorisation (article 28a(3)). The effect in practice is that third country authorities must be given adequate assurances as to the nature of the product and the quality of its manufacture in the light of the common procedures of the Community Directives and the requirements of the World Health Organisation. Where a product is manufactured in the Community purely for export to third countries, with the result that no marketing authorisation has been obtained, the manufacturer must explain that fact. Article 28a does not apparently consider the possibility that a product might be manufactured in one Member State, say Ireland, for marketing in another Member State, say Germany. If article 28a(3) applies in such a case (for example, where the Irish manufacturer, with an authorisation in Germany but not in Ireland, also wished to export the product to the United States) then the explanation would be different from the case where no marketing authorisation had been obtained anywhere within the Community. If the reason why no marketing authorisation is available is that authorisation has been refused then that must also be explained.

Article 29 sets out the Member States' duties and powers in respect of the suspension or revocation of manufacturing authorisation. Article 29(1) requires the Member States to suspend or revoke such authorisation "for a category of preparations or all preparations where any one of the requirements laid down in article 17 is no longer met". That is an equivalent provision to article 11 of Directive (EEC) 65/65 in respect of marketing authorisations[2]. Article 29(2) complements article 28 (relating to the prohibition to supply or withdrawal from the market of a product that no longer satisfies the requirements for marketing authorisation) by giving the Member States the power to suspend manufacture or imports of products, or to suspend or revoke manufacturing authorisation "for a category of preparations or all preparations where articles 18, 19, 22 and 27 are not complied with". Article 28(2) had empowered the Member States to act against "batches" of products; the references to "a category of preparations" has a slightly different focus, apparently permitting the Member States to suspend or revoke a manufacturer's authorisation in respect of one product while maintaining his authorisation in respect of another product.

---

1.   See article 4(2) of Directive (EEC) 65/65 and Part 2, Section B of the Annex to Directive (EEC) 75/318.
2.   See Chapter 11 post.

10.4 Information exchange : Chapters VI and VII of Directive (EEC) 75/319

Chapter VI of Directive (EEC) 75/3 i 9 is entitled "Miscellaneous provisions". Article 30 concerns the exchange of information between the national competent authorities of the Member States : Member States are required to take all appropriate measures to ensure that the authorities exchange information in a way appropriate "to guarantee that the requirements for the authorisations referred to in article 16 or marketing authorisations are fulfilled". In respect of manufacturing authorisations, the individual Member States have direct responsibility under article 18 for ensuring that the requirements of article 17 are satisfied and it is not clear what specific information could be provided by another Member State that would assist the particular authority in making its decision concerning authorisation.

The second paragraph of article 30 is a separate but related provision requiring the Member States, "[u]pon reasoned request", to send the reports referred to in article 26 (of inspections of manufacturing facilities by the national authorities) to the competent authorities of another Member State. The paragraph also provides a mechanism for the resolution of differences of opinion between the Member States : if, after considering the reports, the second Member State cannot accept the conclusions reached by the competent authorities of the first Member State, the second State is required to inform the authorities of the first State of the reasons for its different conclusions and is permitted to request further information. The Member States concerned are required to "use their best endeavours to reach agreement" but they are required to inform the Commission "in the case of serious differences of opinion". The Directive does not specify what steps the Commission is empowered or required to take in order to resolve the difference of opinion between the two States. In the absence of such provisions, the Commission's general supervisory powers under article 169 of the EC Treaty would permit intervention if it was persuaded that one or other Member State was in contravention of its obligations under the Directive. In addition, in so far as the dispute concerned marketing rather than manufacturing authorisation, articles 11 and 12 of the Directive might be relevant to resolve the difference of opinion[1].

Articles 31 and 32 are general provisions equivalent to articles 12 and 21 of Directive (EEC) 65/65 and articles 67 and 68 of Regulation (EEC) 2309/93 in respect of marketing authorisation. Article 31 relates to the procedural safeguards for persons concerned by the operation of the Directive. Five categories of decision are identified : all decisions under article 18 (issuing manufacturing authorisation)[2], 28 (prohibiting the supply of a product or withdrawing it from the market) and 29 (suspending or revoking marketing authorisation); and negative decisions under article 5(b) (refusal of permission to have certain stages of manufacture or control carried out by third parties) and 11(3) (a negative decision of the CPMP in respect of a product referred to it by two Member States in disagreement over marketing authorisation). The party concerned by each of those decisions must be notified of the decision and must also be informed of his legal remedies and the time limits for such remedies in the event that he contests the decision.

Article 32, like article 21 of Directive (EEC) 65/65 and article 68 of Regulation (EEC) 2309/93, prohibits the taking of any decision concerning suspension of manufacture or third country importation, prohibition of supply or withdrawal from the market of a [medicinal product] except on the grounds set out in articles 28 and 29 of the Directive.

---

1.   See section 5.4 ante.
2.   Unlike the equivalent provision of Directive (EEC) 65/65, article 5, which concerns grounds for refusal of marketing authorisation, article 18 is positively phrased. However, it is clear as a matter of common sense and from the other examples in article 31 that the rights of the applicant arise in the case of a negative decision.

Only one of the implementing and transitional provisions of Chapter VII had any bearing on manufacturing authorisation. Article 39(1) gave an extra year to comply with the requirements of Chapter IV to those undertakings which were already authorised under article 16 before the time for implementation of the Directive had expired under article 38. That provision has long since ceased to have any significance.

10.5   Principles of good manufacturing practice : Directive (EEC) 91/356[1]

Commission Directive (EEC) 91/356 laying down the principles and guidelines of good manufacturing practice for medicinal products for human use is the first Directive to have been enacted by the Commission pursuant to its powers under article 2(b) of Directive (EEC) 75/318[2]. Recital 7 of Directive (EEC) 91/356 states that it was adopted in accordance with the opinion of the Committee for the Adaptation to Technical Progress of the Directives on the Removal of Technical Barriers to Trade in the Proprietary Medicinal Products Sector, the Committee established by article 2b of Directive (EEC) 75/318, indicating that the procedure described at article 2c(3)(a) of Directive (EEC) 75/318 was followed. Directive (EEC) 91/356 was also adopted pursuant to article 19a of Directive (EEC) 75/319 (introduced by Directive (EEC) 89/341), which required a directive to be adopted setting out the "principles and guidelines of good manufacturing practice". Article 19a also provided for the adoption of "detailed guidelines in line with those principles" and those guidelines were adopted before the Directive and are referred to at recital 3 thereof. They form Volume IV of the Commission's publication "*The Rules Governing Medicinal Products in the European Community*"[3].

Chapter I of the Directive, articles 1 to 5, is entitled "General Provisions". Article 1 defines the scope of the Directive as laying down "principles and guidelines of good manufacturing practice for medicinal products for human use whose manufacture requires the authorisation referred to in article 16 of Directive (EEC) 75/319". Article 2 is the definitions section : "medicinal product" is defined in accordance with article 1(2) of Directive (EEC) 65/65[4] and "manufacturer" and "qualified person" are defined in accordance with articles 16 and 21 respectively of Directive (EEC) 75/319[5]. Article 2 defines "pharmaceutical quality assurance" as :

"the sum total of the organised arrangements made with the object of ensuring that medicinal products are of the quality required for their intended use"

and "good manufacturing practice" as :

"the part of quality assurance which ensures that products are consistently produced and controlled to the quality standards appropriate to their intended use".

Article 3, first paragraph, refers back to article 26 of Directive (EEC) 75/319[6], requiring the Member States to use the "repeated inspections" provided for in article 26 to ensure that manufacturers respect the principles and guidelines of good manufacturing practice. The Directive is a somewhat unusual piece of legislation in that it expressly refers to administrative guidelines and requires, at article 3, second

---

1.   OJ L193 7.7.91 p30. See Appendix 9 post.
2.   See section 4.2 ante.
3.   EC Commission, Office for Official Publications of the European Communities, Luxembourg, 1989.
4.   See Chapter 2 ante.
5.   See sections 10.1 and 10.2 ante.
6.   See section 10.3 ante.

paragraph, that the Member States interpret the principles and guidelines laid down by the Directive in the light of the administrative document issued by the Commission. The effect is thereby to give the Commission's guidelines a quasi-legislative status despite the fact that none of the requisite procedures for the adoption of legislation has been followed for those guidelines.

Articles 4 and 5 impose four separate obligations on the manufacturer of medicinal products :

(1) to "ensure that the manufacturing operations are carried out in accordance with good manufacturing practice and with the manufacturing authorisation" (article 4, first paragraph);

(2) to "ensure that [medicinal products imported from third countries] have been manufactured by manufacturers duly authorised and conforming to good manufacturing practice standards, at least equivalent to those laid down by the Community" (article 4, second paragraph);

(3) to "ensure that all manufacturing operations subject to an authorisation for marketing are carried out in accordance with the information given in the application for marketing authorisation as accepted by the competent authorities" (article 5, first paragraph); and

(4) regularly to "review their manufacturing methods in the light of scientific and technical progress" and to submit applications to the competent authorities for any necessary modifications to the marketing authorisation dossier (article 5, second paragraph).

The first two obligations simply lay down the fundamental purpose of the Directive, supplementing the requirements imposed on the manufacturer by article 17 of Directive (EEC) 75/319 by requiring him not only to have the necessary equipment and personnel but also to comply with good manufacturing practice as defined. The third and fourth obligations supplement obligations imposed on the "person responsible for placing the medicinal product on the market" under Directive (EEC) 65/65 by requiring the manufacturer to provide a further guarantee that the actual product produced conforms to the product described in the application for marketing authorisation. The final obligation, to amend manufacturing practice in the light of technical advances and to seek approval for such amendments, corresponds to article 9a of Directive (EEC) 65/65. Especially when the holder of the marketing authorisation under article 3 of Directive (EEC) 65/65 is the same person as the holder of the manufacturing authorisation under article 16 of Directive (EEC) 75/319, many of those obligations will collapse into one another[1].

Chapter II of the Directive, articles 6 to 14, entitled "Principles and Guidelines of Good Manufacturing Practice", is identically structured to the Commission's "Guide to Good Manufacturing Practice" :

Article 6 : "Quality management" (Chapter 1 of the Guide);
Article 7 : "Personnel" (Chapter 2);
Article 8 : "Premises and equipment" (Chapter 3);
Article 9 : "Documentation" (Chapter 4);
Article 10 : "Production" (Chapter 5);
Article 11 : "Quality control" (Chapter 6);

---

1.   It is also relevant to note that many of the detailed requirements of the Annex to Directive (EEC) 75/318, which in principle relate to initial marketing authorisation, in practice lay down rules for the proper manufacture of medicinal products.

Article 12 : "Work contracted out" (Chapter 7);
Article 13 : "Complaints and product recall" (Chapter 8);
Article 14 : "Self-inspection" (Chapter 9).

As with the Annex to Directive (EEC) 75/318, the detail of the administrative requirements laid down by Directive (EEC) 91/356 and the Commission's "Guide" are outside the scope of this work. The Guide in particular is specifically intended to provide "a common agreed basis throughout [the] EEC for maintaining good manufacturing practices in the Pharmaceutical Industry".

The only principle that requires specific comment here is article 6, "Quality Assurance". Article 6 provides :

> "The manufacturer shall establish and implement an effective pharmaceutical quality assurance system, involving the active participation of the management and personnel of the different services involved".

That principle is wider than simply good manufacturing practice and thus apparently places a manufacturer of medicinal products under a general obligation to ensure the quality of those products. No guidance is given as to what that means in practice, whether the manufacturer is required to do anything to satisfy the obligation that goes beyond the more specific requirements laid down by the other guidelines in articles 7 to 14[1].

Articles 7 to 14 lay down more or less detailed guidelines under the various headings and those statements of good practice are amplified in the Commission's "Guide". There are also a number of cross-references to the requirements of Directive (EEC) 75/319[2]. The overall effect is of a further layer of complexity in the regulatory regime as the detailed requirements of the Directive and the "Guide" are laid across the requirements of Chapters IV and V of Directive (EEC) 75/319, which are themselves closely related to obligations imposed by Directive (EEC) 65/65 and the Annex to Directive (EEC) 75/318 in respect of initial authorisation.

10.6 Manufacture of products authorised at the Community level : Regulation (EEC) 2309/93[3]

Articles 16 to 18 of Regulation (EEC) 2309/93 lay down the rules for the control of manufacture of products enjoying a marketing authorisation granted in accordance with the Regulation. The principle behind those rules is simple : the Member State authorities which granted authorisation to a manufacturer under article 16 of Directive (EEC) 75/319 are also the relevant "supervisory authorities" under articles 16 and 17 of the Regulation. However, the Regulation does not make it clear whether articles 16 and 17 are of general application to all medicinal products or

---

1. "Quality Assurance ... incorporates Good Manufacturing Practice plus other factors outside the scope of this Guide": the Commission's Guide at page 15. No explanation is given of those "other factors" or their relevance to the specific subject matter of the Directive and the Guide. Examples might be the matters considered in Chapters 13 to 16 post: wholesale distribution, prescription, labelling and packaging, and advertising.
2. Article 9(1) refers to article 22(2) of Directive (EEC) 75/319 in respect of certificates of conformity for production batches; article 11(2) refers to article 5(b) of Directive (EEC) 75/319 in respect of authorisation of outside laboratories to perform quality control testing; article 12(4) refers to article 26 of Directive (EEC) 75/319 in respect of inspections of manufacturing sites; and article 13 refers to article 33 of Directive (EEC) 75/319 in respect of the communication of information after the recall of a medicinal product.
3. OJ L214 24.8.93 p1. See Appendix 5 post.

whether their effect is limited to products authorised at the Community level. The latter seems more plausible : article 17(1) refers to verification by the "supervisory authorities ... on behalf of the Community" and the literal wording of articles 16 and 17 would seem to have no purpose unless it applies only to the newly authorised products; if those articles were to refer to all products authorised under Directive (EEC) 65/65, they would to some extent merely duplicate the existing provisions of Directive (EEC) 75/319, but they would also conflict with those provisions in certain respects[1]. The following discussion assumes that articles 16 and 17 apply only to Community authorised products[2].

Article 16 of the Regulation to a large extent simply extends the scope of articles 16 and 22(1)(b) of Directive (EEC) 75/319 to the case of Community authorised products, giving the title of "supervisory authorities" to the national competent authorities where (i) the article 16 authorisation has been granted or (ii) the initial controls over products imported from third countries have been carried out. The second paragraph of article 16 exempts imported products from controls in the importing country where :

"appropriate arrangements have been made between the Community and the exporting country to ensure that those controls are carried out in the exporting country and that the manufacturer applies standards of good manufacturing practice at least equivalent to those laid down by the Community".

Article 3(2) of Directive (EEC) 93/39 amended Directive (EEC) 75/319 in similar terms, thus co-ordinating the regimes for nationally authorised and Community authorised products and bringing both into conformity with the requirements of article 4 of Directive (EEC) 91/356[3].

The third paragraph of article 16 simply permits one Member State to request assistance from another Member State or the Agency.

Article 17(1) gives the "supervisory authorities" the responsibility (i) for verifying on behalf of the Community that either the person responsible for placing the product on the market or the manufacturer or the importer from third countries satisfies the requirements of Chapter IV of Directive (EEC) 75/319 and (ii) for exercising supervision over such persons in accordance with Chapter V of that Directive. The reference to "the person responsible for placing the product on the market" is surprising in respect of Chapter IV of Directive (EEC) 75/319 which applies only to manufacturers and importers, but it will often be the case that the holder of a marketing authorisation and a manufacturing authorisation are the same person.

Article 17(2) and (3) provide for inspections to be carried out at the request of the Commission in certain circumstances. Article 17(2) relates to products manufactured within the Community where there is a difference of opinion between Member States as to whether the persons specified in article 17(1) are satisfying the requirements of Chapter IV of Directive (EEC) 75/319 and that difference of opinion has been notified to the Commission in accordance with article 30(2) of Directive (EEC) 75/319. The Commission may, after consultation with the Member States concerned :

"request an inspector from the supervisory authority to undertake a new inspection of the aforementioned person, the manufacturer or the importer; the

---

1.   In particular, the powers of inspection granted to the Commission are more extensive under the Regulation than under the Directive.
2.   The effect is to take the opening words of article 15(1) of the Regulation ("After an authorisation has been issued in accordance with this Regulation") as governing the whole of Title II, Chapter 2 of the Regulation.
3.   See section 10.5 ante.

inspector in question may be accompanied by an inspector from a Member State which is not party to the dispute and/or by a rapporteur or expert nominated by the [CPMP]".

Again it is odd that reference is made not only to the manufacturer and the importer of the product but also to the holder of the marketing authorisation.

Article 17(3) is subject to arrangements between third countries and the Community made in accordance with article 16 of the Regulation. The Commission is otherwise authorised to require a third country manufacturer to submit to an inspection by "appropriately qualified inspectors from the Member States, who may, if appropriate, be accompanied by a rapporteur or expert nominated by the [CPMP]". The Commission may act either on its own initiative or at the reasoned request of a Member State or of the CPMP. The report of such inspectors is to be made available to the Commission, the Member States and to the CPMP.

Articles 16 and 17 form part of Title II, Chapter 2, of Regulation (EEC) 2309/93. Articles 15 and 18 of the Regulation are considered in Chapter 11 in respect of supervision.

Chapter 11 : The Supervision Of Authorised Products

11.1 The original rules : Chapter III of Directive (EEC) 65/65[1]

Chapter III of Directive (EEC) 65/65 consists of two articles, 11 and 12, and is entitled "Suspension and revocation of authorisation to market medicinal products." Article 12 is in fact a general provision relating not only to supervision but also to the original authorisation process and imposing certain procedural guarantees on the Member States where they take negative decisions under articles 5, 6 and 11 of the Directive[2]. Article 11 is therefore the only article in Directive (EEC) 65/65 devoted to the topic of supervision.

Article 11 is a sister article to article 5 of the Directive[3]. Whereas article 5 lays down the basic criteria for refusal of authorisation, where a product fails to satisfy one of the three criteria of quality, safety or efficacy, article 11 applies those criteria on a continuing basis to authorised products. The Member States are required by article 11 to suspend or revoke a marketing authorisation where a product :

> "proves to be harmful in the normal conditions of use, or where its therapeutic efficacy is lacking, or where its qualitative and quantitative composition is not as declared. Therapeutic efficacy is lacking when it is established that therapeutic results cannot be obtained with the proprietary product."

The criteria are identical to those laid down in article 5, but their application is clearly different in the context of general supervision of a product on the market. That must apply not only to the criterion of therapeutic efficacy (in relation to quality, the testing of manufacturing facilities and supervision of distribution are two important continuing obligations[4]) but article 11 lays down a short "definition" of lack of efficacy. It is not easy to see how it could subsequently be shown, of a product which had established its efficacy for the purposes of authorisation, that therapeutic results could not be obtained with that product : the only possibility appears to be that there had been an error in the original assessment. In addition, as a matter of commercial reality, a product that was ineffective would fall into disuse and would be withdrawn by the manufacturer. In practice, therefore, it is much more likely that the authorities would be called on to act where an unanticipated adverse effect emerged in use or where the product was found to differ in production from the product that had received authorisation.

In relation to qualitative control, a further paragraph was added to article 11 by Directive (EEC) 83/570 equivalent to the second paragraph of article 5, requiring authorisation to be suspended or revoked in four specific cases :

(1) where the particulars supporting the original application required by articles 4 and 4a of the Directive[5] are incorrect;

---

1.   OJ L22 9.2.65 p369. See Appendix 1 post.
2.   See section 3.6 ante.
3.   See section 3.2 ante.
4.   See Chapters 10 and 13.
5.   See section 3.4 ante.

(2) where those particulars have not been amended in accordance with article 9a[1];

(3) when the controls referred to in article 8 have not been carried out; or

(4) when the controls referred to in article 27 of Directive (EEC) 75/319 have not been carried out.

Article 9a of Directive (EEC) 65/65 requires that the person responsible for placing a medicinal product on the market must update his control methods, as provided for in article 4(7) of the Directive, in the light of scientific progress. Article 9a was slightly amended and expanded by Directive (EEC) 93/39 to cover not only control methods but also manufacturing methods[2]. Article 8 requires the Member States to ensure that the controls have been carried out in accordance with the original application; and article 27 of Directive (EEC) 75/319 requires the Member States to ensure that the persons responsible for marketing and manufacturing the product prove that those controls have been carried out in respect of both the finished product and at an intermediate stage of manufacture[3].

Article 11 was not amended by Directive (EEC) 93/39 and remains the sole general article in relation to supervision contained in Directive (EEC) 65/65[4]. Like article 5, article 11 is governed by article 21 of the Directive, which requires that a marketing authorisation shall not be refused, suspended or revoked except on the grounds set out in the Directive[5]. The Member States therefore have no discretion as to the criteria they apply, though those criteria themselves give the Member State authorities a wide margin of appreciation[6].

It should be noted that Regulation (EEC) 2309/93 contains no precisely equivalent provision to article 11 of Directive (EEC) 65/65 (nor to article 11 of Directive (EEC) 92/27, which permits suspension of authorisation if labelling or a package leaflet fails to comply with the requirements of the Directive[7]. It seems clear that article 11 of Directive (EEC) 65/65 cannot apply in relation to Community authorisations, although the wording of article 11 is unlimited and has not been amended by Directive (EEC) 93/39 : it has never been open to one national authority to revoke or suspend an authorisation granted by another national authority, and for a national authority to revoke or suspend a Community authorisation would be even less appropriate.

The only applicable provision in the Regulation is article 18, which applies on its face only to the supervision of products, in particular of their manufacture, provided for by Chapter V of Directive (EEC) 75/319, discussed below. However, article 18 is very general in its terms and it seems likely that in practice it would be

---

1.   See section 3.6 ante.
2.   See section 8.2 ante.
3.   See Chapter 10 ante.
4.   Supervision and authorisation overlap at the moment of renewal of a marketing authorisation. The requirements for renewal are laid down in article 10 of Directive (EEC) 65/65, now amended by article 1(9) of Directive (EEC) 93/39 : see sections 3.6 and 8.2 ante.
5.   See section 3.2 ante.
6.   The scope of articles 11 and 21 was considered by the European Court of Justice in Case C-83/92 *Pierrel v Ministero della Sanita*, judgment of 7 December 1993 (not yet reported in the ECR; (1993) Transcript 7 December, OJ C18 21.1.94 p3). The Court ruled that the effect of article 21 in this context was that a marketing authorisation could only be revoked or suspended for the reasons set out in Directive (EEC) 65/65 or in other applicable provisions of Community law. In particular, it was incompatible with the Directive for such an authorisation to lapse if it had not been made use of within a specified period.
7.   See section 15.5 post.

used where a Member State, the Commission or the CPMP considered that the revocation or suspension of an authorisation was appropriate. Article 18 is considered in detail at section 11.5 below.

11.2 Consultation of the CPMP at the option of the Member States : articles 11 and 12 of Directive (EEC) 75/319[1]

Articles 11 and 12 of Directive (EEC) 75/319 were discussed in Chapter 5 above as part of the general discussion of Chapter III of the Directive and the CPMP's role in the "multi-State" procedure. Although articles 11 and 12 are somewhat unclear in their terms, they are potentially important provisions permitting unresolved disputes between the national authorities or issues of general Community importance to be referred to the CPMP for an opinion. Article 11 applies where differing decisions have been reached both in respect of original authorisation and in respect of suspension and revocation, whereas article 12 applies prior to an individual national authority's decision to grant, refuse, suspend or revoke an authorisation. In practice, therefore, both articles regularly involve examination of products that are already marketed in one or more States of the Community.

The Commission's latest Report on the Operation of the CPMP[2], includes at Annex 3 thereto all the opinions issued by the CPMP in 1991 and 1992 on matters referred under articles 11 or 12. Those opinions are called "pharmacovigilance" opinions by the CPMP and in practice they regularly involve a "benefit/risk" analysis in relation to a product currently marketed in one or more Member States conducted in the light of differences of view between the Member States as to adverse reactions to the product. They thus demonstrate the inevitable overlap between issues of supervision and of pharmacovigilance and thus the artificiality of the division between Chapters 11 and 12 of this work. The nature of the opinions also serves to demonstrate the level of detail at which the supervisory authorities are obliged to work, considering precise amendments to the wording of the summary of product characteristics or to the appropriate pack sizes that should be permitted for the product.

11.3 Post-authorisation supervision : Chapters V and VI of Directive (EEC) 75/319

Directive (EEC) 75/318 relates solely to the substantive requirements of the authorisation procedure and does not make any provision for post-authorisation supervision. In·practice, the detailed requirements of the Annex to that Directive will form the basis for the assessments required under article 11 of Directive (EEC) 65/65[3].

By contrast, Directive (EEC) 75/319 has a whole Chapter, Chapter V (articles 26 to 29) entitled "Supervision and sanctions"[4]. In addition, certain of the articles in Chapter VI, entitled "Miscellaneous provisions" are essentially concerned with supervision.

---

1. OJ L147 9.6.75 p13. See Appendix 3 post.
2. SEC(93) 771.
3. Part 4H of the Annex, entitled "Post-marketing experience", relates to experience in other countries prior to authorisation in the country to which the current application relates.
4. Chapter V was not amended by Directive (EEC) 93/39 but a further Chapter, Chapter Va, was added in relation to "pharmacovigilance", as to which see Chapter 12.

The title of Chapter V is somewhat misleading : the Chapter follows immediately after Chapter IV of the Directive, which established the Community procedures for authorisation of manufacture of medicinal products discussed in Chapter 10 and the regime of supervision naturally relates as much to supervision of good manufacturing practice as to supervision of the product itself. Article 5 of Directive (EEC) 75/319[1] provides for initial verification that manufacturers and importers are capable of manufacture in accordance with the requirements of article 4, points (4) and (7), of Directive (EEC) 65/65; and the provisions of Chapter V of Directive (EEC) 75/319 are intended to lay down procedures for continuing supervision of manufacture of the product as well as of the product itself. In so far as Chapter V is specifically concerned with manufacturing supervision it is considered at section 10.3 above.

Article 26 consists of three paragraphs. The first provides :

> "The competent authority of the Member State concerned shall ensure, by means of repeated inspections, that the legal requirements governing medicinal products are complied with."

That is an entirely general provision and the idea of "inspections" appears at first sight to be unrestricted. In fact, however, the second and third paragraphs of article 26 make it clear that the inspections are of manufacture and must lead in each case to a report on whether the manufacturer "complies with the principles and guidelines of good manufacturing practice laid down by Community law." The remainder of article 26 is therefore considered at section 10.3.

Article 27 was referred to in article 11 of Directive (EEC) 65/65 and is a general requirement that the person responsible for marketing a product and the person responsible for its manufacture should provide proof of the controls carried out on both the finished product and at an intermediate stage of the manufacturing process, "in accordance with the methods laid down for the purposes of marketing authorisation." Those are continuing obligations to conform to the requirements laid down in outline in article 4 of Directive (EEC) 65/65 and in greater detail in the Annex to Directive (EEC) 75/318 and the associated guidelines.

Article 28 is another general provision which supplements article 11 of Directive (EEC) 65/65. Article 11 requires the Member States to revoke or suspend authorisation for a product that ceases to satisfy the Community criteria; Article 28(1) requires the Member States to take active steps to ensure that the supply of such products is prohibited and the product is withdrawn from the market in four specific circumstances. Articles 28(1)(a), (b) and (c) reflect the traditional criteria of safety, efficacy and quality restated in the same words as in articles 5 and 11 of Directive (EEC) 65/65. Articles 28(1)(d) is similar to the second paragraphs of articles 5 and 11, but the wording is not identical :

> "the controls on the finished product and/or on the ingredients and the controls at an intermediate stage of the manufacturing process have not been carried out or if some other requirement or obligation relating to the grant of the authorisation referred to in article 16 has not been fulfilled."

The effect of that provision is close to adding a fourth criterion for continuing marketing authorisation, that the manufacture of the product complies with good manufacturing practice (the wording clearly refers back to article 27). Article 28 is expressly stated to be "[n]otwithstanding the measures provided for in article 11 of Directive (EEC) 65/65" and it appears that article 28(d) does not correspond to article 11. It opens the possibility that the supply of a product might be prohibited

---

1.   See section 5.3 ante.

and the product withdrawn from the market without marketing authorisation being withdrawn, and thus without infringing article 21 of Directive (EEC) 65/65[1].

That possibility is made clearer by article 28(2), which permits the national competent authority to :

> "limit the prohibition to supply the product, or its withdrawal from the market, to those batches which are the subject of dispute."

If the Member State took such a step it clearly might be a one-off administrative measure required, for example, because of industrial sabotage of a particular manufacturer or by corruption of a single batch of the product caused by an accident.

Articles 28a and 29 are concerned with continuing supervision of manufacture and are considered in section 10.3.

Chapter VI was considered in part at section 5.5. It is hard to classify the provisions, which are indeed miscellaneous. Articles 30 and 31 are principally concerned with manufacturing authorisation and are considered at section 10.4 ante; Articles 32 and 33 are partly concerned with manufacture and partly with general supervision; and Article 34 excludes certain products from the scope of the Directive, as to which see section 5.5. Articles 35 to 37 are amending provisions incorporated in Directive (EEC) 65/65.

Article 32 corresponds to article 21 of Directive 65/65 and provides, inter alia, that no decision concerning prohibition of supply or withdrawal from the market of a medicinal product may be taken except on the ground set out in article 28[2]. Article 33 lays down various requirements in relation to the transmission of information. Article 33(1) requires the Member States to inform the CPMP forthwith of :

> "decisions authorising marketing, refusing or revoking a marketing authorisation, cancelling a decision refusing or revoking a marketing authorisation, prohibiting supply, or withdrawing a product from the market, together with the reasons on which such decisions are based."

Those decisions are decisions taken under both Directives (EEC) 65/65 and 75/319 and the provision is intended to give the CPMP a general role as a repository of information. There is no requirement that the CPMP should be informed of decisions to suspend authorisation taken pursuant to article 11 of Directive (EEC) 65/65[3]. In its original setting in 1975, the provision had only a limited purpose as the CPMP had no significant role in co-ordinating Member States' conduct unless the Member States chose to use the procedures laid down in articles 11 and 12 of the Directive[4]. The requirement gains credibility in the context of the new Agency.

Article 33(2) imposes a similar requirement on the "person responsible for the marketing of a medicinal product". He is required to inform "the Member States concerned" (in practice, those who have granted an authorisation either to market or to manufacture the product) :

---

1. See article 6(d) of Directive (EEC) 92/25, discussed at section 13.4 post, for an important requirement imposed on wholesale distributors of medicinal products, that they should have an "emergency plan" for the recall of a product where necessary.
2. Article 32 makes equivalent provision in the case of refusal of manufacturing authorisation : see section 10.4 ante.
3. Contrast the position under Directive (EEC) 87/22 described at section 11.4 post.
4. See 5.4 and 11.2 ante.

"of any action taken by him ... to withdraw a product from the market, together with the reasons for such action if the latter concerns the efficacy of the medicinal product or the protection of public health".

The Member States are required to pass that information on to the CPMP. The effect of article 33(1) and (2) in combination is to provide a simple system of "pharmacovigilance" where either the supplier or the national competent authority has come to the conclusion that the product's failure to satisfy the Community criteria, in particular those of safety and efficacy, has become sufficiently serious to warrant withdrawal from the market. In such cases, there is a requirement that the CPMP shall be informed and thus indirectly the information will be passed to all the Member State representatives on the CPMP.

Article 33(3) requires the Member States "forthwith" to bring to the attention of the World Health Organisation "appropriate information about action taken pursuant to paragraphs 1 and 2 which may affect the protection of public health in third countries" and to send a copy of such information to the CPMP. The provision again clearly intends to give the CPMP a co-ordinating role in the transmission of information by the Member States which will become more significant if the Agency is given increased administrative resources and a more active co-ordinating role[1].

Article 33(4) requires the Commission to publish annually a list of the medicinal products which are prohibited in the Community. In the context of article 33, the reference must be to those products that have been the subject of one of the negative decisions mentioned at article 33(1) taken pursuant to article 5 or 11 of Directive (EEC) 65/65 or article 28 of Directive (EEC) 75/319. Given that article 3 of Directive (EEC) 65/65 contains a general prohibition on the marketing of an unauthorised medicinal product, there must be other products which have never been the subject of the Community authorisation procedures which are in fact prohibited but which the Commission could not sensibly be expected to identify.

11.4   Compulsory consultation of the CPMP : article 2(4) and article 4(2) of Directive (EEC) 87/22[2]

Articles 11 and 12 of Directive (EEC) 75/319 introduced a voluntary system of consultation of the CPMP available to the Member States where there were differences of opinion or where a point of general Community interest arose. Directive (EEC) 87/22 was intended to give the CPMP a more active role in relation to a limited class of products. Article 1 of the Directive contains a general statement that the Member States are required to refer matters within the scope of the Directive to the CPMP for an opinion before taking a decision "on a marketing authorisation or on the withdrawal or, subject to article 4(2), suspension of a marketing authorisation". In practice, the requirement is considerably qualified in relation to initial authorisation[3] but it is compulsory in relation to the withdrawal and suspension of products which have been subject to the Directive (EEC) 87/22 "concertation" procedure[4] and where the CPMP has issued a favourable opinion.

Article 2(4), and article 4(2) operate together in relation to such products. The national competent authorities are under an absolute obligation to "refer the matter to the CPMP for a new opinion" before deciding on the withdrawal of the marketing authorisation of the product; and they are under a qualified obligation to

---

1.   See section 7.5 ante.
2.   OJ L15 17.1.87 p38.
3.   See section 6.3 ante.
4.   See section 6.4 ante.

refer the matter before deciding to suspend the authorisation. The qualification, introduced by article 4(2), is that :

"in cases of urgency, the Member States may suspend the marketing authorisation in question without waiting for the opinion of the [CPMP] provided that they forthwith inform the Committee thereof, indicating the reasons for the suspension and justifying the urgency of this measure."

The procedures for the issue of CPMP opinions are described in Chapter 6.

Directive (EEC) 87/22 will be repealed with effect from 1 January 1995[1] but the system of compulsory consultation will be preserved and expanded by the new system.

11.5   Supervision of Community authorised products : articles 15 and 18, Chapter 2, Title II of Regulation (EEC) 2309/93[2]

The new "centralised" procedures for the grant or refusal of a Community authorisation based on the opinion of the CPMP are contained in Title II, Chapter 1 of Regulation (EEC) 2309/93 and were described in Chapter 7. Title II, Chapter 2, Articles 15 to 18 is entitled "Supervision and sanctions" but the reference to "sanctions" is somewhat misleading. The wording corresponds to that of Chapter V of Directive (EEC) 75/319 and, like that Chapter, Chapter 2 of Title II of the Regulation is concerned with supervision of both marketing and manufacture and with variation, suspension or withdrawal of authorisation where necessary. Penalties for infringement of the Regulation are in fact dealt with at article 69 of the Regulation and are left largely to the discretion of the Member States.

Unlike Directive (EEC) 65/65, Regulation (EEC) 2309/93 contains no general provision equivalent to article 11 of Directive (EEC) 65/65 laying down criteria for suspension or withdrawal of authorisation. Article 3 of Directive (EEC) 65/65 as amended by Directive (EEC) 93/39 provides that products which have been authorised at the Community level may be marketed in each Member State but there is no equivalent provision for withdrawal. Presumably article 11 does not apply to centrally authorised products (there is nothing in the text of Directive (EEC) 65/65 to limit the Member States powers under article 11 but it would be absurd for the Member States to be able, other than in exceptional circumstances, to suspend or withdraw a product which had been specifically authorised at the Community level)[3] and it would have been natural to include a parallel provision in the new Regulation (as article 11 of the Regulation corresponds to article 5 of Directive (EEC) 65/65 in relation to criteria for initial authorisation)[4].

Articles 67 and 68 of the Regulation apply to decisions to "vary, suspend, withdraw or revoke" marketing authorisations as well as to decisions to grant or refuse such authorisation. In each case, the decisions must "state in detail the reasons on which they are based" and must be "notified to the party concerned" (article 67). They

---

1.   See section 8.6 ante.
2.   OJ L214 24.8.93 p1. See Appendix 5 post.
3.   In exceptional circumstances, the Member States can suspend authorisation : see article 18(4) of the Regulation but article 18(4) would be unnecessary if article 11 of Directive (EEC) 65/65 applied to centrally authorised products.
4.   The nearest equivalent is the reference in article 18, second para, to article 28 of Directive (EEC) 75/319 but article 28 does not refer to withdrawal of marketing authorisation but only to prohibition of supply and withdrawal of the product itself. The Community's power to suspend or withdraw an authorisation once granted is apparently to be implied from the general scope of the Regulation (compare article 68 of the Regulation, considered below in that connection).

must not be taken "except on the grounds set out in this Regulation" (article 68(1)) or "except in accordance with the procedures set out in this Regulation" (article 68(2)). The procedures for such decisions are set out in articles 15 to 18 but no specific grounds for those decisions are included in the text of the Regulation and it is left to the Commission, the CPMP and the Member States to derive those grounds by analogy with those applicable to initial authorisation.

Article 15 of Regulation (EEC) 2309/93 relates to variations of Community marketing authorisations. Article 15(1) to (3) impose various continuing obligations on the person responsible for placing the medicinal product on the market once initial authorisation has been granted :

(1) He must take account of technical and scientific progress in relation to the methods of production and control provided for in article 4, points (4) and (7), of Directive (EEC) 65/65 and make any necessary amendments to those methods; that provision is equivalent to article 9a of Directive (EEC) 65/65 in relation to nationally authorised products[1].

(2) He must apply for approval for those amendments in accordance with the Regulation (article 15(1)).

(3) He must "forthwith" inform the Agency, the Commission and the Member States of "any information which might entail the amendment of the particulars and documents referred to in articles 6 or 9 or in the approved summary of product characteristics" (article 15(2)). Article 6 refers to the usual particulars required under articles 4 and 4a of Directive (EEC) 65/65[2], the detailed requirements of the Annex to Directive (EEC) 75/318, the expert reports required under article 2 of Directive (EEC) 75/319 and the special information required in respect of "genetically modified organisms"[3]. Article 9 refers to the draft product characteristics described in article 4a of Directive (EEC) 65/65, conditions or restrictions on supply or use of the product, and the draft text of the labelling and packaging leaflet proposed by the applicant for authorisation.

(4) Specifically, he must "forthwith" inform the Agency, Commission and Member States of :

> "any prohibition or restriction imposed by the competent authorities of any country in which the medicinal product is placed on the market and of any other new information which might influence the evaluation of the benefits and risks of the medicinal product concerned." (article 15(2)).

"Any country" clearly imposes a general world wide obligation to report prohibitions or restrictions back to the Community authorities. The use of the expression "any other new information" puts the holder of a marketing authorisation under a virtually unlimited obligation to keep the authorities informed, subject only to a minimal test of possibly influencing the authorities' assessment of benefit and risk.

(5) He must make an application to the Agency where he wishes to amend any of the information and particulars referred to in articles 6 and 9 of the Regulation[4] (article 15(3)).

---

1.   Compare also article 5, second para, of Directive (EEC) 91/356 which contains a similar provision in respect of manufacturing techniques : see section 10.5 above.

2.   See section 3.4 ante.

3.   See section 7.4 ante.

4.   See point (3) ante.

Article 15(4) requires the Commission to consult the Agency and to adopt "appropriate arrangements for the examination of variations to the terms of a marketing authorisation". Article 15(4) is equivalent to the new article 15 of Directive (EEC) 75/319[1]. In each case, the Commission is required to set up "a notification system or administrative procedures" relating to minor variations and to define precisely the concept of a "minor variation"; and the Commission is required in each case to use the less restrictive of the two adoption procedures laid down by the new legislation, in the case of Regulation (EEC) 2309/93 by article 72[2] and in the case of Directive (EEC) 93/39 by article 35a[3].

Articles 16 and 17 relate essentially to manufacturing supervision and are considered in section 10.6 above.

Article 18 is of general application and comes into effect in three situations :

(1) where the competent authorities of any Member State holds that a manufacturer or an importer from third countries fails to satisfy the requirements of Chapter IV of Directive (EEC) 75/319 relating to manufacture (article 18(1), first sub-paragraph);

(2) where a Member State or the Commission considers that one of the measures envisaged in Chapter V or Va of Directive (EEC) 75/319 should be applied in respect of the product concerned; and

(3) where the CPMP has given an opinion under article 20 of the Regulation to the same effect as (2) (article 18(1), second sub-paragraph).

In the first situation the Member States are required forthwith to inform the CPMP and the Commission, "stating their reasons in detail and indicating the course of action proposed". In the second and third situation, "the same shall apply", but it clearly makes no sense for the Commission or the CPMP to inform themselves of their own views so the effect must be that they are required to inform one another.

As has already been mentioned, the Regulation contains no equivalent provision to article 11 of Directive (EEC) 65/65 laying down general criteria for withdrawal of marketing authorisation but only article 18, which is triggered by the events set out above. Chapter V of Directive (EEC) 75/319 (referred to in the second situation above) was not amended by Directive (EEC) 93/39 and its provisions are considered at sections 10.3 and 11.3 ante. Article 20 of the Regulation and the new Chapter Va of Directive (EEC) 75/319 are both concerned with the new procedures introduced in respect of "pharmacovigilance" and are discussed in Chapter 12. In summary, articles 28 and 30 of Directive (EEC) 75/319 provide for the prohibition of supply and the withdrawal from the market of a product and for the revocation or suspension of manufacturing authorisation for the product; Article 29h of the new Chapter Va of Directive (EEC) 75/319 provides for cases where a Member State considers that marketing authorisation should be varied, suspended or withdrawn as a result of adverse reaction reports in relation to a product; and article 20 of the Regulation provides for CPMP opinions "on the measures necessary to ensure the safe and effective use of such medicinal products." In the last case, the scope of the CPMP's opinions is governed by article 5 of the Regulation, which provides in particular for opinions concerning variation, suspension or withdrawal of an authorised product and pharmacovigilance.

---

1.   See section 8.3 ante.
2.   See section 7.6 ante.
3.   See section 8.3 ante.

Where the article 18 procedure is brought into effect, article 18(2) requires the Commission "forthwith" to examine the reasons advanced by the Member State concerned and to request the opinion of the CPMP "within a time limit which it shall determine having regard to the urgency of the matter." Those are highly compressed provisions which again take no account of the cases set out in article 18(1) where either the Commission itself or the CPMP has activated the article 18 procedure. Where the Commission itself is the initiator of the procedure, it is not clear whether a CPMP opinion is required to confirm the Commission's view. The structure of the Regulation would suggest that the CPMP should express a view, as it is the CPMP not the Commission that is entrusted with the task of formulating opinions on such matters. Where the CPMP has already given its opinion under article 20, there is clearly no need for it to give a second opinion on the same subject[1].

Article 18(2) further requires that, "[w]henever practicable, the person responsible for placing the medicinal product on the market shall be invited to provide oral or written explanations". Cases where it is not "practicable" for the person responsible for the product to be asked to give evidence are likely to arise where it is necessary to act very quickly in the light of exceptionally severe adverse reactions to the product. That is confirmed by the second paragraph of articles 18(3) and (4).

Article 18(3) requires the Commission to prepare a draft Decision which is to be adopted in accordance with article 10 of the Regulation, the article governing the taking of decisions to grant or refuse initial authorisation[2], but the second sub-paragraph relates to article 18(4) and provides that :

"where a Member State has invoked the provisions of [article 18(4)], the time limit provided for in article 73 shall be reduced to 15 calendar days."

Article 73 is the procedural section laying down the more restrictive of the two procedures to be followed in adopting decisions under the Regulation and is described at section 7.3 above. In fact, two time limits are referred to in article 73, one for the preparation of an opinion on the draft decision by the Standing Committee on Medicinal Products for Human Use, the other for the Council to act in response to a proposal from the Commission. In addition, article 10(3) modifies the article 73 procedure to permit Member States to comment on the draft decision within 28 days. The effect of the second sub-paragraph of article 18(3) must be to reduce the period within which the Council must act, to 15 days, failing which the Commission must adopt its own proposal : the first time limit is at the discretion of the Commission in any event, and the time limit for Member State submissions does not appear in article 73 itself. It must be implicit in article 18(3) that where the time limit for the article 73 opinion is reduced to less than 28 days the Member States' rights to comment are curtailed or eliminated.

Article 18(4) concerns the exceptional case where "urgent action is needed to protect human or animal health or the environment"[3]. In such cases, each Member State is given the power by article 18(4) to suspend the use on its territory of a medicinal product which has been authorised in accordance with the Regulation. That is clearly an exceptional power in that it permits the Member States individually to override the collective Community decision to authorise the product. In such cases, the Member State concerned must "inform the Commission and the other Member States no later than the following working day of the reasons

---

1.   Article 20 itself provides for the adoption of measures proposed in a CPMP opinion using the article 18 procedure. That cannot imply a second opinion on the CPMP's own opinion.
2.   See section 7.3 ante.
3.   It should be compared to articles 15a and 15b of the newly amended Directive (EEC) 75/319, discussed at section 8.4 ante and summarised at section 11.6 post.

for its action". The article 18(2) and (3) procedures are then immediately put into operation and the Council's time for action in the event of a difference of opinion between the Standing Committee and the Commission is reduced to 15 days as described above. Article 18(5) extends the power granted by article 18(4) to permit the Member State concerned to maintain the suspension of the product in question until the procedure initiated under article 18(3) has resulted in "a definitive decision". In practice, that means a decision adopted by either the Council or the Commission under article 73.

Article 18(6) corresponds to article 10(4) and simply requires the Agency, upon request, to inform any person concerned of the final decision. In the case of a national suspension under article 18(3), the number of people concerned may be very large but in such cases the Community decision would be likely to attract considerable publicity, particularly if it differed from the national assessment of risk. It should be noted that the article 73 procedure makes it quite possible for the Member State that has acted to suspend the product to be outvoted at each stage and therefore for that State to be bound by the opinion of the Standing Committee and the Commission or by the qualified majority of the Member States. It is only where the Standing Committee does not agree with the Commission *and* where the Member State can achieve a simple majority on the Council that it would be able to block a Commission decision contrary to its own assessment. Article 18 is therefore likely to prove a politically sensitive provision in the rare cases where a product authorised at the Community level is considered by one of the Member States to have serious adverse consequences on health or the environment.

11.6 Amendments to Directives (EEC) 65/65 and 75/319 in respect of supervision : Directive (EEC) 93/39

Only two alterations to Directive (EEC) 65/65 have a bearing on supervisory issues : the new article 9a expands the obligations of the person responsible for placing a medicinal product on the market to update his practice in the light of technical and scientific progress; and article 10 as amended expands the old provisions in respect of renewal of marketing authorisation. Each is discussed more fully at section 8.2 above.

Although Chapter V of Directive (EEC) 75/319, specifically entitled "Supervision and sanctions", is unchanged by Directive (EEC) 93/39, there are several amendments to the Directive which will have an impact on supervision. The majority of those alterations appear in the new Chapter III of the Directive setting out the powers and functions of the CPMP. Those changes were considered in Chapter 8 above and are simply listed here.

Article 8(2) sets out the CPMP's general responsibilities to include the examination of questions relating to "variation, suspension or withdrawal of marketing authorisation" as well as those relating to initial authorisation. Articles 11 and 12 are expanded versions of the provisions of the old Directive and give the CPMP a general consultative role where the Member States differ in their views on supervision or where "the interests of the Community are involved". Articles 13(4) and (5) set out the obligations of the Agency on receipt of a CPMP opinion, not only in respect of initial authorisation but also in respect of suspension, variation or withdrawal of authorisation. Article 15 sets out procedures for the variation of authorisations granted in accordance with the Directive, while article 15a provides for the use of the articles 13 and 14 procedures where a Member State considers that variation, suspension or withdrawal is necessary for the protection of public health, and for temporary suspension by the Member States without prior consultation in urgent cases. Article 15b is an important transitional article, preserving the CPMP's power to supervise products authorised under the old "concertation" procedure of Directive (EEC) 87/22 after the repeal of that Directive.

The new Chapter Va of Directive (EEC) 75/319 entitled "Pharmacovigilance" is considered in Chapter 12, but it is obvious that the issues of pharmacovigilance and supervision are in practice inseparable. Article 29h of the new Chapter Va is in effect a compressed version of article 15a, but applied specifically to the case of adverse reaction reports.

Chapter 12 : Pharmacovigilance

12.1   Introduction : old wine in new bottles

Chapter Va of Directive (EEC) 75/319[1] was introduced by article 3(3) of Directive (EEC) 93/39[2] and sets out a completely new element in the regulatory scheme established by that Directive. Likewise, Chapter 3 of Title II of Regulation (EEC) 2309/93[3] forms a discrete part of the Regulation devoted to the issue of "pharmacovigilance" in respect of products which have been authorised by the Community in accordance with the Regulation.

However, in practice the idea of "pharmacovigilance" is a very natural and obvious one which is fundamental to any regulatory scheme appropriate to the supervision of pharmaceutical products. The Community had, hitherto, naturally and properly focused on the initial authorisation procedures for marketing and manufacture of such products, but the uninformed observer might have considered the most important element in any system of supervision to be the way in which information was conveyed by consumers, pharmacists, doctors and the industry itself to the regulator to ensure that the products were not causing harmful effects in practice. In essence, that is what "pharmacovigilance" involves.

12.2   The general scheme of pharmacovigilance by the Member States : Chapter Va of Directive (EEC) 75/319

Chapter Va, articles 29a to 29i of Directive (EEC) 75/319, was introduced into the Directive by article 2 of Directive (EEC) 93/39, considered more generally in Chapter 8 above. Article 29a of Directive (EEC) 75/319 defines the scope both of Chapter Va and of Chapter 3 of Title II of Regulation (EEC) 2309/93 :

> "In order to ensure the adoption of appropriate regulatory decisions concerning the medicinal products authorised within the Community, having regard to information obtained about adverse reactions to medicinal products under normal conditions of use, the Member States shall establish a pharmacovigilance system. This system shall be used to collect information useful in the surveillance of medicinal products, with particular reference to adverse reactions in human beings, and to evaluate such information scientifically.
>
> Such information shall be collated with data on consumption of medicinal products.
>
> This system shall also collate information on frequently observed misuse and serious abuse of medicinal products."

The two elements in the system are therefore the "collection" and "collation" of information : collection primarily but not solely concerned with adverse reaction

---

1.   OJ L147 9.6.75 p13. See Appendix 3 post.
2.   OJ L214 24.8.93 p22.
3.   OJ L214 28.8.93 p1 See Appendix 5 post.

monitoring in human beings; and collation relating to data on consumption and "frequently observed misuse and serious abuse of medicinal products". The "collation" element in the system is not fully explained by the remaining provisions of Chapter Va but the idea must be to obtain a proper perspective on the adverse reactions reported by comparing the number and seriousness of those reported reactions with the sales volume of the products concerned and with the incidence of use of the product in a manner other than that specified by the manufacturer and approved by the competent regulatory authority.

The concept of "adverse reaction" is central to the idea of a system of pharmacovigilance and article 29b sets out four simple definitions, of "adverse reaction", "serious adverse reaction", "unexpected adverse reaction" and "serious unexpected adverse reaction". Those definitions are cumulative, so that the last is simply defined to mean "an adverse reaction which is both serious and unexpected". Since "reaction" is not defined, the three important concepts under article 29b are "adverse", "serious" and "unexpected".

"[A]dverse reaction" is defined to mean "a reaction which is harmful and unintended and which occurs at doses normally used in man for the prophylaxis, diagnosis or treatment of disease or the modification of physiological function". Given the major difficulties of construction that have arisen in respect of the twofold Community definition of "medicinal product" contained in article 1(2) of Directive (EEC) 65/65[1] it is unfortunate that the definition of "adverse reaction" should involve an amalgamation of the two definitions of "medicinal product" (with alterations and omissions)[2].

"[S]erious adverse reaction" is defined as "an adverse reaction which is fatal, life-threatening, disabling, incapacitating, or which results in or prolongs hospitalisation". That is clearly not a technically precise definition : "fatal" and "life-threatening" are relatively simple criteria to apply; but the remaining adjectives and phrases could cover a wide variety of medical conditions and it is uncertain to what extent they are truly alternative to one another and to what extent they merely serve as general indicators of the type of reactions intended to be identified as "serious". Most medical conditions are to some extent "incapacitating" and could in some circumstances "prolong hospitalisation", at least in the elderly or infirm. The definition only becomes workable if "incapacitating" is interpreted as "seriously or significantly incapacitating" and if such general criteria are applied in the cases of persons who are relatively resistant to disease. It is doubtful whether they are clearer than the expression "serious adverse reaction" itself.

By contrast, the definition of "unexpected adverse reaction" is precise : "an adverse reaction which is not mentioned in the summary of product characteristics". The summary is a fundamental element in the original authorisation process introduced by Directive (EEC) 65/65[3]. All authorised medicinal products marketed in the Community must have such a summary approved by a national (or now the Community) regulatory authority. The definition of "unexpected adverse reaction" requires the relevant authority to compare the information contained in such summaries with information obtained in respect of the product in actual use.

---

1.   See Chapter 2 ante.
2.   It is not clear that "the prophylaxis" of disease is clearer than "the prevention" of disease in Directive (EEC) 65/65, nor that the definition is wide enough to capture the concepts of "restoring" and "correcting" physiological functions in the second Community definition of medicinal product. There is no reason why the definition of "adverse reaction" should be restricted in this context and it is hard to see why the definition did not simply refer to "doses normally used in man of medicinal products as defined by article 1(2) of Directive (EEC) 65/65".
3   See section 3.4.3 ante.

Articles 29c and 29d of Directive (EEC) 75/319, as amended, impose certain obligations on the "person responsible for placing the medicinal product on the market" in respect of adverse reaction monitoring. Article 29c(1), requires that person to "have permanently and continuously at his disposal an appropriately qualified person responsible for pharmacovigilance". Unlike the detailed provisions in respect of the "qualified person" responsible for monitoring manufacture (see articles 21 et seq of Directive (EEC) 75/319), no specific requirements are laid down as to the qualifications of the "qualified person" responsible for adverse reaction monitoring. However, that person's responsibilities are defined at sub-paragraphs (a) to (c) :

"(a) the establishment and maintenance of a system which ensures that information about all suspected adverse reactions which are reported to the personnel of the company, and to medical representatives, is collected and collated at a single point within the Community;

(b) the preparation for the competent authorities of the reports referred to in article 29d, in such form as may be laid down by those authorities, in accordance with the relevant national or Community guidelines;

(c) ensuring that any request from the competent authorities for the provision of additional information necessary for the evaluation of the benefits and risks afforded by a medicinal product is answered fully and promptly, including the provision of information about the volume of sales or prescriptions of the medicinal product concerned".

Paragraph (a) is intended to ensure that each person responsible for the placing on the market of a medicinal product has an efficient, unified and comprehensive system for the reporting of adverse reactions in place : such a system is *not* limited to "serious" or "unexpected" reactions and includes "suspected" as well as confirmed reactions[1]. Paragraph (b) imposes positive obligations to pass certain information on to the relevant competent authorities in accordance with article 29d; and paragraph (c) imposes a general obligation to co-operate fully with those authorities in the provision of information.

Article 29d is in two paragraphs : article 29(1) relates to the recording and reporting of "suspected serious adverse reactions"; and article 29(2) to the recording and periodic reporting of "all other suspected adverse reactions", in each case qualified by the requirement that the reactions should have been "reported to him by a health care professional"[2]. The obligations are imposed on "the person responsible for placing the medicinal product on the market" though article 29c(b) specifies that the reports are to be prepared by the "qualified person" referred to in that article. In the case of "suspected serious adverse reactions", the obligation is to record and report all such reactions "to the competent authorities immediately, and in any case within 15 days of their receipt at the latest".

The requirements in respect of "all other suspected adverse reactions" is less stringent but somewhat more complex : "detailed records" must be kept of such reactions; unless otherwise provided, those records must be submitted to the competent authorities "at least every six months during the first two years following authorisation, and once a year for the following three years"; the competent authorities may impose other requirements as a condition of the granting of

---

1.   Directive (EEC) 92/28, considered in Chapter 16, further specifies the obligations of medical sales representatives and of "the marketing authorisation holder" : see sections 16.4 and 16.5 below.

2.   The expression "health care professional" is not defined in Directive (EEC) 75/319; in Directive (EEC) 92/28 the expression is used to refer to "persons qualified to prescribe or supply [medicinal products]" : see section 16.4 post.

authorisation and may also request that the records should be submitted immediately; after five years, the records are to be submitted every five years together with the application for renewal of authorisation (see article 10 of Directive (EEC) 65/65), or immediately upon request. The records are to be accompanied by "a scientific evaluation".

Articles 29e and 29f impose obligations on the Member States. Article 29e(1) requires the Member States to "take all appropriate measures to encourage doctors and other health care professionals to report suspected adverse reactions to the competent authorities". That Community obligation, to "encourage" such reporting, is clearly a vague and minimal requirement : it would be very difficult to prove that a Member State had failed to comply with the obligation. Article 29e(2) empowers the Member States to "impose specific requirements on medical practitioners, in respect of the reporting of suspected serious or unexpected adverse reactions, in particular where such reporting is a condition of the authorisation". That is the only reference to "unexpected" adverse reactions and the effect of the paragraph is to enable the Member States to lay down national requirements on "medical practitioners" to report adverse reactions which either are "serious" or were not mentioned in the summary of product characteristics approved at the time of marketing authorisation. Such requirements may "in particular" be linked to the imposition of conditions on the marketing authorisation itself.

Article 29f is linked to article 29d(1) and 29e : where reports of suspected serious adverse reactions are made, the Member States are required to ensure that the reports "are immediately brought to the attention of the Agency and the person responsible for placing the medicinal product on the market, and in any case within 15 days of their notification, at the latest". Article 29f is not limited to reports from the person responsible for placing the medicinal product on the market under article 29d(1) or from medicinal practitioners or health care professionals under article 29e and could therefore apparently include also reports from private citizens or reports in the media (though there is no reason why the Agency should not monitor at least the latter for itself).

Article 29g provides for the drawing up of Community guidelines by the Commission :

"In order to facilitate the exchange of information about pharmacovigilance within the Community, the Commission, in consultation with the Agency, Member States and interested parties, shall draw up guidance on the collection, verification and presentation of adverse reaction reports.

This guidance shall take account of international harmonisation work carried out with regard to terminology and classification in the field of pharmacovigilance."

At present, no guidelines have been drawn up pursuant to this provision, although the CPMP had already approved several such guidelines before the adoption of Directive (EEC) 93/39[1].

Article 29h(1) requires a Member State to inform the Agency and the person responsible for the placing the medicinal product on the market "forthwith" where

---

1.	See pp 41-43 of the Commission's report on the Operation of the CPMP of 12.5.93, SEC(93) 771, in respect of : a "rapid alert" procedure operated through the CPMP (CPMP guideline III/3366/91); and "Procedure for causality classification in Pharmacovigilance in the European Community" (Guideline III/3445/91). The last issue, the establishment of a credible causal link between a specific treatment and a specific adverse reaction, is clearly of the greatest importance and, in many cases, involves very difficult questions of scientific proof.

"as a result of the evaluation of adverse reaction reports [the] Member State considers that a marketing authorisation should be varied, suspended or withdrawn". Where the traditional national authorisation procedures established in accordance with Directive (EEC) 65/65 have been followed, the relevant provisions are article 11 of that Directive and article 28 of Directive (EEC) 75/319. Those articles do not include any provision for "variation" of an authorisation (though article 9 of Directive (EEC) 65/65 provides for the updating of control methods). In respect of products authorised under the new "decentralised" procedure introduced by Directive (EEC) 93/29, the new articles 15 to 15b of Directive (EEC) 75/319 apply in respect of "variations". Article 29h does not expressly exclude from its scope products authorised by the Community under the new "centralised" procedure introduced by Regulation (EEC) 2309/93; but the Member States clearly have no power to vary or withdraw an authorisation which they have not granted and their limited powers to suspend such an authorisation, in so far as it applies to their territory, are specifically provided for by article 18(4) of the Regulation.

Article 29h(2) permits the Member States to act in urgent cases to suspend the marketing of a product without informing the Agency, "provided the Agency is informed at the latest on the following working day"[1]. No reason is given in Directive (EEC) 93/39 for the provision of such information to the Agency but article 24(2) of Regulation (EEC) 2309/93 requires the Agency to act, in consultation with the Member States and the Commission, to :

> "set up a data-processing network for the rapid transmission of data between the competent Community authorities in the event of an alert relating to faulty manufacture, serious adverse reactions and other pharmacovigilance data regarding medicinal products marketed in the Community".

That provision is not limited to products authorised in accordance with the "centralised" procedure under the Regulation.

In addition, Chapter V of and Annex III to the Commission's Report on the Operation of the CPMP[2] make it clear that an important part of the CPMP's role under articles 11 and 12 of Directive (EEC) 75/319 has been to give opinions on medicinal products originally authorised in more than one Member State where one of those Member States is led to suspend authorisation because of evidence of adverse reactions[3].

The final article of the new Chapter Va of Directive (EEC) 75/319, article 29i, provides that any amendments required to update the provisions of the Chapter "to

---

1. Compare the Member States' power to suspend products authorised under the "centralised" procedure under article 18(4) of Regulation (EEC) 2309/93 or after the operation of the "decentralised" procedure under article 15a of Directive (EEC) 75/319 as amended. Article 29h cannot limit the Member States' residual powers to suspend national authorisations under article 11 of Directive (EEC) 65/65, although the wording of article 29h appears to be intended to restrict such powers by requiring prior notification to the Agency except in exceptional circumstances. In practice, that will operate as an administrative requirement rather than a material fetter on the Member States' discretion.
2. SEC(93) 991 of 12.5.93.
3. A good example, described at pp45-47 of the Commission Report, is the United Kingdom's unilateral suspension of Triazolam (Halcion), followed by an article 11 reference to the CPMP by France and the Netherlands. In that case, the CPMP issued both a position statement and a final opinion, but the United Kingdom remained the only Member State where the product's authorisation was suspended. In another case, Glafenine, a reference under article 12 by Belgium led ultimately to the withdrawal of the product or the withdrawal or suspension of authorisation in all those Member States where the product had previously been marketed : see pp 44-45 of the Report.

take account of scientific and technical progress" are to be adopted in accordance with the article 37a procedure : that is the less rigorous of the two procedures, requiring the Council to act within three months by qualified majority if legislation proposed by the Commission without the agreement of the Standing Committee on Medicinal Products for Human Use is to be blocked[1].

12.3   Pharmacovigilance for centrally authorised products : Title II, Chapter 3 of Regulation (EEC) 2309/93

The provisions of Title II, Chapter 3 of Regulation (EEC) 2309/93 are a further example of the intricate scheme of regulation now in force at the Community level in respect of pharmaceuticals. Chapter 3 is in certain respects derivative from Chapter Va of Directive (EEC) 75/319, in other respects it is a separate regime applicable only to centrally authorised products and in yet other respects goes beyond the provisions of Directive (EEC) 75/319 by introducing new elements common to all medicinal products.

Article 19 simply provides that the definitions of "adverse reaction", "serious adverse reaction", "unexpected adverse reaction" and "serious unexpected adverse reaction" contained in article 29b of Directive (EEC) 75/319 shall apply for the purposes of the Regulation.

Article 20 provides for the provision of information to the Agency "about suspected adverse reactions to medicinal products which have been authorised by the Community in accordance with this Regulation". The first sentence of the article merely declares that the Agency, "acting in close co-operation with the national pharmacovigilance systems established in accordance with article 29a of Directive (EEC) 75/319", shall receive all such relevant information, without specifying how the information is to be provided. The second paragraph of article 20 requires that "the person responsible for placing the medicinal product on the market and the competent authorities of the Member States" bring all such relevant information "to the attention of the Agency in accordance with the provisions of this Regulation"[2].

The second and third sentences of article 20 are unrelated to the remainder of the article and provide for the CPMP to formulate opinions on "the measures necessary to ensure the safe and effective use of such medicinal products" (i.e. centrally authorised products). Such opinions are said to be in accordance with article 5 of the Regulation, which provides for CPMP opinions, inter alia, on :

> "any question concerning the ... variation, suspension or withdrawal of an authorisation to place a medicinal product for human use on the market arising in accordance with the provision of this Title and pharmacovigilance".

Article 20 further provides that measures proposed by the CPMP are to be adopted in accordance with the procedure laid down in article 18 of the Regulation. Article 18(1), second sentence, expressly provides for the adoption of measures in the light of an article 20 opinion. Article 18 was considered at section 11.5 above in respect of marketing supervision.

---

1.   See section 4.2 ante for the procedure, originally introduced by article 2 of Directive (EEC) 75/318 (OJ L147 9.6.75 p1).
2.   An important element in this process will be the "scientific service in charge of information about the medicinal products which he placed on the market" which a marketing authorisation holder is required to establish by article 13 of Directive (EEC) 92/28 : see section 16.5 post.

Articles 21 and 22 impose detailed requirements on "[t]he person responsible for the placing on the market of a medicinal product authorised by the Community in accordance with the provisions of this Regulation".

The requirements of article 21 in respect of centrally authorised products are almost identical to those of article 29c of Directive (EEC) 75/319 in respect of non-centrally authorised products. Each requires the appointment of "an appropriately qualified person" responsible for the establishment of a unified information system in respect of suspected adverse reactions, the preparation of reports for the competent authorities and for answers to requests from those authorities. The only material differences are that article 21(a) of the Regulation requires information to be "collected, evaluated and collated so that it may be accessed at a single point within the Community" whereas article 29c(a) of the Directive requires that it be "collected and collated at a single point within the Community"; and article 21(b) refers to the preparation of reports "for the competent authorities of the Member States and the Agency in accordance with the requirements of this Regulation" whereas article 29c(b) refers to preparation of reports "for the competent authorities ... in such form as may be laid down by those authorities, in accordance with the relevant national or Community guidelines". The second difference is the more significant in that it reflects the fact that the national authorities retain a margin of discretion in respect of the pharmacovigilance reports which they require, at least in the absence of Community harmonising measures.

Article 22 of the Regulation (like article 29d of Directive (EEC) 75/319 in respect of article 29c(b) of the Directive) sets out detailed requirements in respect of the preparation of the reports referred to in article 21(b).

Article 22(1), first sub-paragraph, imposes requirements on the person responsible for placing the product on the market in respect of "suspected serious adverse reactions occurring within the Community to a medicinal product authorised in accordance with the provisions of this Regulation which are brought to his attention by a health care professional" : he must record all such cases and report them "to the Member States in whose territories the incident occurred, and in no cases later than 15 days following receipt of the information."

Article 22(1), second subparagraph, imposes a general obligation on the person responsible for placing the product on the market to ensure that "all suspected serious unexpected reactions occurring in the territory of a third country, are reported immediately to Member States and the Agency and in no case later than 15 days following the receipt of the information". In its terms, that provision is not limited to centrally authorised products, but it must be qualified in some way, either to centrally or to *centrally and non-centrally* authorised products marketed by the person upon whom the obligation is imposed, and the most natural construction in the context of the Regulation is to *centrally* authorised products[1].

On the other hand, there is no good reason why pharmacovigilance information obtained from third countries should only be important in respect of centrally authorised products and it therefore seems possible that a "purposive" construction, broadening the scope of the provision, would be adopted. It should also be noted that the obligation is in respect of suspected "serious unexpected reactions", the

---

1.   As a matter of pure construction, the most natural reading of "the person responsible for placing *the* medicinal product on the market" (emphasis added) is as a reference back to article 21(1) "[t]he person responsible for the placing on the market of a medicinal product authorised by the Community in accordance with the provisions of this Regulation" and thus to read all of article 22 as limited in scope to such products; but it is notorious that the European Court of Justice and the Commission have never been bound by such verbal niceties and that Community legislation is frequently imprecise in its drafting.

narrowest category of adverse reaction identified by article 29b of Directive (EEC) 75/319. No provision of Directive (EEC) 75/319 relates to that limited category which may also indicate that the second sub-paragraph of article 22(1) of the Regulation should be construed widely, to cover products otherwise within the scope of the Directive.

Likewise, article 22(1), third sub-paragraph, provides that :

> "arrangements for the reporting of suspected unexpected adverse reactions which are not serious, whether arising in the Community or in a third country, shall be adopted in accordance with article 26".

Again, there is no indication of the scope of the subparagraph and no clear reason to limit that scope. The Member States retain a discretion under article 29e of Directive (EEC) 75/319 to require medical practitioners to report "suspected serious or unexpected adverse reactions" but there is no other provision in respect of "unexpected" reactions in the Directive. Article 26 of the Regulation is described below.

Article 22(2) corresponds to article 29d(2) of Directive (EEC) 75/319 in respect of the keeping of records. The first sentence of article 22(2) imposes a general requirement on the person responsible for marketing the product "to maintain detailed records of all suspected adverse reactions occurring within or outside the Community which are reported to him by a health care professional".

The remainder of article 22(2) corresponds precisely to article 29d(2) of the Directive (except that the "competent authorities" of the Directive are replaced by the Community, the Member States and the Agency). Unless the Community has imposed a condition on the original authorisation, records must be submitted (with a scientific evaluation) to the Member States and the Agency, immediately on request or six-monthly for two years, annually for a further three years, and five-yearly thereafter on renewal of the marketing authorisation in accordance with article 13 of the Regulation.

Article 23(1) is linked to article 22(1), first sentence, and requires the Member States, to which the person responsible for marketing a centrally authorised product must report all suspected serious adverse reactions occurring within a particular Member State's territory within 15 days, themselves to record and report all such incidents "immediately to the Agency and the person responsible for placing the medicinal product on the market, and in no case later than 15 days following the receipt of the information." Article 23 therefore imposes a reciprocal obligation on the Member States in respect of the person responsible for marketing the product, to inform him of any suspected serious adverse reaction reports of which he may hitherto be unaware, in addition to an obligation to keep the Agency informed.

Article 23(2) requires the Agency to inform "the national pharmacovigilance systems", set up in accordance with article 29a of Directive (EEC) 93/39, presumably in practice the relevant section of the national competent authorities. That is an important part of the new Agency's role in establishing a structure for co-operation between the national and Community authorities whereby information is passed up to the Agency from the national level and then passed back down to other national authorities which would not necessarily obtain such information without the Agency's assistance. It is notable that the Agency is not required to provide such information to the national authorities within any particular period of time.

Articles 24 and 25 impose three important obligations on the Community authorities. Article 24(1) requires the Commission, "in consultation with the

Agency, Member States and interested parties" to "draw up guidance on the collection, verification and presentation of adverse reaction reports". That corresponds to article 29g of Directive (EEC) 75/319.

Article 24(2) provides that the Agency, "in consultation with the Member States and the Commission", shall :

> "set up a data-processing network for the rapid transmission of data between the competent Community authorities in the event of an alert relating to faulty manufacture, serious adverse reactions and other pharmacovigilance data regarding medicinal products marketed in the Community".

A "rapid alert" system has been operation since 1979 through the CPMP[1]. The coming into existence of the Agency should enable that system to be placed on a more permanent footing.

Article 25 requires the Agency to collaborate with the World Health Organisation on "international pharmacovigilance". The Agency is required to :

> "take the necessary steps to submit promptly to the World Health Organisation appropriate and adequate information regarding the measures taken in the Community which may have a bearing on public health protection in third countries"

and to send a copy thereof to the Commission and the Member States. The importance of that provision will clearly depend on the credibility of the Agency, which will in turn depend on the level of co-operation and resources granted to the Agency by the Member States.

Article 26 provides for the amendment of Title II, Chapter 3 "to take account of scientific and technical progress" : as in the case of amendments pursuant to articles 29i and 37a of Directive (EEC) 75/319, the less restrictive procedure is adopted, under article 72 of the Regulation, whereby the Council can only block a Commission proposal that has not been approved by the Standing Committee on Medicinal Products for human use by qualified majority within three months of the submission of the proposal[2].

1.　　　See p42 of the Commission's Report on the Operation of the CPMP of 12 May 1993, SEC(93) 771.
2.　　　See section 7.6 ante for the procedure.

PART V : THE MARKETING OF AUTHORISED PRODUCTS - THE RATIONAL USE PACKAGE

Chapter 13 : Directive (EEC) 92/25[1] - The Wholesale Distribution of Authorised Products

13.1   The scheme of the Directive : the recitals

The recitals to Council Directive (EEC) 92/25 on the wholesale distribution of medicinal products for human use explain the essential purpose of the Directive, to facilitate the free movement of medicinal products for human use as part of the 1992 Programme by harmonising the diverse national rules governing the wholesale distribution of such products, in the light of the fact that "many operations involving the wholesale distribution of medicinal products for human use may cover several Member States simultaneously" (recitals 1 and 2)[2]. Recital 3 sets out the specific purpose of the rules, "to exercise control over the entire chain of distribution of medicinal products, from their manufacture or import into the Community through to supply to the public, so as to guarantee that such products are stored, transported and handled in suitable conditions"; it is also stated that the new rules will "considerably facilitate the withdrawal of defective products from the market and allow more effective efforts against counterfeit products". It is thus made clear that the aim is to close a possible loophole in the Community regime by enabling the competent authorities to regulate not only the initial authorisation of the marketing and manufacture of a product, and to withdraw those authorisations where necessary, but also to monitor the distribution of the product.

Recitals 4, 5 and 6 summarise the actual terms of the Directive :

(1)   wholesale distributors (but not pharmacists or others authorised to supply medicinal products directly to the public who limit themselves to that activity) are to obtain a special authorisation; and pharmacists and others are to keep records of "transactions in products received" (recital 4);

(2)   the Member States are required to impose minimum conditions on authorisations of wholesale distributors and to recognise authorisations granted by other Member States (recital 5);

(3)   an exemption is granted to those Member States which impose "public service obligations" on "wholesalers who supply medicinal products to pharmacists and on persons authorised to supply medicinal products to the public"; they are permitted to impose such obligations on wholesalers in other Member States :

> "on condition that they do not impose any obligation more stringent than those which they impose on their own wholesalers and provided that such obligations may be regarded as warranted on grounds of public health

---

1.   OJ L113 30.4.92 p1. See Appendix 10 post.
2.   Recital 1 is the standard 1992 Programme recital, which also appears as recital 1 to Directives (EEC) 92/26, 92/27/, 93/39 and 93/40. It is noteworthy that it does not appear in Regulation (EEC) 2309/93, whose legal basis was article 235 of the EC Treaty rather than article 100a : see Chapter 7 ante; nor in Directive (EEC) 92/28, which was not originally part of the 1992 harmonisation package: see Chapter 16.

protection and are proportionate in relation to the objective of such protection" (recital 6)[1].

In summary, the Directive is a "minimum requirements" Directive, permitting the Member States to impose more stringent requirements on wholesalers seeking authorisation, subject to the general rules under articles 30 to 36 of the EC Treaty and subject to the requirement of mutual recognition in respect of an authorisation granted by another Member State at least in respect of the minimum Community law requirements imposed by the Directive. The mutual recognition obligation is qualified by the Member States' right to impose higher obligations in respect of its own territory, particularly in respect of "public service obligations"; that right is in turn governed by rules which reflect the general Community law principles of non-discrimination and proportionality and more specifically article 36 of the EC Treaty.

13.2   Scope and definitions : Article 1

Article 1 of the Directive defines the scope of the Directive : article 1(1) defines "medicinal products" by reference to Chapters II to V of Directive (EEC) 65/65, which are themselves governed by articles 1 and 2 of that Directive[2]; the Directive is to cover "the wholesale distribution in the Community" of such products. Article 1(2) sets out two definitions :

"wholesale distribution of medicinal products shall mean all activities consisting of procuring, holding, supplying or exporting medicinal products, apart from supplying medicinal products to the public; such activities are carried out with manufacturers or their depositories, importers, other wholesale distributors or with pharmacists and persons authorised or entitled to supply medicinal products to the public in the Member State concerned,

public service obligation shall mean the obligation placed on wholesalers to guarantee permanently an adequate range of medicinal products to meet the requirements of a specific geographical area and to deliver the supplies requested within a very short time over the whole of the area in question."

Wholesale distribution is clearly deliberately widely defined, to cover all activities between (but excluding) manufacture within or import into the Community and final supply to the end consumer. It is notable that the definition includes distribution leading to export out of the Community.

13.3   Authorisation as a wholesale distributor : Articles 2 and 3

Article 2 is a parallel provision to article 3 of Directive (EEC) 65/65 and is expressed as being without prejudice to that article. Whereas article 3 of Directive (EEC) 65/65 prohibits the marketing within a Member State of any medicinal product within the scope of Chapters II to V of that Directive that has not been issued with an authorisation by that Member State (or, from 1 January 1995, by the Community), article 2 of Directive (EEC) 92/25 requires the Member States to take "all appropriate measures to ensure that only medicinal products in respect of which a marketing authorisation has been granted in accordance with Community law are distributed on their territory". The effect of that provision appears to be that the Member States are required to prohibit the distribution on their territory of any product that has not obtained either a Community authorisation or a national authorisation from at least one Member State. It is not entirely clear how article 2

---

1.   See article 7, which is not in fact limited to "public service obligations."
2.   See Chapter 2 and section 3.3 ante.

would apply, for example, where a product that was authorised in France, but not in Ireland or the United Kingdom, was to be distributed in Ireland. The natural interpretation of the provision is that the Irish authorities would be entitled to permit distribution within Ireland where it formed part of a chain of distribution leading to supply to end consumers in France; whereas it would not be so entitled where the distribution was undertaken for the purposes of supply in Ireland itself or in the United Kingdom. In respect of distribution for the purposes of supply within Ireland, article 3 of Directive (EEC) 65/65 would also apply to the Irish authorities, but in respect of distribution in Ireland for the purposes of supply within the United Kingdom it would be necessary to interpret article 2 broadly to find that no marketing authorisation had been granted "in accordance with Community law" by the United Kingdom authorities and in respect of the marketing of the product in the United Kingdom even though such an authorisation had been granted by the French authorities and in respect of the marketing of the product in France.

Article 3 sets out the essential structure of the authorisation process for wholesale distribution. Article 3(1) imposes the basic obligation on the Member States to ensure that such distribution is subject to "the possession of an authorisation to engage in activity as a wholesaler in medicinal products, stating the place for which it is valid". Given the general structure of the Directive it would be natural to expect that authorisations would be general in their scope, applying at least to substantial areas of a Member State and frequently permitting cross-border trade. However, the wording of article 3(1), and in particular the reference to "the place for which it is valid", is reminiscent of that of Chapter IV of Directive (EEC) 75/319, in particular article 18(3), where manufacturing authorisation is limited to specific premises and specific products[1]. In the case of distribution as against manufacture, authorisation must at least permit the goods to be moved, and in the case of high value, low bulk products such as pharmaceuticals it would be natural to grant authorisation for a large territory.

Article 3(2) and (3) concern the relationship between authorisation of wholesale distribution and authorisation of persons (i) to supply the public with medicinal products (article 3(2)) and (ii) to manufacture medicinal products (article 3(3)). In some Member States, wholesale distributors can also supply the public with medicinal products; in those States, article 3(2) requires that such persons obtain authorisation in accordance with article 3(1). By contrast, possession of manufacturing authorisation under article 16 of Directive (EEC) 75/319 is stated by article 3(3) to include authorisation as a distributor for the products covered by that authorisation . However, the second sentence of article 3(3) makes it clear that the converse is not true : possession of a wholesale distribution authorisation does not give dispensation from Chapter IV of Directive (EEC) 75/319, "even where the manufacturing or import business is secondary".

The scope of a wholesale distribution authorisation becomes particularly acute where article 3(3) is relied on. As stated above, article 18(3) of Directive (EEC) 75/319 limits the scope of manufacturing authorisations to specific premises and specific products. Literal interpretation of article 3(3) would render it meaningless as it would be limited to distribution within the authorised premises. On the other hand, no guidance is given as to any geographical limitation of such an authorisation, apparently implying that, as a matter of Community law at least, a person authorised to manufacture a specific product is entitled to distribute that product throughout the Community. It is unclear whether, by similar reasoning, such an interpretation could be applied to article 3(1) of the Directive and thus generally to distribution authorisations. The Directive as currently drafted gives very little attention to the movement of medicinal products.

---

1.   See Chapter 10 ante.

Article 3(4) requires each Member State, at the request of the Commission or any other Member State, to supply "all appropriate information concerning the individual authorisations which they have granted under [article 3(1)]". Article 3(5) requires checks to be carried out "on the persons and establishments authorised to engage in the activity of wholesaler in medicinal products" and provides that "the inspection of their premises shall be carried out under the responsibility of the Member State which granted the authorisation". That provision tends to confirm that the principal focus of the Directive is similar to that of Chapter IV of Directive (EEC) 75/319 in respect of manufacture, on the premises where distribution is principally organised and carried out, rather than on the transport of the goods from those premises to their final destination.

Article 3(6) and (7) are very general provisions in respect of the suspension or revocation of the article 3(1) authorisation. Article 3(6) merely provides that the authorisation granted by a Member State shall be suspended or revoked by that Member State "if the conditions of authorisation cease to be met" and requires the Member State to inform the other Member States and the Commission thereof. Article 3(7) requires each Member State other than the authorising Member State to inform the Commission and the authorising Member State if it considers that the conditions of authorisation are not, or are no longer, met and requires the authorising Member State to take "the measures necessary", and to inform the Commission and the first Member State "of the decisions taken and the reasons for those decisions". It is noteworthy that no mechanism is established for the reconciliation of differing views between the Member States or between a Member State and the Commission; also that there is no question of involvement by the European Agency established by Regulation (EEC) 2309/93. The matter appears to remain entirely within the discretion of the authorising Member State, subject only to the general Community rules applicable to such matters[1].

13.4   Procedures and criteria for authorisation : Articles 4 to 12

Article 4 provides minimal procedural requirements modelled on those imposed in respect of marketing authorisations by articles 7 and 12 of Directive 65/65. Article 4(1) requires that the Member States ensure that applications for article 3(1) authorisations are processed within 90 days of their receipt; however, that period may be suspended, where the competent national authority exercises the power granted by the second sub-paragraph of article 4(2) by requiring the applicant to supply "all necessary information concerning the conditions of authorisation," until the additional data is supplied. Article 4(2) requires that the reasons for any refusal, suspension or revocation of an authorisation shall be stated in detail and that the party concerned by such a negative decision shall be notified and shall be informed "of the redress available to him under the laws in force and of the time limit allowed for access to such redress".

Article 5 imposes three "minimum requirements" which must be satisfied in order to obtain an article 3(1) authorisation :

"(a)   they must have suitable and adequate premises, installations and equipment so as to ensure proper conservation and distribution of the medicinal products;

1.·   For example, the Commission could bring article 169 proceedings against a Member State that had authorised distribution by a company which did not satisfy the minimum requirements of articles 5 and 6.

(b)   they must have staff, and in particular a qualified person designated as responsible, meeting the conditions provided for by the legislation of the Member State concerned;

(c)   they must undertake to fulfil the obligations incumbent on them under the terms of article 6."

Those are highly general provisions in respect of premises and personnel and leave the Member States with a wide margin of appreciation as to the minimum standards to be satisfied : sub-paragraph (a) at least imposes a criterion to be applied, albeit highly general; whereas sub-paragraph (b) leaves it open to the individual Member States to set their own standards, requiring them only to have some applicable conditions imposed by national legislation. The reference in sub-paragraph (a) to "installations and equipment" is presumably wide enough to cover transport equipment, but the focus is again on the fixed premises used for the storage of the products prior to distribution.

Article 6 imposes a further seven "minimum requirements" on those who obtain article 3(1) authorisations. Article 6(a) requires that the premises, installations and equipment referred to in article 5(a) must be "accessible at all times to the persons responsible for inspecting them", in practice the relevant national competent authorities. The operation of that requirement in practice casts light on the difficulties of interpretation of the Directive previously alluded to. A Community-wide distributor will naturally have premises in several Member States; if a single Member State's article 3(1) authorisation is to be valid throughout the Community then there is the prospect of, for example, French inspectors being granted access to premises in Germany or Greece for the performance of their task under article 6(a). That does not appear to be a practical possibility, with the result that a series of national authorisations will often be necessary; but if that is correct, then it is hard to see what remains of mutual recognition, since an application to the French authorities in respect of premises in France can hardly bind the German or Greek authorities in respect of completely distinct, and possibly far less satisfactory, premises in Germany or Greece.

Article 6(b) and (c) impose limitations on the persons from whom and to whom medicinal products may be supplied : they may only be obtained from persons themselves authorised under article 3(1) or who are exempt under article 3(3); and they may only be supplied to persons authorised under article 3(1) or to persons authorised or entitled to supply such products to the public. The effect of those provisions is to ensure that there is a complete chain of authorised distributors from the manufacturer or importer to the final supplier of the product to the public.

Article 6(d) is a distinct, and isolated, provision of considerable importance not only in respect of wholesale distribution but also in respect of the more general Community rules relating to the withdrawal of a product from the market. Each authorised distributor is required to have :

"an emergency plan which ensures effective implementation of any recall from the market ordered by the competent authorities or carried out in co-operation with the manufacturer or holder of the marketing authorisation for the product concerned".

The detailed rules in respect of supervision and pharamacovigilance were discussed previously in Chapters 11 and 12. Article 6(d) is intended to ensure that a mechanism is in place to give effect to decisions taken under those rules.

Article 6(e) and (f) provide for the keeping of records in respect of "any transaction in medicinal products received or dispatched". The records must be kept "either in the form of purchase/sales invoices, or on computer, or in any other form" and must include the following minimum information : the date; the name of the product; the quantity received or supplied; and the name and address of the supplier or consignee, as appropriate. Those records must be kept available to the competent authorities, for inspection purposes, for five years.

Article 6(g) simply requires that a holder of an article 3(1) authorisation comply with "the principles and guidelines of good distribution practice for medicinal products as laid down in article 10". Article 10 requires the Commission to publish guidelines on good distribution practice in consultation with the CPMP and the Pharmaceutical Committee. The latter Committee was created by Council Decision (EEC) 75/320[1] to examine problems arising as a result of approximation and harmonisation of Community pharmaceutical legislation. In practice, it meets much less frequently and is of less day to day importance than the CPMP. The procedure envisaged is similar to that provided for under article 19a of Directive (EEC) 75/319 in respect of good manufacturing practice, though with no provision for a Commission Directive on good wholesale distribution practice to correspond to Directive (EEC) 91/356. The Commission has now published the envisaged guidelines.

Article 7 is the "mutual recognition" provision :

"With regard to the supply of medicinal products to pharmacists and persons authorised or entitled to supply medicinal products to the public, Member States shall not impose upon the holder of an authorisation referred to in article 3(1) which has been granted by another Member State, any obligation, in particular public service obligations, more stringent than those they impose on persons whom they have themselves authorised to engage in equivalent activities.

The said obligations should, moreover, be justified, in keeping with the Treaty, on grounds of public health protection and be proportionate in relation to the objective of such protection."

The article does not expressly require the Member States to recognise authorisations granted by other Member States, unlike recital 5, which states that "each Member State must recognise authorisations granted by other Member States". The mutual recognition obligation appears to be limited to those matters which are specified by the Directive : it would not be open to a Member State to require a distributor to produce evidence of such matters which were in effect already certified by another Member State. In addition, article 7, unlike recital 6, is not limited to extra "public service obligations" (as defined at article 1(2)) which appear only to be an example of the type of extra obligation that could be imposed. For the reasons already given, it is doubtful whether the mutual recognition will have much effect in practice as each Member State not only (i) retains the power to impose further restrictions on authorisations granted by other Member States, subject to general principles of Community law, but will also (ii) frequently be required to issue a separate authorisation in respect of facilities, owned by the person involved within that Member State, which were not within the scope of the original authorisation. It is only where the wholesaler supplies directly to another wholesaler within the second Member State, or to an authorised end supplier in that State, that the Directive is likely to limit the powers of the Member States. However, even in those cases, the second Member State will retain control over the second wholesaler or the end supplier.

---

1.   OJ L147 9.6.75 p23.

Article 8(1) is misplaced in the Directive and in fact imposes an eighth requirement on the holder of an article 3(1) authorisation, relating to supplies to persons "authorised or entitled to supply medicinal products to the public in the Member State concerned". The "authorised wholesaler" must enclose a document with all such supplies that makes it possible to ascertain : the date of the supply; the name and pharmaceutical form of the product; the quantity supplied; and the name and address of the supplier and consignor.

However, article 8(2) requires the Member States to impose a distinct obligation on "persons authorised or entitled to supply medicinal products to the public" : such persons must be able to "provide information that makes it possible to trace the distribution path of every medicinal product". That is an extremely vague requirement and it is far from certain that the persons involved will be in any position to satisfy the requirement in practice except by referring the matter up the distribution chain to their immediate suppliers. If such an obligation is in practice to be enforced directly on the end supplier, it would clearly have been desirable to impose far stricter requirements on the wholesaler to supply detailed information to the final supplier as to the origins of the products supplied.

Article 9 is likewise misplaced, since it sets out four specific categories of product where the Member States are permitted to apply more stringent requirements in respect of wholesale distribution. It therefore complements the general provisions of Article 7 and further limits any harmonisation of the measures in force in the Member States. The four categories are : "narcotic or psychotropic substances within their territory[1]"; blood products governed by Directive (EEC) 89/381[2]; immunological products governed by Directive (EEC) 89/342[3]; and radiopharmaceuticals governed by Directive (EEC) 89/343[4]. The last three categories are the products finally brought within the scope of Directive (EEC) 65/65 and Directive (EEC) 75/319 by the "extension Directives". Article 9 should be contrasted with the specially simplified rules laid down for homeopathic products by Directive (EEC) 92/73[5].

Article 10 was considered in relation to article 6(g) above.

Article 11 requires the Member States to implement the Directive by 1 January 1993.

---

1.   The words "within their territory" appear to be misplaced : they would naturally qualify the words "wholesale distribution" in the introductory words to article 9. There can be no possible justification for permitting the Member States to impose more stringent requirements on the distribution of narcotics and psychotropics only within their territory while imposing such restrictions on the distribution of the other products identified by article 9 throughout the Community.

2.   OJ L181 28.6.89 p44.

3.   OJ L142 25.5.89 p14.

4.   OJ L142 25.5.89 p16.

5.   See Chapter 9 ante.

Chapter 14 : Directive (EEC) 92/26[1] -
The Classification of Authorised Products

14.1   The need for the Directive : the recitals

Council Directive (EEC) 92/26 concerning the classification for the supply of medicinal products for human use has a simple purpose : to lay down certain basic principles to be followed by the Member States and by the Community in classifying medicinal products as "subject to medicinal prescription" or not so subject. The need for such a Directive is explained in the recitals.

Recitals 1 to 5 state the background to the Directive. Recital 1 refers to the 1992 Programme in general terms. Recital 2 notes the considerable variations in the conditions for the supply of medicinal products between the Member States, and in particular the differences between the States with regard to the question of which products can be sold without prescription. Recital 3 cross refers to Directive (EEC) 92/28[2], which "specifies what medicinal products may be advertised to the public", and states that :

"in view of the development of means of communication, the conditions governing the supply of medicinal products to the public should be harmonised."

The recital is not very explicit, but the control over the advertising of medicinal products introduced by Directive (EEC) 92/28 is in part based on the distinction between prescription only and non-prescription products (see in particular article 3(1)); and recital 3 implies that the development of cross-border advertising through advances in telecommunications necessitates common classification of medicines if the provisions of Directive (EEC) 92/28 are to be properly effective.

Recital 4 consists of three separate propositions, the third of which, the need to harmonise the conditions governing the supply of medicinal products to the public, is supposed to be some sort of logical consequence of the first two. The first point is that "persons moving around within the Community have the right to carry a reasonable quantity of medicinal products lawfully obtained for their own use"; and the second point is that "it must also be possible for a person established in one Member State to receive from another Member State a reasonable quantity of medicinal products intended for his personal use." For example, a United Kingdom citizen must be permitted to bring personal supplies of a product into France, whether or not he or she obtained those supplies from a source that would have been lawful in France, and he must also be able to establish himself or herself in France and continue to obtain supplies from the United Kingdom for his or her personal use in France. Recital 4 derives from those facts that it is important that the conditions of supply in France and the United Kingdom should be harmonised but it is not easy to discover any logical basis for that conclusion rather than for the conclusion that such trans-border transactions should be permitted under the national laws of the Member States. The background to recital 4 seems to be the restrictive rules in force in Germany in respect of the import of pharmaceuticals for

---

1.   OJ L113 30.4.92 p5. See Appendix 11 post.
2.   OJ L11 17.1.92 p38. See Appendix 13 post.

personal use. The German restrictions have been condemned in two separate judgments of the European Court of Justice[1] but recital 4 in effect expresses the hope that the difficulties which have arisen could be eradicated if harmonised standards were adopted.

Recital 5 makes a much more straightforward point, that under the Future System proposals certain products will be authorised by the Community on a Community-wide basis. For that purpose at least, it is necessary to lay down a classification of medicinal products to be applied to those products. On the other hand, it is not obvious that such classification needs to be generally applied to products which continue to be marketed and authorised on a national basis. In addition, article 8 states that the Directive is addressed to the Member States, not to the Community institutions, in accordance with article 189 of the EC Treaty so that the Directive is clearly not itself binding on the institutions. The terms of article 3(1) to (4) are incorporated by reference into the Community authorisation procedure by article 9(3)(b) of Regulation (EEC) 2309/93[2] but there is no reason why they could not have been included within the terms of that Regulation.

Overall, in fact, the justifications for the Directive offered by recitals 1 to 5 are weak, and it is easy to see why that should be so : the supply of medicinal products to end consumers is essentially a local matter conducted within the individual Member States; the examples given in recital 4 are obviously of marginal significance; and there is therefore no obvious reason why the current national rules should not continue in force. It is only where mandatory Community rules come into force whose application is affected by the legal classification of medicinal products, as is the case with the new rules on advertising and with marketing authorisations at a Community level, that there is a need for common rules.

That lack of justification is reflected in the minimal degree of harmonisation in fact required. Recital 6 makes it clear that the Directive constitutes only "an initial step" establishing harmonised "basic principles applicable to the classification for the supply of medicinal products in the Community or in the Member State concerned". It also states that those principles are based on :

"principles already established on this subject by the Council of Europe as well as the work of harmonisation completed within the framework of the United Nations, concerning narcotic and psychotropic substances".

Those references are not explained in the Directive, but they refer :

(1) in respect of the Council of Europe, to the Resolution of the Committee of Ministers (Partial Agreement in the Social and Public Health Field), AP (89) 3, on the classification of medicines which are obtainable only on medical prescription; this Resolution sets out a detailed list of such products;

(2) in respect of the United Nations, to the Single Convention on Narcotic Drugs 1961 and the Convention on Psychotropic Substances 1971.

Recital 7 makes it clear that the classification of a medicinal product in accordance with the Directive does not affect "the national social security arrangements for reimbursement or payment for medicinal products on prescription". That would

---

1.   Case 215/87 *Schumacher v Hauptzollamt Frankfurt* [1989] ECR 617 and Case C-62/90 *Commission v Germany* [1992] ECR I-2575, require the free movement of such products, at least where the products in question were obtained from a pharmacist in the home State and, if a prescription-only product, had been prescribed by a medical doctor.

2.   OJ L214 24.8.93 p1. See Appendix 5 post.

apply not only to national classifications made for the purposes of national marketing authorisation but also to classifications made for the purposes of Community wide authorisation : see also article 1 of Regulation (EEC) 2309/93 and article 3 of Directive (EEC) 65/65[1], as amended by Directive (EEC) 93/39[2]. In the present state of development of the Community, nothing obliges a Member State to pay for any particular treatment, regardless of the procedure of authorisation of the product concerned and regardless of that product's classification.

14.2   Scope and definitions : article 1

Article 1 defines the scope of the Directive. Article 1(1) states the subject matter of the Directive to be a twofold classification of medicinal products for the purpose of supply for human use in the Community : "medicinal products subject to medical prescription" (referred to in this Chapter as "prescription only products"); and "medicinal products not subject to medical prescription" (referred to in this Chapter as "non-prescription products"). Article 1(2) defines the two essential terms used in the Directive : "medicinal product" and "medicinal prescription." "Medicinal product" is defined by reference to article 1 of Directive (EEC) 65/65, discussed in Chapter 2 above; it should be noted that there is no limitation on the "medicinal products" subject to Directive (EEC) 92/26, so that it differs in that respect from the other Rational Use Directives which are all limited in their scope to products falling within the scope of Chapters II to V of Directive (EEC) 65/65, in practice products subject to industrial manufacture and therefore to marketing authorisation under article 3 of Directive (EEC) 65/65.

"Medical prescription"[3] is defined to mean :

> "any prescription issued by a professional person qualified to prescribe medicinal products".

That definition clearly does not attempt to define the term "prescription" and the definition of "medical" is unexpected. It would have been natural to expect that a "medical prescription" would be a prescription *of medicinal products* but that does not form part of the definition[4]. Instead the definition relates to all prescriptions, not limited to prescriptions of medicinal products, which are "issued" by a specific category of persons. Clearly a doctor is the paradigm case of "a professional person qualified to prescribe medicinal products" but the definition is sufficiently broad and general to permit other categories of professional to be authorised by the individual Member States to prescribe medicinal products. The only other purpose of the definition appears to be to exclude "prescriptions" made by persons who do not enjoy the relevant qualifications under national law. The Directive does not attempt to specify which persons should be regarded as so qualified.

14.3   Classification and classification criteria : articles 2 to 4

Article 2(1) requires the competent national or Community authorities to classify medicinal products, on the grant of marketing authorisation, into prescription only and non-prescription products, applying the criteria laid down in article 3 of the

---

1.   OJ No 22 9.2.65 p369/65. See Appendix 1 post.
2.   OJ L21424.8.93 p22.
3.   There is a misprint in the Official Journal text, where the definition is said to be of "medicinal prescription."
4.   The fact that the definition is sufficiently broad to include, e g, prescription of a wheelchair or a sling does not matter for the purposes of the Directive which is in practice solely concerned with the classification of medicinal products.

Directive. Article 2(2) grants the competent authorities the power to sub-categorise prescription only products into three further sub-classifications :

"(a) medicinal products on renewable or non-renewable medical prescription;

(b) medicinal products subject to special medical prescription;

(c) medicinal products on restricted medical prescription, reserved for use in certain specialised areas."

No further guidance is given in the Directive as to when category (a) would be appropriate; presumably a product should be categorised as "non-renewable" where there was a known or possible risk of adverse effects in the event that the product was taken over a prolonged period without proper medical supervision. Categories (b) and (c) are subject to article 3(2) and (3) discussed below. It should be noted that the Member States (and the Community authorities) have only a limited discretion : they can either make only a twofold classification or they can make that classification with three specified sub-categories in respect of prescription only products. They cannot apparently pick and choose within the sub-categories, nor can they adopt further categories of their own invention[1].

Article 3 sets out criteria for the operation of the system of classification introduced by article 2. Article 3(1) gives four alternative criteria for classification as prescription only medicinal products, requiring products to be so classified if any one of the following criteria is satisfied in respect of them :

"— ... likely to present a danger either directly or indirectly, even when used correctly, if utilised without medical supervision, or

— ... frequently and to a very wide extent used incorrectly, and as a result ... likely to present a direct or indirect danger to human health, or

— [they] contain substances or preparations thereof the activity and/or side effects of which require further investigation, or

— ... normally prescribed by a doctor to be administered parenterally."

Nothing in article 3(1) restricts any further criteria which a competent authority may apply, so that the criteria specified are in practice "minimum requirements."

Article 3(2) and (3) set out "factors" to be taken into account by Member States which provide for the sub-categories of "products subject to special medical prescription" and "restricted prescription" respectively, in accordance with article 2(2)(b) and (c)[2]. The factors to be taken into account in respect of "special prescription" are that the product :

"— ... contains, in a non-exempt quantity, a substance classified as a narcotic or a psychotropic substance within the meaning of the international conventions in force (United Nations Conventions of 1961 and 1971), or

— ... is likely, if incorrectly used, to present a substantial risk of medicinal abuse, to lead to addiction or be misused for illegal purposes, or

---

1. However, article 3(4) extends the discretion of the competent authorities by permitting specific exceptions to be granted for particular products: see below.
2. The possibility of such classifications being granted by the Community itself is provided for by article 13(3) of Regulation (EEC) 2309/93, which permits products to be "authorised only for use in hospitals or for prescription by some specialists." The Regulation does not expressly provide for category (a) under article 2(2) of the Directive but the CPMP is given wide powers by article 9(3)(b) of the Regulation to suggest "conditions or restrictions which should be imposed on the supply or use of the medicinal product concerned." The CPMP's discretion in this regard appears to be unfettered, unlike that of the competent national authorities.

— ... contains a substance which, by reason of its novelty or properties, could be considered as belonging to that group as a precautionary measure."

No guidance is given as to the significance of classification as a "special prescription" product, whether the product's availability is limited to special sales outlets or is administered by medical practitioners directly, or whether only a limited class of medical practitioners are permitted to prescribe such products, or practitioners generally but only under special conditions. Those issues are again left to the national (or Community) competent authorities.

Article 3(3) sets out the factors to be taken into account in classifying a product as "subject to restricted prescription." The product :

"... because of its pharmaceutical characteristics or novelty or in the interests of public health, is reserved for treatments which can only be followed in a hospital environment,

... is used in the treatment of conditions which must be diagnosed in a hospital environment or in institutions with adequate diagnostic facilities, although administration and follow-up my be carried out elsewhere, or

... is intended for outpatients but its use may produce very serious side-effects requiring a prescription drawn up as required by a specialist and special supervision throughout the treatment."

This category appears to be a matter of common sense : certain treatments are so serious or complex that they can only sensibly be administered under constant medical supervision and with immediate access to specialist facilities and staff.

Article 3(4) and (5) significantly qualify the scheme established by article 2 and article 3(1) to (3). Article 3(4) permits the relevant competent authority to "waive application" of paragraphs (1) to (3) of article 3 having regard to :

"(a) the maximum single dose, the maximum daily dose, the strength, the pharmaceutical form, certain types of packaging; and/or

(b) other circumstances of use which it has specified".

In practice, that provision would give the Member States a wide discretion to permit specific medicinal products to be supplied without prescription, or on an ordinary doctor's prescription, under specified conditions. That discretion would operate at the time of issue of the product's marketing authorisation and would offer the possibility of a far wider range of classifications than article 2 appears to permit.

Article 3(5) limits the discretion of a competent authority that chooses to operate the simplest system of categorisation of medicinal products in accordance with article 2(1), merely distinguishing prescription only and non-prescription products. Such an authority is required nonetheless to take into account the factors (referred to as "criteria" at article 3(5)) set out at article 3(2) and (3), in deciding whether or not a product should be supplied only on prescription. It is not easy to see how a product to which any of those factors applied could fail to be caught in any event by at least one of the criteria set out in article 3(1). That may imply that the authorities are in practice encouraged by the Directive to operate the more complex scheme described in article 2(2) and article 3(2) and (3).

Article 4 simply states that "[m]edicinal products not subject to prescription shall be those which do not meet the criteria listed in article 3." Strictly, only article 3(1) contains "criteria" to determine whether or not a medicinal product is subject to medical prescription, but article 4, like article 3(5), appears to treat all the criteria/factors as equally applicable to the issue of whether or not a product should be subject to prescription. The significance of article 4 lies in the fact that it appears to preclude the possibility, left open by article 3, of other criteria being applied to a product by a competent authority in addition to those laid down in article 3. Article 4 does therefore ensure that a significant degree of harmonisation will in practice be achieved in the administrative practices of the various authorities.

14.4   Administrative provisions : articles 5 to 8

Article 5 imposes certain administrative obligations on the competent authorities. Article 5(1) requires those authorities to draw up, and to update annually, a list of prescription only products, specifying the category of classification if necessary, that is, where the discretion granted by article 2(2) is exercised. Article 5(2) requires them to "examine and, as appropriate, amend the classification of a medicinal product, by applying the criteria listed in article 3" either (i) when the product's marketing authorisation is renewed after five years, in accordance with article 10 of Directive (EEC) 65/65 (or article 13(1) of Regulation (EEC) 2309/93), or (ii) when new facts are brought to their notice. The Directive does not specify any transitional measures but the effect of article 5 will be that the provisions of article 2 will gradually be brought into operation in respect of products which have been issued with marketing authorisations prior to the coming into effect of the Directive as each product's authorisation is renewed after the expiry of the relevant five-year period.

Article 6(1) further requires that the lists referred to in article 5(1) shall be communicated by the Member States to the Commission, and, on request, to the other Member States, within two years of the adoption of the Directive, that is, by 31 March 1994. Article 6(2) requires that the Member States shall communicate changes to the list to the Commission and to the other Member States. Article 6(2) does not limit the obligation to supply information only to those Member States that request it but it would seem pointless to supply information of changes to a list where the list itself had not been supplied. With regard to products authorised under the new Regulation (EEC) 2309/93 procedures, article 9(3)(b) and article 10 of the Regulation ensure that the Commission and the Member States would be aware of the classification of each individual product at the time of authorisation by the Community. There is no obligation on the Community to compile or supply a list of the classification of such products to the national authorities but it is clearly important that those authorities should know the conditions under which the products are to be supplied to the public.

Article 6(3) provides for the Commission to submit a report to the Council on the application of the Directive within four years of its adoption, that is, by 31 March 1996, accompanied, if necessary by "appropriate proposals".

Article 7 requires the Member States to implement the Directive by 31 January 1993 though, as stated above, the Directive will have no immediate effect on products which were already authorised prior to that date. The Member States will only be required to give effect to the Directive in respect of such products when their authorisations fall to be renewed after five years[1].

---

1.   See article 5 discussed above.

Chapter 15 : Directive (EEC) 92/27[1] - Labelling and Package Leaflets for Authorised Products

15.1   Introduction : the recitals

Although many foods and cosmetics provide some guidance as to their nutritional contents and as to how they should be consumed or applied on their outer packaging, failure to abide by those instructions does not normally have disastrous consequences and, particularly in the case of foods, consumption of excessive quantities of a food rarely causes any lasting damaging consequences[2]. By contrast, the correct use of a medicinal product is in general essential for its effectiveness and incorrect use can have immediate and drastic harmful effects.

In addition, the existence of the various Community languages and the considerable diversity of approaches to the marketing of medicinal products between the Member States has meant that divergences in labelling and package leaflets is a significant impediment to free trade in such products[3].

As a result, the provision of adequate information on the labelling and outer packaging of such products and the harmonisation of national rules have always been concerns of the Community. Minimum requirements were imposed on the Member States by Chapter IV of Directive (EEC) 65/65[4] and further requirements, particularly in respect of package leaflets, were introduced by articles 6 and 7 of Directive (EEC) 75/319[5]. Those rules thus formed an integral part of the initial authorisation process introduced by those Directives in respect of the marketing of medicinal products within the Member States of the Community.

Recitals 2, 3 and 4 of Council Directive (EEC) 92/27 on the labelling of medicinal products for human use and on package leaflets make it clear that the Directive is intended (i) to supplement the previous Community rules and to give details in respect of the presentation of the information that has to be included, and (ii) to bring the provisions on labelling and package leaflets into a single text[6].

Recital 1 contains standard 1992 Programme wording in respect of the creation of the internal market, while recitals 5 and 6 set out the principles upon which the Directive is based :

---

1.   OJ L113 30.4.92 p8. See Appendix 12 post.
2.   These remarks are true only at a high level of generality. There are obvious counter-examples, such as frozen meats or foods for young children, where detailed instructions are necessary as to proper preparation.
3.   The difficulties that have arisen in respect of intellectual property rights, and their interaction with the Community rules on competition and free movement of goods, fall outside the scope of this work. They are considered in detail in the standard works on those subjects identified in Chapter 1.
4.   OJ L22 9.2.65 p369. See Appendix 1 post.
5.   OJ L147 9.6.75 p13. See Appendix 3 post.
6.   Article 13 of the Directive in fact repeals articles 13 to 20 of Directive (EEC) 65/65 and articles 6 and 7 of Directive (EEC) 75/319, so Directive (EEC) 92/27 is a rare phenomenon, a true consolidated piece of legislation enacted by the Community.

"Whereas the provisions governing the information supplied to users should provide a high degree of consumer protection, in order that medicinal products may be used correctly on the basis of full and comprehensible information;

Whereas the marketing of medicinal products whose labelling and package leaflets comply with this Directive should not be prohibited or impeded on grounds connected with the labelling or package leaflet."

The Directive is thus presented as a true harmonisation measure, setting high common standards in all Member States and giving the Member States no discretion to apply different standards, even if those standards would imply a higher degree of consumer protection, where the terms of the Directive are satisfied. The extent to which variations will remain is discussed below.

Given the links between the Directive and Directives (EEC) 65/65 and 75/319, the inclusion of the Directive in the Rational Use package is particularly misleading. The Directive in fact forms an integral part of the Future System package, and is referred to in both Regulation (EEC) 2309/93[1] (at article 9(1) and (3)(c), and article 11) and in Directive (EEC) 65/65 as amended (at article 4, point 11). In fact, articles 10 and 11 of Directive (EEC) 92/27 represent a serious anomaly in the Future System regime, in that they contradict the specific wording of article 21 of Directive (EEC) 65/65, which requires that a marketing authorisation "shall not be refused, suspended or revoked except on the grounds set out in [Directive (EEC) 65/65]." Articles 10 and 11 of Directive (EEC) 92/27 provide for such steps to be taken where the rules laid down by the Directive have not been followed[2].

Directive (EEC) 92/27 consists of four Chapters : I. Scope and definitions; II. Labelling of medicinal products; III. Package leaflets; and IV. General and final provisions. Chapters II and III, in particular articles 2, 3 and 7, consist of extensive lists of information that must be included on immediate labelling and package leaflets respectively.

15.2 Scope and definitions : Chapter I, article 1

Article 1 consists of two paragraphs. Article 1(1) states the scope of the Directive :

"This Directive deals with the labelling of medicinal products for human use and leaflets inserted in packages of such products, to which Chapters II, III, IV and V of Directive (EEC) 65/65 apply."

The scope of the Directive is thus determined by article 1(2) and article 2 of Directive (EEC) 65/65[3] and is the same as that of Directives (EEC) 92/25 and 92/28[4]. The most important categories of product excluded from the scope of the

---

1. OJ L214 24.8.93 p1. See Appendix 5 post.
2. That anomaly was considered in passing by the European Court of Justice in Case C-83/92 *Pierrel v Ministero della Sanita*, (not yet reported in the ECR; (1993) Transcript 7 December, OJ C18 21.1.94 p3). The Court considered that article 21 cannot be limited to its literal wording but must be extended to apply to all applicable provisions of Community law. That is obviously a highly unsatisfactory and uncertain state of affairs : the specific case of Directive (EEC) 92/27 is exceptional, in that the Directive replaces the provisions of Directive (EEC) 65/65 itself in respect of labelling, but the Court does not restrict its finding to such a case. The true answer is of course that the legislation was drafted without sufficient consideration of the effects of consolidation. For the wording of article 21, see section 3.2 ante.
3. See Chapters 2 and 3 ante.
4. OJ L113 30.4.92 pp1-4, 13-18. See Appendices 10 and 13 and Chapters 13 and 16.

Directive are in practice products prepared by pharmacists specifically for their own patients[1].

Article 1(2) sets out a series of definitions, each of which requires brief discussion :

> "— *name of the medicinal product* means the name given to a medicinal product, which may be either an invented name or a common or scientific name, together with a trade mark or the name of the manufacturer; the invented name shall not be liable to confusion with the common name;
> — *common name* means the international non-proprietary name recommended by the World Health Organisation, or, if one does not exist, the usual common name".

The name of a medicinal product is clearly very important not only for the identification of a product by a doctor, pharmacist or, in the case of non-prescription products, by the consumer, but also for the marketing of a product. There are also a variety of different categories of name, of which the most important appear to be[2] :

(1) a brand name for a specific product, of which examples would be products such as "Disprin", "Savlon", "Strepsil";

(2) a brand name for a range of products, such as "Sudafed" available in tablet form or in solution;

(3) well-known and simple scientific names, such as "Aspirin", "Paracetamol" or "Milk of Magnesia";

(4) less well-known but commercially recognised "generic" names such as "cimetidine" or "acyclovir";

(5) simple descriptive names, such as "Bronchial Cough Mixture".

Further complications of great commercial and practical significance arise from : any associated name of a well-known manufacturer or retailer ("Beechams Powders", "Boots' Bronchial Cough Mixture"); any associated trade mark (for example, the sword within a circle surrounding the name "Disprin"); and the details of the presentation of the product (for example, "Savlon" in a pale blue tube with clear white lettering). The definitions of "name of the medicinal product" and "common name" are not so wide as to cover the detailed presentation of the product but they are intended to cover all the major categories of name and to include names incorporating references to the manufacturer of the product or, as is very common, involving the use of trade marks.

The general definition of "name of the medicinal product" envisages two possible types of name : an "invented" name or a "common or scientific" name. Invented names clearly correspond to categories (1) and (2) identified above, names such as "Disprin" or "Sudafed". "Common or scientific" appears from the wording of the

1.   See article 2(3) and article 1(4) and (5) of Directive (EEC) 65/65, discussed in Chapter 3. Somewhat anomalously, article 13 of Directive (EEC) 92/27 repeals all the articles, 13 to 20, of Chapter IV of Directive (EEC) 65/65, so that the reference in article 1(1) of Directive (EEC) 92/27 to Chapter IV of Directive (EEC) 65/65 is simply to the heading, "Chapter IV : Labelling of medicinal products."

2.   In what follows, as an aid to clarity, some elementary examples are given of medicinal products likely to be familiar to consumers in the United Kingdom (none of the references should be taken as any form of recommendation or criticism of any particular product or its labelling or package leaflet).

definition to refer to two alternative formulations of the same type of name, and the difference between them is explained by the definition of "common name". Some medicinal products, particularly those with only a single active ingredient, have an established name. Examples are very widely used products such as "aspirin" or "paracetamol"; likewise "cimetidine" is the name given to the medicinal compound originally marketed as "Tagamet"; and "acyclovir" is the active ingredient in the product marketed as "Zovirax". The definition of "common name" specifies that such names shall be those recommended by the World Health Organisation. Other products, in particular those which are neither sold under a brand nor consist of a single active ingredient, are sold under simple descriptive names, such as "Bronchial Cough Mixture" (a hybrid would be "Soluble Aspirin"). Such names are examples of the second limb of the definition of "common name", the "usual common name" to be used in the absence of a WHO recommendation.

It thus appears that "scientific" is not truly an alternative to "common" name but rather a sub-category of "common name". It should be noted that even the internationally recognised WHO name is likely to be an abbreviated version at best of a chemically accurate name specifying the actual composition of the compound in question.

The general definition of "name of the medicinal product" includes not only the name itself, whether invented or common, but also "a trade mark or the name of the manufacturer". The definition is misleadingly drafted. The idea must be that *if* a name consists of or involves the use of a trade mark (as in the case of "Disprin" and the associated sword within a circle) then that trade mark forms part of the name for the purposes of the Directive. Likewise, if a manufacturer links his name with the name of the product then that also forms part of the name (as in "Boots' Bronchial Cough Mixture). It would be entirely contrary to normal practice in the industry or commercial practice generally to require manufacturers (as article 2 of the Directive would do in the case of the "name" if the wording was taken literally) to call all their products by trade marked names and to add their own name to the name of the product[1].

The definition of "name" finally requires that "the invented name shall not be liable to confusion with the common name". The purpose of that requirement is clearly to prevent the owner of intellectual property rights over the "invented name" - used to market the product during the period of patent protection - to retain extensive rights (and in particular trade mark rights) over a scientifically (as against commercially) recognised name after the period of such protection. The effect is thus to permit the emergence of generic competitors using the common name to compete with the established brand of the original manufacturer. Implementation of such a requirement is clearly a highly subjective matter and there are as yet few principles developed at the level of Community law[2].

---

1.   It should be noted that the name may include the name of the manufacturer (ie the person authorised under article 16 of Directive (EEC) 75/319) not the name of the "person responsible for placing the medicinal product on the market (ie the person authorised under articles 3 and 4 of Directive (EEC) 65/65).

2.   Though see Advocate-General Jacobs' discussion of confusingly similar names in his Opinion in Case C-10/89 SA CNL-SUCAL NV v HAG GF AG ("Hag II") [1990] ECR I-3711, paras 33 to 36 at 3738-2741. Given the notoriously restrictive rules applied by the German Courts in trade mark cases, manufacturers obviously consider the matter carefully : and see now Case C-317/91 *Deutsche Renault AG v AUDI AG,* judgment of 30 November 1993 (not yet reported in the ECR; (1993) Transcript 30 November, OJ C1 4.1.94 p8). The difficult issues which arise in relation to parallel imports and market partition, where a manufacturer uses a *different* trade mark and get up for essentially identical products marketed in different Member States, fall outside the scope of this work. See the standard works on EC competition law cited in Chapter 1 for discussion of those issues.

"— *strength of the medicinal product* means the content of the active ingredient expressed quantitatively per dosage unit, per unit of volume or weight according to the dosage form".

That definition is straightforward : for a product in tablet form, the strength of the product will be the quantity of active ingredient in each tablet (for example, each Disprin tablet contains "Aspirin Ph. Eur. 300mg"); for a product in solution, the strength will be the quantity of active ingredient in a small measure of the product (for example, one teaspoonful of Boots' Bronchial Cough Mixture contains : "Ammonium Chloride B.P. 150 mg ... Ammonium Carbonate 100 mg ... Guaisphenesin 32.5 mg."); whereas the strength of ointments, because they are not administered in precise volumes, is expressed as a percentage (for example, Zovirax contains "Acyclovir 5% w/w").

"— *immediate packaging* means the container or other form of packaging immediately in contact with the medicinal product,
— *outer packaging* means the packaging into which is placed the immediate packaging".

These are self-evident definitions, but they have considerable importance in the Directive because of the difficulties that arise where a small "immediate" package is used that is capable of being removed from the outer packaging, in particular in the case of tablets packaged in "blister packs". Most medicinal products sold directly to the public comprise a cardboard box containing either a glass or plastic container of liquid, a metal or plastic tube of ointment or tablets contained either loose within a plastic or glass container or individually packaged in a foil blister pack. The inner container is inevitably smaller than the outer container with the result that less information can be fitted on that inner container. However, the outer container is often thrown away soon after purchase (the same is true of the package leaflet) so that the immediate packaging is particularly important as the sole item that is virtually guaranteed to be present at the time when the product is finally prepared for administration to the patient.

"— *labelling* means information on the immediate or outer packaging,
— *package leaflet* means a leaflet containing information for the user which accompanies the medicinal product".

The definition of "labelling" is surprising : one would naturally consider "labelling" to mean either the same as "label" or else the process of attaching a label to something, but the Directive states that "labelling means information". The thrust of the definition is that "labelling" for the purposes of the Directive comprises not merely the attaching of a name or label to a medicinal product but the entire process of affixing the necessary written text (or other pictorial representation) to the packaging of the product to enable it to be used safely and effectively by consumers of that product. The definition of "package leaflet" is self-explanatory.

The final definition is of "manufacturer" and makes reference to articles 16 and 22 of Directive (EEC) 75/319[1]. In summary, article 16 imposes the fundamental Community requirement that manufacturers and importers of medicinal products obtain national authorisation from the relevant competent authorities, whereas article 22 concerns batch inspections of manufactured products. The definition of manufacturer at article 1 of Directive (EEC) 92/27 states that he is the person "on behalf of whom the qualified person has performed the specific obligations laid down in article 22 of [Directive (EEC) 75/319]". That is strange wording for a definition (for all other purposes, the manufacturer is sufficiently identified by article 16 of Directive (EEC) 75/319 alone) but the purpose of the "definition"

---

1.   See Chapter 10 ante.

appears to be to draw attention to the fact that, in the context of labelling and package leaflets, it is crucial that the actual product contained in the specific packaging (upon which the information contained in such labelling and such leaflets is printed) (i) conforms to the information stated on the labelling or leaflet and (ii) is of the requisite quality.

15.3   Labelling : Chapter II, articles 2 to 5

Article 2(1) contains a list of fourteen particulars which "shall appear on the outer packaging of medicinal products or, where there is no outer packaging, on the immediate packaging". Those particulars are set out at Appendix 12 hereto, but in summary they concern : (a) the name of the product; (b) a statement of the active ingredients; (c) the pharmaceutical form of the product (tablets, ointment, etc) and contents; (d) the excipients; (e) the method and route of administration; (f) a warning to keep the product out of the reach of children; (g) other necessary special warnings; (h) the month of expiry; (i) any special storage precautions; (j) any special disposal precautions; (k) the name and address of the holder of the marketing authorisation; (l) the number of the marketing authorisation (in the United Kingdom, the product licence number); (m) the manufacturer's batch number; and (n) instructions on the use of the product if intended for self-medication.

Article 2(1)(b), (c), (f), (h), (k), (l) and (m) are straightforward and mandatory, not only in the sense that article 2 itself is in mandatory terms but also because the wording of the particulars is unconditional. Particular (e) only requires the route of administration of a product to be specified "if necessary"; (g) only requires a special warning "if this is necessary for the medicinal product concerned"; (h) requires special storage precautions, "if any", to be stated; (i) requires special disposal precautions for unused products or waste materials to be stated "if appropriate"; and (n) gives no guidance on when a product is to be regarded as used for "self-medication". The last case is different from the others in that it is essentially a definitional matter : it does not appear to correspond to the distinction between "prescription only" and "non-prescription" products established by Directive (EEC) 92/26; if that is correct then it must presumably be a matter of common sense to determine whether a product is administered (in general at least) at home by patients themselves or whether it is normally administered only under medical supervision (for example specialist anaesthetic products only used in practice in hospitals)[1].

In the other cases, a degree of discretion is granted in determining whether or not particular information must be present on the packaging of a product but no guidance is given as to how or by whom that discretion is to be exercised. The labelling of a product is finalised under Directive (EEC) 65/65, and now Regulation (EEC) 2309/93, after the detailed exchange of information specified by articles 4, 4a and 4b of Directive (EEC) 65/65, between the applicant for marketing authorisation and the relevant competent authority. Point 9 of article 4 and article 4a set out in considerable detail information that is to be given to the competent authorities in the form of a "summary of product characteristics" and "specimens or mock-ups of the sales presentation of the product", including details of such matters as special precautions for use, storage and disposal. It is clearly at that stage that the detailed application of article 2 of Directive (EEC) 92/27 will fall to be determined, ultimately by negotiation between the applicant and the relevant authority.

Article 2(1)(a) is more complex, requiring the following information to appear :

---

1.   Article 12(1) provides for Commission guidelines on "particular information needs relating to self-medication" but not for any specification of the meaning of "self-medication."

"the name of the medicinal product followed by the common name where the product contains only one active ingredient and if its name is an invented name; where a medicinal product is available in several pharmaceutical forms and/or several strengths, the pharmaceutical form and/or strength (baby, child or adult as appropriate) must be included in the name of the medicinal product".

The use of the words "followed by" would suggest that the "invented" name and the common name of a product with only a single active ingredient should appear one after the other, eg "Disprin Aspirin" or "Sudafed Pseudoephedrine Hydrochloride BP", but that is clearly not the practice of the industry and would be commercially ridiculous. Given that particular (b) requires that the active ingredients of the product must be stated in the labelling, it is hard to see what purpose is served by this further requirement in the case of products with only a single active ingredient. If "followed by" merely means that, as is natural, the "invented" name appears on the front of the packaging and the common name appears either lower down on the front or on the back of the packaging, the requirement apparently adds nothing to particular (b)[1].

Particular (a) also introduces a further classification, not otherwise present in the Community pharmaceutical legislation and in particular not contained in Directive (EEC) 92/26 on the classification of medicinal products, between "baby", "child" and "adult" products. Given that Directive (EEC) 92/27 is intended to be a comprehensive harmonisation Directive, it is not satisfactory to have such a classification introduced without any criteria laid down at the Community level as to the basis upon which a product is to be classified in this respect[2].

Article 2(1)(d) concerns excipients, and requires that those excipients are listed which are "known to have a recognised action or effect and included in the guidelines published pursuant to article 12". The first part of this wording is redundant since it is not an alternative to the second part and article 12(1), fifth indent, specifies "the list of excipients which must feature on the labelling of medicinal products and the way these excipients must be indicated". In the absence of such guidelines (which article 12(1) requires the Commission to publish "as necessary"), the first sentence of particular (d) appears to have no effect.

Article 2(1)(d) has one specific requirement : "if the product is injectable, or a topical or eye preparation, all excipients must be stated". In that context, "topical" means that the product is applied to a specific part of the body. It is easy to see that there should be specific requirements in respect of sensitive parts of the body such as the eye or the rectum; it is less easy to see why it is necessary to identify *all* the excipients in, for example, athlete's foot solution or cream. The requirement does not appear to be observed in practice, at least in the case of common household products available in the United Kingdom.

Article 2(2) permits the outer packaging (and therefore, presumably, the immediate packaging where there is no outer packaging : see article 2(1)) to include :

---

1.   It is now common practice, at least for products containing aspirin and paracetamol, to have a statement in bold print stating "CONTAINS ASPIRIN/PARACETAMOL" on the outer packaging. That might suggest that particular (a) only applies in this respect in the case of products containing generally known products (it is hard to see how it would assist the consumer to have a complex scientific name stated twice on the packaging) but the wording does not support such an interpretation.
2.   It is a further minor anomaly that particular (a) requires that this classification be included in the name of the product where several strengths are available, whereas the definition of the "name of the medicinal product" in article 1 makes no mention of this possibility.

"symbols or pictograms designed to clarify certain information mentioned in paragraph 1 and other information compatible with the summary of the product characteristics which is useful for health education, to the exclusion of any element of a promotional nature."

This provision is straightforward in relation to "symbols or pictograms", permitting them for clarification purposes. That appears to exclude, for example, a picture of a sad face beside the symptoms that the product is intended to combat and a picture of a happy face beside the beneficial effects claimed for the product. The general provision in respect of "other information" is more problematic : there is clearly room for argument concerning the meaning of the expressions "useful for health education" and "any element of a promotional nature". Claims that a product acts "fast" or that it avoids certain side-effects normally associated with a particular type of treatment are clearly intended as attractive marketing features of the product. Likewise, claims that a product contains an "improved formula" or has a "new improved taste" are commonplace and hard to characterise as excluding "any element of a promotional nature." On the other hand, if the claims are true, then it can be argued that it is "useful for health education" that consumers are made aware of these facts. There is considerable scope for disputes between regulatory authorities and applicants for authorisation as to the precise interpretation of article 2(2).

Article 3 sets out special rules in respect of immediate packaging. Article 2(1) had specified that the particulars set out therein must appear on immediate packaging where there was no outer packaging. Article 3(1) further requires that those particulars appear on "immediate packaging other than those referred to in paragraphs 2 and 3." Article 3(2) applies to "immediate packaging which take the form of blister packs and are placed in an outer packaging that complies with the requirements laid down in article 2". It thus appears that if a product was issued in a blister pack *without* an outer packaging (which may be unlikely in practice) then article 2 would apply to the pack. Where article 3(2) applies, only four particulars are required to be present : the name of the product "as laid down in article 2(a)" (the reference is clearly to article 2(1)(a)); the name of the holder of the marketing authorisation; the expiry date; and the batch number. Strict observation of the requirements of article 3(2) would require considerable changes in the manufacturing practices of pharmaceutical companies, many of which have hitherto been content simply to affix the name of the product, perhaps with the logo of the company, in a recurrent pattern onto the foil backing of the pack. If article 2(1)(a) is to be applied strictly to blister packs, so that it will be necessary in future to state the common name of a product with only one active ingredient, the pharmaceutical form of a product which is available in several forms, and the classification as baby, child or adult strength where different strengths are available, then further complexity will be added.

Article 3(3) concerns "small immediate packaging units on which the particulars laid down in article 2 cannot be displayed"[1]. It appears that article 3(3) applies to packaging units whether or not they are placed in an outer packaging unit and, if so, whether or not that outer packaging complies with article 2. No guidance is given to the Member States to enable them to determine whether or not the particulars laid down in article 2 can or cannot be displayed on a particular "unit", but article 4(1) of the Directive requires that the particulars on labelling should be "easily legible" and article 12(1), third indent, provides for the possibility of the Commission issuing guidelines on "the legibility of particulars on the labelling and package leaflet." In practice, there must be specified minimum sizes for lettering and for spacing between words and lines and also specified proportions of the

---

1.   Obvious examples would be small sachets of powder.

surface area of the packaging unit in question, allowance being made for the presence of the brand or trade mark of the product and, perhaps, bar coding.

Where article 3(3) applies, the following particulars must be given : the name of the product and, if necessary, the strength and the route of administration; the method of administration; the expiry date; the batch number; and the contents by weight, volume or unit. It is not clear why neither the name of the holder of the marketing authorisation nor the name of the product has to conform to article 2(1)(a) of the Directive. In those respects, article 3(3) is less demanding that article 3(2) in respect of blister packs. By contrast, it is not clear why blister packs do not have to specify the strength or contents of the units contained in each "blister"; though it may be thought that the method of administration of the contents of a blister pack will always be the same, which will not be true of the contents of a "small immediate packaging unit".

Article 4(1) requires that "the particulars referred to in articles 2 and 3 shall be easily legible, clearly comprehensible and indelible". Legibility has already been considered in respect of article 3(3) and article 12(1) : in practice, the only issues likely to arise in respect of an industrially produced product are the size of the print and the spacing between words and lines. Comprehensibility presumably refers primarily to the content of the information rather than its presentation and must relate to the needs of the patient : for example, it must be easy to understand how to use the product safely and effectively and what to do if the product proves unsatisfactory in use. Indelibility is only normally a problem in respect of the batch number and the expiry date, which must be changed with each batch and each month respectively. That problem is overcome in practice by the use of punched lettering or, less satisfactorily, by ink stamping of individual products. The greatest problems are likely to arise in respect of the new requirements that all blister packs and small packaging units should bear the expiry date and batch number of the product in question.

Article 4(2) concerns the language in which the particulars are to be given. They must appear "in the official language or languages of the Member State where the product is placed on the market". That requirement, apart from the difficulties it causes in Belgium, where all products must automatically carry twice as much written material (other than names and dates) as in other Member States, is clearly a severe impediment to the free movement of pharmaceuticals between the Member States. However, article 4 contains no qualification of the requirement (for example, to limit the requirement to the most generally understood languages within the Community) and the safety aspect of the pharmaceutical legislation makes it difficult to see how the requirement could be limited.

Instead, the second sentence of article 4(2) makes it clear that nothing (except physical space on the packaging) prevents the particulars "from being indicated in several languages, provided that the same particulars appear in all the languages used". The equivalent provision in respect of package leaflets, article 8, is of some importance, because in that case space is less limited; in the case of labelling, the suggestion appears to be of no general significance. The only way in which the problem could be significantly reduced in the foreseeable future would seem to be to introduce a category of fundamental information that must be given in each official language of the Member States where the product is to be marketed and to qualify that requirement in respect of less fundamental information. The other alternative, the extended use of pictograms or non-linguistic symbols common to all Member States, seems unlikely to be of great general assistance. It is only in the case of blister packs covered by article 3(2) that it seems likely that a common finished product will in practice be marketable in each Member State of the Community and even in that case the pack must be placed within outer packaging which will not in general be physically large enough to carry all the information required by article 2 in each official language of the Community.

Overall, therefore, article 4(2) of Directive (EEC) 92/27 seems certain to prove one of the most important continuing obstacles to the creation of a true single market for pharmaceuticals. The effect in practice will be to create the possibility of a limited number of truly integrated markets, in particular, Ireland/the United Kingdom and Austria/Germany, with the remainder of the Community fragmented by the official language or languages used in the various Member States. Whether the difficulties caused by further additions to the list of official languages of the Community will force a more radical solution to be adopted is part of a much wider question concerning the development of the Community.

Article 5 defines the scope of the harmonisation achieved by the Directive in respect of labelling. Article 5(1) provides :

> "Member States may not prohibit or impede the placing on the market of medicinal products within their territory on grounds connected with labelling where such labelling complies with the requirements of this Chapter".

That provision is clearly intended to indicate that, subject to article 5(2), the Member States may not impose higher standards than those laid down in the Directive. However, the normal benefits of harmonisation, mutual recognition followed by the free movement of goods between Member States, will not apparently follow for at least two reasons :

(1)   the language problem just discussed means that the authorisation procedure will normally have to be followed in each Member State where marketing authorisation is sought (the fact that the United Kingdom authorities were satisfied with the English language text of a label will not assist the Portuguese or Greek authorities in assessing the text presented to them in Portuguese or Greek)[1]; and

(2)   the degree of discretion granted to the Member States, in respect of what information is "necessary" or "appropriate", leaves it open that even the United Kindgom and Irish authorities might reasonably differ in their interpretation of articles 2 and 3 (in particular, there might well be differing interpretations of information "useful for health education" or "the exclusion of any element of a promotional nature" under article 2(2)).

Nothing in article 5 indicates that mutual recognition is required under the Directive and it appears highly unlikely that such recognition will in practice be achieved except in limited circumstances[2].

---

1.   A technical difficulty could in theory arise if the pharmaceutical company makes use of the possibility suggested by the second sentence of article 4(2) : if the labelling is in all the languages of the Community, no single national authority may be in a position to determine whether each language version conforms to the requirements of the Directive, in particular the requirement that "the same particulars appear in all the languages used." In addition, where the Member States differ in their interpretation of article 2 in respect of a particular product, the particulars may differ in substance in addition to the different languages in which they are expressed. If that is so, it becomes impossible to have a multi-language version because the versions either differ, infringing article 4(2), or do not reflect the authorisation granted in one or other Member State, infringing article 2.

2.   That pessimistic conclusion does not prevent all progress : where the summary of product characteristics is agreed by more than one national authority it may be a relatively simple matter to adapt labelling and package leaflets approved in one Member State so as to satisfy the requirements of another Member State.

Article 5(2) further qualifies the degree of harmonisation likely to be achieved by permitting the Member States to :

"require the use of certain forms of labelling making it possible to indicate :

— the price of the medicinal product,
— the reimbursement conditions of social security organisations,
— the legal status for supply to the patient, in accordance with Directive (EEC) 92/26,
— identification and authenticity".

Clearly, any variation in the information required to be contained on the packaging is of commercial significance in that it requires an alternative or additional process, however trivial, to be followed. The first three possibilities seem likely merely to add such trivial extra processes to either the manufacture or retail process (nothing indicates at what stage the labelling must conform to the requirements of the Directive, but it is natural to assume, for example, that the price of the product does not have to be indicated until the final point of sale).

The fourth possible additional requirement appears more problematic. Given that the particulars set out in article 2(1) include detailed requirements in respect of the name, the contents, the form, the authorisation number and the batch number of the product and also the name and address of the holder of the marketing authorisation, it is hard to see what further requirements could be imposed in respect of either identification or authentication of the product. One possibility appears to be some external mark of authentication affixed by the national competent authorities either at the point of manufacture or during the distribution of the goods. Further steps to *identify* the product would apparently undermine the harmonisation process completely since the detailed requirements of article 2(1) are fundamentally concerned with the accurate identification of the product[1].

15.4   Package leaflets : Chapter III, articles 6 to 9

The idea of a package leaflet is unproblematic, unlike that of packaging. However, it is practically very unsatisfactory to attach such a leaflet to the outside of the immediate packaging of a product so that in practice a package leaflet normally only makes sense where the product consists of both outer and immediate packaging. Chapter III of the Directive overlaps to some degree with Chapter II in that very similar information (though somewhat more detailed) is required to be present on both the labelling and the package leaflet and a package leaflet is not always necessary where sufficient information is present on the labelling of a product.

Article 6 requires "[t]he inclusion in the packaging of all medicinal products of a package leaflet for the information of users ... unless all the information required by article 7 is directly conveyed on the outer packaging or on the immediate packaging". Article 6 does not expressly require that outer packaging should always be used where a leaflet is necessary, though it could be doubted whether a leaflet attached, for example, to a tube of ointment with a rubber band was "included" in the packaging of the product. Likewise, the expression "directly conveyed" does not expressly require that all the information required by article 7 be stated on the packaging, but it is not easy to see how the information is to be "conveyed" if it is not so stated : one possibility seems to be that the physical form of the packaging

---

1.   Article 7(1)(a) of the Directive does suggest one further element that could be added : "the pharmaco-therapeutic group, or type of activity in terms easily comprehensible for the patient."

may convey information that a leaflet would have to express in words (it would not be necessary for a tube to have "This is a tube" written on it); however, there would not be much more point in the leaflet stating matters that were obvious from the form of the packaging. Another possible explanation for the wording is that article 7 requires not only certain information to be included but also that it should be included in a particular order and that the latest date of revision of the leaflet should be stated; those requirements do not seem appropriate where the information is contained on the labelling.

The effect of article 6 is to make the requirements of article 7, which are mandatory in respect of package leaflets where such leaflets are necessary, optional in respect of labelling. If but only if that option is exercised, so that all the information required by article 7 is present in the labelling, then the obligation to include a leaflet lapses.

One further complication is that the option can be exercised either in respect of the outer or the immediate packaging and article 6 could be construed to mean that *all* the information must be present on the outer packaging or that it must all be present on the immediate packaging. Where there is no outer packaging then article 6 must clearly mean that all the information must be present on the immediate packaging if a leaflet is not to be obligatory; but if there is outer packaging then there seems no reason to prevent some of the necessary information appearing on the outer packaging and other such information appearing on the immediate packaging (the only problem in practice seems to be that referred to above, that the package leaflet and the outer packaging will frequently be thrown away by the consumer, so that information on the immediate packaging is of particular importance).

Article 7(1) states that the package leaflet "shall be drawn up in accordance with the summary of the product characteristics". No reference is made to Directive (EEC) 65/65 but the summary of product characteristics is an essential element of the information required in an application for marketing authorisation in accordance with articles 3 and 4 of that Directive and the detailed information to be included in the summary is contained in article 4a of that Directive (it is also referred to as an essential element in the "dossier" to be presented by an applicant in the Annex to Directive (EEC) 75/318, in particular at section B of Part 1 of the Annex)[1].

In addition to being "in accordance" with the summary of product characteristics prepared for the purposes of initial authorisation, article 7 specifies seven categories of information which must be included and specifies further the order in which they must appear : (a) particulars for the identification of the product; (b) the therapeutic indications (ie the symptoms which the product is intended to relieve); (c) a list of information which is necessary before taking the medicinal product; (d) the necessary and usual instructions for proper use; (e) a description of the undesirable effects which can occur under normal use of the medicinal product and, if necessary, the action to be taken in such a case; (f) a reference to the expiry date contained on the label; (g) the date on which the package leaflet was last revised.

The requirement under article 7(1)(a) very largely corresponds o the particulars set out at article 2(1)(a), (b), (c) and (k) in respect of the labelling. The only differences are that the leaflet is required to state the excipients used in the product in qualitative terms and that it is required to include information in respect of each presentation of the product. The latter requirement implies that the same product leaflet is intended to be used for a medicinal product in each presentation so that it

---

1.   See section 3.4 ante for the details of those requirements.

is a matter for the labelling to identify, for example, whether particular tablets contain 10, 50 or 100 milligrams of a specific active ingredient. That would be another respect in which the information contained on the labelling of a product might be considered to satisfy the requirements of article 6 without including all the information required under article 7 : it would be calculated to confuse the consumer to include information on the labelling of a product which related to a presentation other than that actually contained within the packaging on which the labelling was found.

Article 7(1)(a) imposes two additional requirements to those imposed in respect of the labelling : the leaflet must state "the pharmaco-therapeutic group, or type of activity in terms easily comprehensible for the patient"; and it must state the name and address not only of the holder of the marketing authorisation for the product but also for the manufacturer. Examples of easily comprehensible pharmaco-therapeutic groups are : "clears nasal congestion fast", "soluble pain relief", "relieves colds, flu and a blocked nose fast", "the antiseptic burns cream", "relieves infant colic and griping pain". In practice, such statements normally appear on the labelling immediately adjacent to the name of the product. It is surprising that the information is not required on the labelling, where it is of particular commercial significance for non-prescription products, enabling consumers to identify categories of product which may assist treatment of a particular condition.

Article 7(1)(b) to (f) are closely modelled on points 5 and 6 of article 4a of Directive 65/65/EEC, which specify the clinical and pharmaceutical particulars to be contained in the summary of product characteristics. The order set out in article 4a of Directive (EEC) 65/65 has been changed and the wording is somewhat less technical and fuller in article 7(1). Given that the leaflet is required by article 7 to be "in accordance" with the summary of product characteristics, it would perhaps be desirable if in due course article 4a was updated so that the two lists were in the same form. The following matters are specified (with the reference in Directive (EEC) 65/65 preceding that in Directive (EEC) 92/27) :

— *Therapeutic indications* (reasons for taking the product) : article 4a, point 5.5; article 7(1)(b);

— *Contra-indications* (reasons for not taking the product) : article 4a, point 5.6; article 7(1)(a), first indent;

— *Undesirable effects* : article 4a, point 5.3; article 7(1)(e); (the latter requires also that the leaflet should expressly invite the patient to communicate any other such effect to his doctor or pharmacist, a further element in the pharmacovigilance system described in Chapter 12);

— *Special precautions for use* : article 4a, point 5.4; article 7(1)(c), second indent;

— *Use during pregnancy and breastfeeding* : article 4a, point 5.5; article 7(1)(c), fifth indent (the latter includes further references to children, the elderly and persons with specific pathological conditions);

— *Interactions with other medicinal or non-medicinal products* : article 4a, point 5.6; article 7(1)(c), third indent (the latter specifies alcohol, tobacco and foodstuffs);

— *Dosage and method of administration* : article 4a, point 5.7; article 7(1)(d) (the former specifies that administration to children should be considered where necessary; the latter sets out a series of specific requirements in respect of dosage and mode and frequency of administration, and, where appropriate, in respect of duration of treatment, overdose, failure to take one or more doses, and risk of withdrawal effects);

— *Overdose* : article 4a, point 5.8; article 7(1)(d), fifth indent;

— *Special warnings* : article 4a, point 5.9; article 7(1)(c), fourth indent;

— *Effects on ability to drive and use machinery* : article 4a point 5.10; article 7(1)(c), sixth indent;

— *Shelf life* : article 4a, point 6.2; article 7(1)(f) (the latter is more detailed, requiring a warning against use after the specified expiry date and, if necessary, a warning against visible signs of deterioration);

— *Special precautions for storage* : article 4a, point 6.3; article 7(1)(f), second indent;

Article 4, points 6.1, 6.4, 6.5 and 6.6 of Directive (EEC) 65/65 specify : major incompatibilities, nature and contents of the container, name and address of the holder of the marketing authorisation and special disposal precautions. The name issue is dealt with by article 7(1)(a) of Directive (EEC) 92/27; incompatibilities are only dealt with under the headings of interaction with other products and undesirable effects in normal use (article 7(1)(c), third indent, and article 7(1)(e)); whereas the other information is either contained on the labelling in accordance with articles 2 and 3 of Directive (EEC) 92/27 or is not appropriate (the specifications of the container are clearly appropriate *before* the product is manufactured; it is of no concern to the consumer, provided that its appropriateness and safety have been officially approved).

Apart from the matters already referred to which are dealt with in more detail in Directive (EEC) 92/27 than in Directive (EEC) 65/65, reflecting the fact that the leaflet is intended for use, among others, of people with no medical knowledge, article 7(1)(c), seventh indent, requires that those excipients should be detailed "knowledge of which is important for the safe and effective use of the medicinal product and included in the guidelines published pursuant to article 12." As with article 2(d) of the Directive, since inclusion in the guidelines is necessary for application of article 7(1)(c), seventh indent, the question of which knowledge is "important for the safe and effective use" should never arise as an independent question. It is, however, clearly desirable that such guidelines should be made available as soon as possible.

Article 7(2) is a specific provision relating to the requirement laid down by article 7(1)(b), that the "therapeutic indications" for the use of a product should be included in the leaflet. Article 7(2) permits the competent authorities to decide that :

"certain therapeutic indications shall not be mentioned in the package leaflet, where the dissemination of such information might have serious disadvantages for the patient".

The provision is not very explicit, but the obvious explanation for the exception is for treatments for conditions to which a serious social stigma attaches, which can have major economic disadvantages for an individual or which are viewed with particular fear or lack of understanding by the general public. Examples would be sexually transmitted diseases and might also include conditions such as multiple sclerosis, where the development of the condition is highly uncertain and poorly understood and where the symptoms may in themselves be relatively minor[1].

Article 7(3) corresponds to article 2(2) above, permitting the use of pictograms and symbols for clarification and other information compatible with the summary of product characteristics "which is useful for health education, to the exclusion of any element of a promotional nature". The difficulties likely to arise in interpreting that provision have already been discussed in respect of article 2(2).

Article 8 corresponds to article 4 in respect of labelling. The leaflet must be "written in clear and understandable terms for the patient and be clearly legible in the official language or languages of the Member State where the medicinal product is placed on the market". It may be printed in several languages (which must mean that several language versions may be included in a single leaflet) "provided that the same information is given in all the languages used".

The physical difficulties of including all the necessary information in a confined space which arise in the case of the labelling of medicinal products do not arise in the case of packaging leaflets. It is also much less problematic to insert leaflets in different languages, for the purposes of marketing in different language areas of the Community, into identically labelled finished packages than it is to alter the labelling of those packages. It would therefore have been possible to minimise the information that must be carried on the labelling of a pharmaceutical product but to require either that the leaflet be printed in all languages of the Community (or in each official language of the area within which the product was to be marketed) or that a leaflet in the appropriate language or languages should be inserted before marketing in any particular area. However, that approach has not so far been adopted, presumably because of the practical disadvantages of leaflets as against labelling (that they are not physically tied to the product until the moment of administration, unlike the immediate packaging of a product). In addition, not all such difficulties would be solved by such an approach : it would remain the case that, as with labelling, no single national authority would be able to approve a leaflet in all the languages of the Community and the degree of discretion permitted to the national authorities in authorising both the summary of product characteristics and the information to be included in a leaflet means that this is not, at least at present, merely a problem of translation.

Article 9 corresponds to article 5 in respect of labelling and prevents the Member States from prohibiting or impeding the marketing of medicinal products within their territory "on grounds relating to the package leaflet if the latter complies with the requirements of this Chapter". As with labelling, there is no explicit requirement of mutual recognition and it appears that the discretion permitted to the Member States in determining when the provision of information is necessary or appropriate (and in particular the application of article 7(2) in respect of sensitive therapeutic indications) leaves it open to Member States to apply Chapter III of the Directive in various ways (and the problem of language differences remains). However, unlike in the case of labelling, the Member States are given no discretion to apply criteria other than those set out in Chapter III in determining whether a package leaflet is satisfactory.

---

1.   Article 7(2) is referred to at article 9(3)(c) of Regulation (EEC) 2309/93, where the discretion of the Member States is preserved in respect of the question of therapeutic indications included in a package leaflet even where Community authorised products are concerned : see section 7.3 ante. Compare also the list of "therapeutic indications", contained at article 3(2) of Directive (EEC) 92/28, which may not be included in advertising of medicinal products to the general public : see section 16.3 post.

15.5   General and final provisions : Chapter IV, articles 10 to 15

Articles 10 and 11 set out the administrative procedures to be followed by applicants for marketing authorisation. They are very similar to those contained in Chapter II of Directive (EEC) 65/65 and certain provisions effectively reproduce the terms of the earlier Directive. That is not inappropriate or surprising since the authorisation of the labelling and package leaflet of a product is not in fact an independent activity but merely forms a significant part of the general process of marketing authorisation set out in Directive (EEC) 65/65 (and now also Regulation (EEC) 2309/93, which incorporates the provisions of Directive (EEC) 92/27 by reference at article 9(3)(c) and the second paragraph of article 11).

Article 10(1) is in substance the same as point 9 of article 4 of Directive (EEC) 65/65, which requires, inter alia, that an application for marketing authorisation should be accompanied by "one or more specimens or mock-ups of the sales presentation of the [medicinal] product, together with a package leaflet where one is to be enclosed". Article 10(1) merely interprets "sales presentation" in the terms of Directive (EEC) 92/27 to mean "the outer packaging and the immediate packaging" of the product.

Article 10(2) can be seen as a particular instance of the second paragraph of article 5 of Directive (EEC) 65/65, which provides that market authorisation shall be refused "if the particulars and documents submitted in support of the application do not comply with article 4". Article 10(2) of Directive (EEC) 92/27 provides that authorisation shall be refused "if the labelling or the package leaflet [does] not comply with the provisions of this Directive or if they are not in accordance with the particulars listed in the summary of product characteristics referred to in article 4b of Directive (EEC) 65/65". Article 10(2) goes beyond article 5 of Directive (EEC) 65/65 in so far as the requirements of Directive (EEC) 92/27 go beyond those of article 4 of the earlier Directive. The question of the compatibility with article 21 of Directive (EEC) 65/65 of articles 10 and 11 of Directive (EEC) 92/27 has already been discussed[1].

Article 10(3) requires "[a]ll proposed changes to an aspect of the labelling or to the package leaflet covered by this Directive and not connected with the summary of characteristics" to be submitted to the competent authorities. That is a compressed provision which appears to permit changes to be made without prior approval (i) for purely commercial or aesthetic reasons (such as a new logo for the manufacturing company); and (ii) where such changes are consequential on a change to the summary of product characteristics. Given the close relationship between the information contained in the summary and in the labelling and the leaflet, a literal interpretation of article 10(3) would permit almost all changes to be made without prior approval : there are few changes which are wholly *unconnected* with the summary (examples might be changes to the description of the "pharmaco-therapeutic" group to which the product was stated to belong, or to the symbols or pictograms added for the purposes of clarification). That cannot have been the intention of the legislation and the literal interpretation should therefore be rejected.

Where article 10(3) does apply, an "opposition procedure" applies, whereby the change is permitted unless the competent authorities oppose the change within 90 days "following the introduction of the request". That expression appears to mean that time runs from the date of notification of the proposed change.

Article 10(4) corresponds to article 9 of Directive (EEC) 65/65 and confirms that authorisation of labelling and package leaflets by national competent authorities, or

---

1.   See section 15.1 ante.

changes thereto, "does not alter the general legal liability" of either the manufacturer or the holder of the marketing authorisation.

Article 10(5) is an important exception to both Chapters II and III of the Directive, permitting exemption by the competent authorities for "labels and package leaflets for specific medicinal products from the obligation that certain particulars shall appear", ie the obligations imposed by articles 2, 3 and 7; and also from the obligation "that the leaflet must be in the official language or languages of the Member State where the product is placed on the market". Those exemptions are permitted to be granted "when the product is not intended to be delivered to the patient for self-administration". "Self-medication" is expressly mentioned at article 2(1)(n) but it would clearly be possible to give less elementary information in respect of the use and administration of a product if it was known that the product would be administered in practice only by qualified medical personnel. Article 12(1), second indent, provides for the Commission issuing guidelines on "particular information needs relating to self-medication" : such guidelines would necessarily also indicate what types of information were *not* necessary where self-administration was not a possibility. Similar considerations apply to the relaxation of the requirement in respect of language : there is obviously less risk that a medically trained person would use a medicinal product without either being able to understand the information contained on its labelling or in its package leaflet (or at least having made reasonably careful enquiries as to its properties) than would be the case with a private individual.

Article 11 deals with suspension of marketing authorisation where the provisions of the Directive are not complied with and "a notice served on the person concerned has remained without effect". In such circumstances, article 11(1) permits the national competent authorities to suspend the authorisation "until the labelling and the package leaflet of the medicinal product in question have been made to comply with the requirements of this Directive". It should be noted that the Member States are under no obligation to take any such action and also that they have no power to revoke an authorisation on this basis. In those respects, the Directive has significantly less impact on the conduct of the Member States than article 11 of Directive (EEC) 65/65, which *requires* the Member States either to revoke or suspend an authorisation where the requirements of that Directive cease to be satisfied. Article 11(1) of Directive (EEC) 92/27 also fails to specify any period of time within which the person served with a notice under the paragraph must act, failing which the national authority's power to suspend authorisation becomes effective.

A final problem is that article 9(3)(c) of Regulation (EEC) 2309/93 applies the provisions of Directive (EEC) 92/27 to centrally authorised products. However, it is not clear whether the national authorities' power to suspend authorisation under article 11(1) of the Directive applies in respect of centrally authorised products : given that the Member States are given only a very restricted general power to suspend by article 18(4) of the Regulation, it appears unlikely that any such power was intended to be granted in this relatively minor case (article 18(4) of the Regulation is in fact sufficiently broad in its scope that it could in theory permit suspension in utterly exceptional circumstances of this kind, where a defect in the labelling or package leaflet was so severe that "urgent action [was] essential to protect human or animal health or the environment"[1].

Article 11(2) is a standard Community law provision corresponding with article 12 of Directive (EEC) 65/65. Decisions under article 11(1) to suspend authorisation must state in detail the reasons on which they are based, must be notified to the person concerned, and that person must be informed at the same time of the legal

---

1.   See section 11.5 ante.

remedies available to him and of the time limits for the exercise of those remedies. Oddly, there is no equivalent provision in respect of decisions to refuse authorisation under article 10(2) which would in principle raise the possibility that an application for marketing authorisation could be refused without reasons and without notification to the applicant because of a defect in the labelling or package leaflet. That would be an absurd situation and a Court would be compelled either to find that general principles of Community administrative law required that the normal rules applied even where not specified by legislation or to construe article 12 of Directive (EEC) 65/65 sufficiently broadly that it applied not only to decisions taken pursuant to article 5, 6 or 11 of that Directive, as the wording states, but also to decisions taken pursuant to article 10(2) of Directive (EEC) 92/27. A final possibility would be to find that a refusal based on article 10(2) was in fact taken "pursuant to article 5" of Directive (EEC) 65/65, for the reasons set out above : if that were correct then article 12 of the same Directive would apply directly.

Article 12 provides for the publication of guidelines in the form of a Commission Directive adopted in accordance with article 2c of Directive (EEC) 75/318, ie in the same way as Directive (EEC) 91/356 in respect of good manufacturing practice[1]. No such guidelines have as yet been published but they are to be published "as necessary" by the Commission on the following five topics : special warnings for certain categories of medicinal products (compare article 2(1)(f) and (g) and article 7(1)(c), fourth indent); particular information needs relating to self-medication (compare article 2(1)(n) and article 7(1)(d)); the legibility of particulars on the labelling and package leaflet (compare article 4(1) and article 8); methods for the identification and authentication of products (compare article 5(2)); and the list of excipients which must appear on the labelling of products and the way these excipients must be indicated (compare article 2(1)(d) but also article 7(1)(c), seventh indent). The last case is the most urgent in that the relevant provisions of articles 2 and 7 are, literally at least, unworkable without such guidelines. At the time of writing (15 March 1994), it appears unlikely that the Commission will be able to obtain the necessary support from the Member States for further Directives on these issues, though draft Directives were produced in 1993 on special warnings, legibility and excipients. Preliminary guidelines in respect of excipients are currently subject to consultation.

Article 13 repeals the former provisions of Directive (EEC) 65/65 and 75/319 with immediate effect. Article 14(1) requires the Member States to take the measures necessary to comply with the Directive before 1 January 1993, but article 14(3) further requires that, from *1 January 1994*, the Member States "shall refuse an application for authorisation to place a medicinal product on the market or for the renewal of an existing authorisation, where the labelling and the package leaflet do not comply with the requirements of this Directive". In respect of refusal of an initial application, that provision apparently is intended to mean that article 10(2) was not required to be put into effect until 1 January 1994 (apart from an obvious error in the drafting which makes it necessary that both the labelling *and* the leaflet must be defective before authorisation is to be refused, whereas in fact only one needs to be defective). Article 14 does not make it clear whether refusal is compulsory for *applications* or for *decisions* made after 1 January 1994. Given that nothing prevents the national authorities from applying the rules in advance and that the delay in implementation would be trivial if a Member State incorrectly construed the provision as applying only to applications after 1 January 1994, it seems highly unlikely that the point will fall to be decided.

The provisions in relation to renewal will gradually make existing medicinal products subject to the Directive, and by 1 January 1999 at the latest all products

---

1   See section 10.5 ante and section 4.2 ante in respect of Directive (EEC) 75/318.

will be subject to its requirements. If the Directive is to be strictly implemented, considerable changes will be necessary to manufacturing practices.

Chapter 16 : Directive (EEC) 92/28[1] - The Advertising of Authorised Products

16.1   Introduction : the recitals

The control of the advertising of medicinal products is clearly only one element in the broad issues of consumer protection and unfair competition raised by the marketing of products, particularly in the face of continuing rapid development in telecommunications and broadcasting. However, the marketing of medicinal products raises special problems given the large social and commercial interests involved. In respect of consumers, it is clearly a fundamental element in the protection of public health that consumers should not be misled by inaccurate claims for particular medicinal products or by suppression of information concerning adverse side effects of using such products; the same applies in respect of medical practitioners, but they also require protection from unfair or improper commercial pressure to prescribe particular products. Given the large costs of medicinal products to the national health systems of the Member States, such issues are of major political and commercial significance in so far as they relate to products which are, directly or indirectly, paid for by the national authorities.

The extent to which Council Directive (EEC) 92/28 on the advertising of medicinal products for human use is merely part of a wider Community scheme for the control of advertising within the Community, is reflected in the references contained in the Directive to other Community Directives concerning other aspects of that scheme : Council Directive (EEC) 84/450[2] relating to the approximation of the laws, regulations and administrative provisions of the Member States concerning misleading advertising; and Council Directive (EEC) 89/552[3] on the co-ordination of certain provisions laid down by law, regulation or administrative action in Member States concerning the pursuit of television broadcasting activities. The European Parliament has been strongly critical of the Commission's approach of presenting piecemeal legislation treating specific areas rather than laying down a general framework for the control of advertising[4].

Recitals 1 to 3 are general observations about advertising within the Community. Recital 1 states that the provisions of the Directive are without prejudice to the application of measures adopted pursuant to Directive (EEC) 84/450 in respect of misleading advertising, while recital 3 provides that the principle laid down by Directive (EEC) 89/552, which "prohibits the television advertising of medicinal products which are available only on medical prescription in the Member State

---

1.   OJ L113 30.4.92 p13. See Appendix 13 post.
2.   OJ L250 19.9.84 p17.
3.   OJ L298 17.10.89 p23.
4.   See in particular the Report of the Committee on the Environment, Public Health and Consumer Protection on the Commission proposal for Directive (EEC) 92/28 (EN\RR\109301) in the Explanatory Statement at pp23-30 : "It is regrettable, however, that the Commission is once again proposing a detailed framework directive for a specific group of products without first having proposed framework directives for unfair and comparative advertising. If there were comprehensive legislation on these two areas in the form of a European framework directive, there would be no need for a number of detailed proposals, including some of those in the present text."

within whose jurisdiction the television broadcaster is located", should be made "of general application by extending it to other media". The operation of the principle identified from Directive (EEC) 89/552 (in fact, from recital 30 and article 14 thereof) is far from straightforward : if an Italian company broadcasts from Germany for reception in Denmark, is it the law that those broadcasts may not contain advertisements of products which are prescription-only in Italy, or in Germany? What does it mean for a broadcaster to "fall within the jurisdiction" of a Member State? However, the substantive provisions of Directive (EEC) 92/28 simply ban all advertising of prescription only products, without addressing the question of which Member State's rules are to be applied to determine whether a product is to be regarded as "prescription only" for the purposes of the Directive : for example, if a German pharmaceutical company issued promotional leaflets throughout the Community for a product that was available without a prescription in Germany, could the Greek authorities prohibit the distribution of that leaflet in Greece if the product was available only on prescription in Greece? Indeed, would they be obliged to do so by the Directive? The difficulty of such questions indicates the links that exist between the various elements of the pharmaceutical regime : if Directive (EEC) 92/26 was a more complete harmonisation measure then differences between Member States over the classification of medicinal products would no longer exist and the rules on advertising would no longer raise difficult questions of interpretation, or at least those difficult questions would no longer have to be answered.

Recital 2 sets out the most general justification for the Directive (it should be noted that Directive (EEC) 92/28 differs from the other Rational Use Directives, discussed in Chapters 13 to 15 ante, in that it does not contain the standard 1992 Programme recital) :

> "Whereas all Member States have adopted further specific measures concerning the advertising of medicinal products; whereas there are disparities between these measures; whereas these disparities are likely to have an impact on the establishment and functioning of the internal market, since advertising disseminated in one Member State is likely to have effects in other Member States".

Recital 2 does not explain how advertising within one Member State affects other Member States but a brief explanation is given at recital 1 of Directive (EEC) 84/450 : "since advertising reaches beyond the frontiers of individual Member States, it has a direct effect on the establishment and the functioning of the common market". A more plausible justification for many types of advertising, and for readily transportable goods such as pharmaceutical products in particular, is that advertising within a single Member State is likely to influence movements in the goods advertised across the national borders of the Community where those goods are manufactured or distributed in a Member State other than that in which the advertisement takes place. National restrictions on the advertising of such products will therefore inhibit cross-border trade in the products, and differences in such restrictions will add to the industry's costs, as different marketing campaigns have to be prepared for the different Member States.

Recitals 4 and 5 summarise the provisions of the Directive in respect of advertising to the general public : because such advertising, even of non-prescription products, "could affect public health, were it to be excessive and-ill-considered" it ought therefore, where permitted, to "satisfy certain criteria which ought to be defined". Further, "distribution of samples free of charge to the general public for promotional ends must be prohibited".

Recitals 6 to 10 relate to advertising to "persons qualified to prescribe or supply medicinal products". Recital 6 recognises that advertising "contributes to the information available to such persons" but requires that it should be "subject to strict conditions and effective monitoring, referring in particular to the work carried out within the framework of the Council of Europe". The reference to the Council of Europe is unexplained, but it refers to a number of Resolutions of the Committee of Ministers (Partial Agreement in the Social and Public Health Field), in particular : AP (82) 1 on regulations concerning medicines and the advertising of them to persons qualified to prescribe or supply them; AP (83) 1 on regulations governing the advertising of medicines to the public; AP (84) 2 on the inclusion of packaging leaflets in pharmaceutical specialities and the nature of the information shown on such leaflets; and AP (88) 1 on warning phrases for certain categories of medicaments. The provisions of AP (82) 1 and AP (83) 1 have clearly influenced both the structure and the wording of Directive (EEC) 92/28.

Recital 7 notes the important role of medical sales representatives in the promotion of medicinal products and recognises the need to impose certain obligations on them, in particular the need to give summaries of product characteristics[1] to "the person visited". Recital 8 notes the need for persons qualified to prescribe medicinal products to be able to "carry out these functions objectively without being influenced by direct or indirect financial inducements"[2]. Recital 9 recognises the reasonableness of supplying samples of medicinal products free of charge, to enable persons prescribing or supplying such products to "familiarise themselves with new products and acquire experience in dealing with them", but only "within certain restrictive conditions". Finally, recital 10 states a very general need for such persons to "have access to a neutral, objective source of information about products available on the market", while recognising that the provisions to be introduced to meet that need is a matter for the Member States "in the light of their own particular situation".

It emerges from recitals 6 to 10 that the concept of "advertising" in Directive (EEC) 92/28 is intended to be a broad one. Given that medicinal products perform a crucial social function, it is appropriate to consider advertising in the broad context of the supply of information both to the consumer and to the medical professional. It would perhaps have avoided misunderstanding if the Directive had been entitled "on the supply of information concerning medicinal products for human use by advertising and other means" (though such a title would have overlapped to some degree with the terms of Directive (EEC) 92/27[3]).

Recitals 11 and 12 concern respectively monitoring and the supply of accurate information by manufacturers and importers of medicinal products. Monitoring is required by recital 11 to be "effective" and "adequate" and reference is made to "the monitoring mechanisms set up by Directive (EEC) 84/450". That Directive falls outside the scope of this work but, in summary, articles 4 to 6 of Directive (EEC) 84/450 require that persons having a legitimate interest in prohibiting misleading advertising should be enabled to have recourse to the courts and/or to an administrative body with effective powers to prevent or terminate such advertising, optionally supplemented by self-regulation. Article 12 of Directive (EEC) 92/28 to a large extent reproduces this regulatory scheme with appropriate amendments. Recital 12 merely states that manufacturers and importers should "set up a

---

1.   See section 3.4.3 ante.

2.   The Report of the European Parliament (EN\RR\109301) includes in its Opinion at p44 one spectacular example of such an inducement : "a three day cruise on the Rhine for a number of prominent rheumatologists" forming part of a campaign which is stated to have cost the British National Health Service £13.5 million, "more than the product's developments costs". The Report further states that "[i]n 1988, in the United Kingdom, it was demonstrated that the pharmaceutical industry spent 80 times more than the National Health Service on information to doctors". The question of inducements is therefore not a trivial one.

3.   See Chapter 15 ante.

mechanism to ensure that all information supplied about a medicinal product conforms with the approved conditions of use". The recital is badly drafted since no such obligation is in fact imposed by the Directive on manufacturers and importers and "the approved conditions of use" is a strange expression, which it would have been natural to replace with "the approved summary of product characteristics"[1]. Article 13 of the Directive, which appears to correspond to recital 12, in fact imposes various obligations on the holder of a marketing authorisation.

The substantive provisions of Directive (EEC) 92/28, which are extremely diverse and disjointed, consisting largely in lists of obligations and prohibitions, fall into four Chapters : I Scope, definitions and general principles; II Advertising to the general public; III Advertising to health professionals; and IV Monitoring of advertising.

16.2 Scope, definitions and general principles : Chapter I, articles 1 and 2

Article 1 defines the scope of the Directive by specifying the meaning of four separate concepts : medicinal products for human use; name (and common name) of such products; summary of product characteristics; and advertising. Article 1(1) specifies that the Directive concerns the advertising of medicinal products for human use and uses the same definition as Directives (EEC) 92/25 and 92/27, referring back to Chapters II to V of Directive (EEC) 65/65 and thus indirectly to article 1(2) and article 2 of the same Directive[2]. Article 1(2), states that the definitions of name and common name shall be those laid down by Directive (EEC) 92/27, in fact by article 1(2) thereof[3]; and that "the summary of product characteristics shall be the summary approved by the competent authority which granted the marketing authorisation in accordance with article 4b of Directive (EEC) 65/65"[4].

Article 1(3) and (4) set out an inclusive definition of "advertising" and list seven specific activities that fall within the scope of the definition and four activities that fall outside it. Advertising is said to include :

> "any form of door-to-door information, canvassing activity or inducement designed to promote the prescription, supply, sale or consumption of medicinal products".

In common sense terms, the legislator envisages the following persons as the targets of this marketing activity : the doctor deciding which product to prescribe for a particular ailment; the pharmacist deciding which product to recommend to a prospective purchaser; the consumer deciding which product to choose and the consumer deciding which product, of those in his possession at any given time, to consume (and also deciding in what quantities and at what intervals to consume the product).

The seven activities identified as constituting advertising for the purposes of the Directive are : advertising of medicinal products to the general public and to persons qualified to prescribe or supply such products (article 1(3), first and second indent); visits by medical sales representatives to persons qualified to prescribe

---

1.　　The second "general principle" of the Directive, article 2(2), in fact requires that all advertising complies with "the particulars listed in the summary of product characteristics"; and see also article 1(2). Compare the wording of article 2(2), article 7(1) and 7(3) of Directive (EEC) 92/27 concerning the accuracy of the information contained in labelling and package leaflets.

2.　　See Chapter 2 and section 3.2 ante.

3.　　See section 15.2 ante.

4　　See section 3.4.3 ante.

such products (article 1(3), third indent); the supply of samples and "the provision of any inducements to prescribe or supply medicinal products by the gift offer or promise of any benefit or bonus, whether in money or in kind, except when their intrinsic value is minimal" (article 1(3), fourth and fifth indents); and the sponsorship of promotional meetings or scientific congresses attended by persons qualified to prescribe or supply medicinal products, and in the latter case the payment of related travelling and accommodation expenses (article 1(3), sixth and seventh indents). In relation to the first two instances, it is not entirely clear whether the general examples of what constitutes advertising for the purposes of the Directive are intended to specify the meaning of "advertising" in those indents. Given that there is no strict definition of the term, it does not in practice matter : television or newspaper advertisements are not directly identified by article 1(3) but they both clearly fall within the scope of the Directive. More difficult issues might arise where, for example, sponsorship of more subtle kinds than those identified by article 1(3), sixth and seventh indents were involved, in particular the grant of research finance to medical practitioners or academics. Another example might be charitable donations, either of money or of medicinal products, to the victims of plague or famine. Although the last two instances given in article 1(3) might cast some doubt on the matter, and the Directive does not say so expressly, in practice it is clear from the examples given and from the wording of article 1(3) as a whole that general advertising by pharmaceutical companies is not the target of the Directive, which concerns advertising *of medicinal products*, eg Zovirax or Disprin, not of manufacturers, eg Wellcome or Reckitt and Colman[1].

Article 1(4) gives four specific examples of activities which are not covered by the Directive. The first is labelling and package leaflets, now dealt with in detail by Directive (EEC) 92/27[2]. It is clear from the two Directives that the Community is not, at least not yet, concerned to control the design of the packaging of medicinal products but only the information of potential significance to a purchaser relating to those products (though practical defects in the packaging design would be of concern at the time of the initial application for marketing authorisation). The second, third and fourth indents of article 1(4) specify three other matters :

"—   correspondence, possibly accompanied by material of a non-promotional nature, needed to answer a specific question about a particular medicinal product;
—   factual, informative announcements and reference material relating, for example, to pack changes, adverse-reaction warnings as part of general drug precautions, trade catalogues and price list, provided they include no product claims;
—   statements relating to human health or diseases, provided there is no reference, even indirect, to medicinal products."

Of these, the first is relatively straightforward : it is not advertising for a pharmaceutical company to reply to a written enquiry concerning one of its products and its reply may include "material of a non-promotional nature". The only difficulty is the meaning of "non-promotional" : if an article in a medical journal contained an answer to the specific enquiry but also contained strong praise of the product in question, it might be a difficult question whether the company should simply state the answer or whether it could reasonably include a copy of the entire article. Similarly, the second example, factual announcements and reference material, does not constitute advertising so long as "no product

---

1.   "Advertising" was defined by article 2(2) of Directive (EEC) 84/450 to mean : "the making of a representation in any form in connection with a trade, business, craft or profession in order to promote the supply of goods or services, including immovable property, rights and obligations".
2.   See Chapter 15 ante.

claims" are included. "Claims" in this context must mean positive statements about the product, presumably including not only the three criteria by the Community, quality, safety and efficacy, but also value for money.

Obviously, the second and third indents permit reference to be made to particular medicinal products; but the fourth indent covers a quite different activity, the issuing of statements by pharmaceutical companies of an entirely general kind. If a company wishes to make such statements, they will constitute advertising for the purposes of the Directive if they contain any reference to medicinal products. It thus appears that a pharmaceutical company with a very successful product on the market for the treatment of stomach ulcers could issue a health information leaflet concerning diet and lifestyle calculated to reduce the risk of stomach ulcers without falling within the scope of the Directive. It could not, however, make any reference to its successful product, nor could it make any (possibly disparaging) reference to products supplied by competitors, even in an indirect form.

Article 2 of the Directive sets out three general principles to be followed by the Member States and those responsible for the advertising of medicinal products within the Community. Article 2(1) prohibits the advertising of any medicinal product which has not received a marketing authorisation "granted in accordance with Community law". That provision confirms the fundamental importance of marketing authorisation in the Community regime and must now be read in the light of the newly amended article 3 of Directive (EEC) 65/65 to refer not only to national authorisations granted in accordance with that Directive but also Community authorisations granted in accordance with Regulation (EEC) 2309/93[1].

Article 2(2) requires that "[a]ll parts of the advertising of a medicinal product must comply with the particulars listed in the summary of product characteristics". That requirement also emphasises the importance of initial marketing authorisation, since one fundamental element of that authorisation process is the completion of an approved summary of product characteristics[2].

Article 2(3) imposes two further obligations on advertising of medicinal products. Such advertising :

> "—   shall encourage the rational use of the medicinal product, by presenting it
>   objectively and without exaggerating its properties,
> —   shall not be misleading."

The expression "rational use" has given its name to the entire package of legislation considered in Chapters 13 to 16. In the context of article 2(2), the expression appears primarily to refer to the state of mind of a person administering a medicinal product (possibly to himself or herself), that he or she should have a proper and accurate appreciation of the properties of the product and of the appropriate circumstances for that product's use. In a secondary sense, which has given its name to the four Rational Use Directives, "use" is taken in an extended sense to include all stages after manufacture but in particular the choices of doctors, pharmacists and consumers in prescribing, recommending or choosing particular products. It is obviously highly doubtful whether so vague a criterion could sensibly be applied in practice to control advertising except in blatant cases of frivolous or inaccurate claims.

"Misleading advertising" is not defined in the Directive but recitals 1 and 10 refer to Directive (EEC) 84/450 and that Directive contains, at article 2(2), a definition of "misleading advertising" :

---

1.   See Chapters 3, 7 and 8 ante.
2.   See section 3.4.3 ante.

"any advertising which in any way, including its presentation, deceives or is likely to deceive the persons to whom it is addressed or whom it reaches and which, by reason of its deceptive nature, is likely to affect their economic behaviour or which, for those reasons, injures or is likely to injure a competitor".

Given the close links between Directives (EEC) 84/450 and 92/28 in respect of the control of misleading advertising (see recital 10 and article 12 of Directive (EEC) 92/28), it seems likely that the earlier definition would be closely considered in any legal proceedings relating to allegedly misleading advertising under Directive (EEC) 92/28.

16.3   Advertising to the general public : Chapter II, articles 3 to 5

Article 3 sets out a variety of rules concerning the prohibition and authorisation of advertising to the general public; article 4 imposes positive obligations in respect of such advertising; and article 5 consists of a list of twelve types of material which may not be contained in such advertising.

Article 3(1) specifies three categories of medicinal products the advertising of which shall be banned by the Member States; and article 3(3) specifies a fourth category the advertising of which *may* be banned. The first category is those products which are available only on medical prescription in accordance with Directive (EEC) 92/26, as to which see Chapter 14. The second category is those products which "contain psychotropic or narcotic substances, within the meaning of the international conventions". That provision is likely in many cases to be subordinate to the first indent, given that, at article 3(2) of Directive (EEC) 92/26, the presence of such substances (in a non-exempt quantity) was a factor to be taken into account by the Member States not only in making a product subject to medicinal prescription but subject to "special" medical prescription in accordance with article 2(2)(b) of that Directive[1]. It is only where such substances are present in an exempt quantity that medicinal products containing them are at all likely to be *available* without a medical prescription.

The third category of excluded products is defined by reference to article 3(2), products which "may not be advertised to the general public in accordance with [article 3(2)]". On its face, that would naturally mean "those products which article 3(2) prohibited" but in fact article 3(2) is a permissive provision and the third indent of article 3(1) therefore must refer to those products that do not fall within the terms of article 3(2). The overall effect of article 3(1) is therefore that *only* those products which :

— fall within the scope of article 3(2); and

— are not prescription only; and

— do not contain psychotropic or narcotic substances;

may be advertised within the Community.

Further, article 3(2), first sub-paragraph, specifies those products which may be advertised to the general public, namely those which :

---

1.   Article 3(2) of Directive (EEC) 92/26 specifies the international conventions referred to, to be the "United Nations Conventions of 1961 and 1971" : see section 14.3 ante.

"by virtue of their composition and purpose, are intended and designed for use without the intervention of a medical practitioner for diagnostic purposes or for the prescription or monitoring of treatment, with the advice of the pharmacist, if necessary."

As drafted, it appears that a product must be *both* designed for use without a doctor *and* either for diagnostic or monitoring purposes. If that were correct, then the limitation in terms of purpose would be highly restrictive and, in terms of the definition of medicinal products contained in article 1(2) of Directive (EEC) 65/65 and discussed in detail in Chapter 2, only those products which may be administered to human beings with a view to making a medical diagnosis, ie the first limb of the second definition[1] would be within the scope of article 3(3) of Directive (EEC) 92/28. All products which have the properties of preventing or treating disease or which may be administered with a view to restoring, correcting or modifying physiological functions in human beings (or are presented as such) would then fall outside the scope of article 3(2).

Nothing in the Directive suggests that so restrictive an approach was intended and it therefore appears that article 3(2) specifies three alternatives : (i) use without a doctor, (ii) diagnostic purposes or (iii) prescription/monitoring purposes, any one of which suffices to permit a product to be advertised. In effect, a comma is missing after "medical practitioner". If that is correct, then medicinal products which are designed to treat rather than diagnose or monitor a medical condition may only be advertised if they satisfy the requirements of article 3(1) and also are designed for use "without the intervention of a medical practitioner" but "with the advice of a pharmacist, if necessary". Those products which do not necessarily involve the expert assistance of medical practitioners are, to that extent, more akin to ordinary consumer products and it is therefore not surprising that the advertising of such products is permitted subject to appropriate controls.

Article 3(2) second sub-paragraph, is completely unrelated to the first sub-paragraph, and consists of a list of therapeutic indications (ie human ailments), the mention of which in advertisements to the general public the Member States are required to prohibit[2] : tuberculosis; sexually transmitted diseases; other serious infectious diseases; cancer and other tumoral diseases; chronic insomnia, and diabetes and other metabolic illnesses. No explanation is given of this provision either in the recitals to the Directive or in the main text; in the original Commission proposal[3] reference was made to the fact that certain indications were not suitable for self-medication, but that does not appear in the final text. The justification for the provision may therefore be the same as for article 7(2) of Directive (EEC) 92/27, that there might be serious personal disadvantages for a patient in having it widely known that a particular product was used to treat serious conditions such as those specified.

Article 3(3) permits the Member States "to ban on their territory the advertising to the general public of medicinal products the cost of which may be reimbursed". That provision is likely to cause problems in practice, since it, like the provision on "prescription only" products, gives no guidance as to the operation of the Directive in respect of cross-border advertising. Nothing in the Directive makes it clear whether a Member State faced with such cross-border advertising, in particular by

---

1. See section 2.5.4 ante.
2. The provision should be compared to article 7(2) of Directive (EEC) 92/27, which permits the national authorities to decide that certain therapeutic conditions not be mentioned in package leaflets "where the dissemination of such information might have serious disadvantages for the patient". No examples are given of such "indications" but it is natural to suppose that the examples listed here would also be likely candidates under article 7(2).
3. COM(90) 212 final-SYN 273 (OJ C163 4.7.90 p10).

satellite television, could prevent the advertising of medicinal products whose costs were not able to be reimbursed in the country of origin of the advertisement (or in respect of which the country of origin did not choose to exercise the power granted under article 3(3)) but which were able to be reimbursed in the Member State where the broadcast could be received.

It might be thought that, at least in respect of cross-border television advertising, the position would be resolved by Directive (EEC) 89/552; and article 3(5) states that the prohibition contained in article 3(1) "shall apply without prejudice to articles 2, 3 and 14 of Directive (EEC) 89/552". However, no reference is made to article 3(3) of Directive (EEC) 92/28 and it thus appears that the Member States' powers under article 3(3) are unfettered by Directive (EEC) 89/552.

Indeed, the text of Directive (EEC) 89/552 itself tends to support such an interpretation. Article 14 of that Directive contains a further specific prohibition in respect of television advertising of medicinal products available only on prescription "in the Member State within whose jurisdiction the broadcaster falls". That prohibition is now displaced by the general prohibition contained in the first indent to article 3(1) of Directive (EEC) 92/28, although that general provision gives no guidance as to how it is to be applied where a product advertised in several Member States is not "prescription only" in all of them. At least in respect of television advertising, article 14 will apparently still apply, with the difficulties of interpretation mentioned above in respect of recital 3 to Directive (EEC) 92/28. In respect of national conditions of reimbursement for *non-prescription* products, article 14 of Directive (EEC) 89/552 does not apply, so it would be necessary to apply articles 2 and 3 of that Directive directly. Article 2 in particular requires each Member State to ensure that television broadcasts for which it has responsibility "comply with the law applicable to broadcasts intended for the public in that Member State" and further requires the other Member States to ensure freedom of reception and not to restrict retransmission of such broadcasts "for reasons which fall within the fields co-ordinated by this Directive", subject only to very limited exceptions. The scope of each Member State's responsibility under article 2 is far from clear but it does appear that the conditions of reimbursement of a medicinal product are clearly not "within the fields co-ordinated" by Directive (EEC) 89/552. If that is correct then the Member States should remain free to exercise the power granted by article 3(3) of Directive (EEC) 92/28 in respect of television broadcasts, notwithstanding the provisions of Directive (EEC) 89/552.

Article 3(4) exempts from the prohibition imposed by article 3(1) : "vaccination campaigns carried out by the industry and approved by the competent authorities of the Member States". That provision gives the Member States a further discretion to permit advertisements for any type of medicinal product as part of a "vaccination campaign". The effect would be that the general prohibition would be suspended in respect of the product or products in question for the period of the campaign.

Article 3(6) requires the Member States to "prohibit the direct distribution of medicinal products to the public by the industry for promotional purposes". It should be noted that this prohibition does not apply (i) where the distribution is not "by the industry", eg where the national health service effects the distribution, or (ii) where the distribution is not "for promotional purposes". The second point is made explicit in article 3(6), which permits the Member States to "authorise such distribution in special cases for other purposes". "Other purposes" are not defined but they would naturally be taken to include informational purposes and the avoidance of serious threats to public health.

Article 4 applies in the limited number of cases where advertising to the general public of a medicinal product is permitted by article 3. Article 4(1) imposes two positive obligations on advertising to the general public. The first obligation (article

4(1)(a)) is to set out the advertisement "in such a way that it is clear that the message is an advertisement and that the product is clearly identified as a medicinal product". In practice, this requirement is likely to raise difficulties of interpretation similar to those raised by the "presentation" criterion for a medicinal product[1]. Not all such advertisements will include a notice stating "this is an advertisement for a medicinal product". Article 4(1)(b) specifies three items of minimum information to be included in the advertisement : (i) the name of the product, as well as the common name if the product contains only one active ingredient (for a similar requirement in respect of labelling and package leaflets, see article 2(1)(a) and article 7(1)(a) of Directive (EEC) 92/27, discussed in Chapter 15), (ii) the information necessary for correct use of the product (that is a highly compressed provision which leaves it wholly unclear how much information must in practice be included: compare the detailed requirements of articles 2 and 7 of Directive (EEC) 92/27 in respect of labelling and package leaflets), (iii) an "express, legible[2] invitation to read carefully the instructions of the package leaflet or on the outer packaging, according to the case" (that indicates that less information is required to be included in an advertisement, though not how much less; article 6 of Directive (EEC) 92/27 provides for the circumstances in which a package leaflet is not obligatory[3]). The overall effect of article 4(1)(b) is highly restrictive and would make any advertising other than written advertisements virtually impossible.

Article 4(2) qualifies article 4(1) by granting the Member States a discretion to decide that the advertising of a medicinal product to the general public may include only the name of the product "if it is intended solely as a reminder". There are many medicinal products which have been on the Community market for many years but for an advertisement to be intended "solely" as a reminder, it appears that the advertisement would have to be targeted at a limited class of consumers who were known by the supplier to have purchased the product in the past. The obvious examples of such persons would be people with an established need for a particular treatment such as diabetes sufferers for insulin. It is therefore hard to see how article 4(2) could apply to advertisements "to the general public" in an unrestricted sense, since the advertisement would not be a reminder to all members of the public possibly exposed to the advertisement. "General public" must here be used in contrast with "health care professionals" and to apply without regard to the size of the class to which such a "reminder" is addressed.

Article 5 prohibits the inclusion of twelve types of material in the advertising of medicinal products to the general public. The full text of article 5 is set out in Appendix 13 hereto. The prohibited material falls into five categories :

— material which "gives the impression" or "suggests" that something is the case (article 5(a), (b), (c), (d), (g) and (h));

— material which is directed at a particular class ("exclusively or principally at children", article 5(e));

— material which "refers to" or "mentions" certain matters (article 5(f), (j) and (l));

— material which "could lead to" an unfortunate result ("erroneous self-diagnosis", article 5(i)); and

— material which "uses", ie contains certain material ("pictorial representations", article 5(k))

---

1. See section 2.4 ante.
2. Article 4(1)(b) does not apparently contemplate oral advertising, for example on the radio. A "purposive" construction might interpret "legible" to mean "readily intelligible" in such cases.
3. See section 15.3 ante.

The matters which must not be "suggested" are that : "a medical consultation or surgical operation is unnecessary, in particular by offering a diagnosis or by suggesting treatment by mail" (article 5(a)); "the effects of taking the medicine are guaranteed, are unaccompanied by side effects or are better than, or equivalent to, those of another treatment or medicinal product" (article 5(b)); "the health of the subject can be enhanced by taking the medicine" (article 5(c)); "the health of the subject could be affected by not taking the medicine", subject to article 3(4) in respect of vaccination campaigns (article 5(d)); "the medicinal product is a foodstuff, cosmetic or other consumer product" (article 5(g)); and "the safety or efficacy of the medicinal product is due to the fact that it is natural" (article 5(h)). In general, these diverse prohibitions are relatively easy to understand but certain comments are required. In respect of article 5(a) it should be noted that there is no positive Community obligation, either in Directive (EEC) 92/27 in respect of labelling and package leaflets or in Directive (EEC) 92/28 in respect of advertising,, that a consumer should be advised to consult a doctor if symptoms persist[1]. Article 5(b) clearly prohibits comparative advertising of medicinal products, but it is less clear that an advertisement cannot make *any* claims in respect of the avoidance of unwanted side-effects, for example "does not cause drowsiness"; the wording of 5(b) is ambiguous in that respect. Article 5(c) and (d) refer to "the health of the subject" : it is on its face strange that no claims can be made for medicinal products in respect of beneficial or adverse effects on health; however, in context, the expression must refer to the general health of the patient, not to the fact that the product has a specific effect on a specific ailment. Article 5(g) is strictly redundant, since article 4(1)(a) imposes a positive obligation clearly to identify a product as a medicinal product and, as a matter of Community law, that identification takes priority over any other classification[2]; however, it is a further protection of the consumer that a product cannot be jointly classified (for example, as a foodstuff and a medicinal product), since the consumer will not normally be aware of the legal position. Article 5(h) is an anomalous provision reflecting the scientific priorities of the Community : a product is authorised as safe and efficacious on the basis set out in Directive (EEC) 65/65 and Regulation (EEC) 2309/93; consumers should not be led to believe that "natural" products have any special claim to such properties under the Community regime.

Article 5(e) is easy to understand but would not necessarily be easy to apply in practice : an advertisement which concerns a childhood ailment will not necessarily or even normally be principally directed at children; whether it is so directed can presumably only be determined by the style of the advertising and the context in which it normally appears (an advertisement in an academic medical journal would never be so directed).

Article 5(f), (j) and (l) respectively concern references : "to a recommendation by scientists, health professionals or persons who are neither of the foregoing but who, because of their celebrity, could encourage the consumption of medicinal products"; "in improper, alarming or misleading terms, to claims of recovery"; and to the fact that "the medicinal product has been granted a marketing authorisation". Paragraph (f) prohibits recommendations by, for example, sports stars or television presenters; because of its limitation to celebrities, it would not apparently prevent, for example, a very tall, athletic or handsome person from being used to advertise a particular product. Such examples would, however, be prohibited under paragraph (j) if they gave a misleading impression of a recovery resulting from consumption of a particular product; there is clearly room for dispute as to the meaning of "improper" and "alarming" in the context of claims to recovery. Finally, the prohibition on the mention of the grant of a marketing authorisation prevents the

---

1   Though there is such a requirement in respect of homeopathic products : see article 7(2) of Directive (EEC) 92/73 and section 9.4 ante.

2.   See section 2.3.2 ante.

misleading impression being given that it is a special mark of distinction for a product to be so authorised, whereas in fact no medicinal product can be marketed (or, by article 2(1) of the Directive, advertised) if it has not received marketing authorisation.

Article 5(i) is intended to identify a particular category of misleading advertising which could have serious consequences in the case of a medicinal product. The paragraph prohibits "a description or detailed representation of a case history" which "could ... lead to erroneous self diagnosis". The provision is again hard to apply in practice because even the most accurate and illuminating examples can be misinterpreted. It is clearly not intended to prohibit the use of all such descriptions and representations, so that in practice it appears that it must be intended to impose high standards if such techniques are used. One possibility to reduce the risk of error by the consumer would be to give a warning against the literal application of the example to different facts without taking medical advice.

Article 5(k) prohibits the use "in improper, alarming or misleading terms [of] pictorial representations of changes in the human body caused by disease or injury, or of the action of a medicinal product on the human body or parts thereof". As with article 5(j), the difficulty in practice is likely to arise in defining "improper" and "alarming" in this context.

16.4   Advertising to health professionals : Chapter III, articles 6 to 11

Articles 6 to 11 set out, in some detail and reasonably clearly, Community rules in respect of five separate matters : "advertising of a medicinal product to persons qualified to prescribe or supply such products" (article 6); "documentation relating to a medicinal product which is transmitted as part of the promotion of that product to persons qualified to prescribe or supply it" (article 7); medical sales representatives (article 8); "pecuniary advantages or benefits in kind" and "hospitality" (articles 9 and 10); and "[f]ree samples" (article 11).

Article 6(1) imposes two positive obligations in respect of material to be included in any advertising to persons qualified to prescribe or supply medicinal products : "essential information compatible with the summary of product characteristics"; and "the supply classification of the medicinal product". No guidance is given as to the meaning of "essential information" in this context, by contrast with the detailed guidance in respect of labelling and package leaflets in Directive (EEC) 92/27. However, the six categories of information set out in article 7 of that Directive in respect of package leaflets indicates the type of information required : identification of the product; therapeutic indications; information necessary before taking the product; instructions for use; possible undesirable effects; the expiry date; and the date of revision of the leaflet. The detail of those requirements is discussed in Chapter 15. The needs of health professionals are clearly different from those of consumers in respect of information and that would have to be taken into account in assessing what information was "essential" to them. The information must be compatible with the summary of product characteristics[1].

The requirement that the "supply classification" of the product must be included in advertising to health professionals is a clear reference to Directive (EEC) 92/26, discussed in Chapter 14. A health professional must know whether an advertised product is non-prescription or prescription only and, where such categories are applied by the Member State in which he or she works, if the product is subject to renewable or non-renewable, special or restricted prescription[2].

---

1.   See section 3.43 ante.
2.   See articles 2 and 3 of Directive (EEC) 92/26 (OJ L113 30.4.92 p5).

Article 6(1), second paragraph, permits the Member States additionally to require such advertising to include "the selling price or indicative price of the various presentations and the conditions for reimbursement by social security bodies". article 6(2) is parallel to article 4(2) in respect of advertising to the general public and permits the Member States to decide that advertising to health professionals is exempt from the requirement of article 6(1) "if it is intended solely as a reminder". A "reminder" in this context must refer to advertising designed to lead to repeat orders of products previously supplied to the doctor or pharmacist in question.

Article 7 demonstrates that article 6 is not limited to advertising in documentary form, as article 7 lays down rules in respect of "documentation relating to a medicinal product which is transmitted as part of the promotion of that product to persons qualified to prescribe or supply it". Article 7(1), requires such information to "include as a minimum the particulars listed in article 6(1)" and to "state the date on which [the documentation] was drawn up or last revised". Article 7(2) requires that the documentation be "accurate, up-to-date, verifiable and sufficiently complete to enable the recipient to form his or her own opinion of the therapeutic value of the medicinal product concerned". In general, it would seem that a product leaflet produced in accordance with the requirements of article 7 of Directive (EEC) 92/27 would fulfil the majority of the requirements of article 7(1) and (2) of Directive (EEC) 92/28; however, it would not give sufficient information for a doctor or pharmacist to form his or her own opinion of the product and article 7(3) provides for the provision of information of a kind that would not appear in a product leaflet : "[q]uotations as well as tables and other illustrative matter taken from medical journals or other scientific works"; article 7(3) requires such information to be "faithfully reproduced and the precise sources indicated."

Article 8 imposes certain obligations on pharmaceutical companies which employ medical sales representatives and on those representatives themselves. The representatives must :

— "be given adequate training by the firm which employs them"; and

— "have sufficient scientific knowledge to be able to provide information which is precise and as complete as possible about the medicinal products which they promote" (article 8(1));

those are extremely vague requirements which would require detailed implementation by the Member States if they were to be effectively enforceable.

They must also, during each visit :

— "give the person visited, or have available for them, summaries of the product characteristics of each medicinal product they present together, if the legislation of the Member State so permits, with details of the price and conditions for reimbursement referred to in article 6(1)" (article 8(2));

— "transmit to the scientific service referred to in article 13(1) any information about the use of the medicinal products they advertise, with particular reference to any adverse reactions reported to them by the persons they visit" (article 8(3)).

The representatives are thus required to provide essential information both to health professionals and from health professionals as part of their work. The "scientific service" referred to is discussed below in respect of article 13 of the Directive : the information passed back from health professionals to pharmaceutical companies is clearly a very important element in the "pharmacovigilance" system discussed in

Chapter 12 and medical sales representatives are required by article 8(3) to perform a significant part in that process.

Articles 9 and 10 relate to inducements to health professionals of all kinds : pecuniary advantages, benefits in kind and hospitality. Article 9(1) lays down the basic rule that no such advantages or benefits "may be supplied, offered or promised to such persons unless they are inexpensive and relevant to the practice of medicine or pharmacy". That is clearly a strict rule with only a minor exception. The much more significant exception in financial terms is the provision of hospitality at sales promotion meetings and meetings held for "purely professional and scientific purposes". That is dealt with at article 9(1) and article 10. In each case, such hospitality is permitted but "must always be reasonable in level and remain subordinate to the main purpose [or scientific objective] of the meeting and must not be extended to other than health professionals". Promotional extravaganzas are thus outlawed by the Directive.

Article 9(3) imposes a prohibition on persons qualified to prescribe or supply medicinal products, not to "solicit or accept any inducement prohibited under [article 9(1) or contrary to [article 9(2)]".

Article 9(4) contains an important exception, that "[e]xisting measures or trade practices in Member States relating to prices, margins and discounts shall not be affected by [article 9]". The topic of price control and reimbursement is discussed briefly in Chapter 1 ante but it is clearly an important area where Member States' practices are widely divergent and which the Community has so far not sought to control to any degree. Pharmacists in particular are retailers as well as health professionals and they therefore depend in part on their margins on resale for their livelihood, subject to the special rules brought into force in the Member States to reflect the artificiality of a market in which the consumer does not generally pay the true cost of the product purchased and frequently pays nothing at all. Article 9(4) confirms that such practices do not constitute "pecuniary advantages" within the scope of article 9(1).

Article 11 concerns free samples. Article 11(1) provides that they are to be provided "on an exceptional basis only to persons qualified to prescribe them" ie not to pharmacists, and subject to seven conditions. Only "a limited number of samples for each medicinal product each year on prescription" may be supplied : article 11(1)(a). That is unclear, but appears to indicate that samples may only be provided of prescription only products; no definition is given of "a limited number" but that is a matter to be specified in implementing legislation; the appropriate number of samples would vary with the nature and cost of the product concerned. Article 11(1)(b) requires that any supply of samples "must be in response to a written request, signed and dated, from the recipient"; and article 11(1)(c) requires those supplying the samples to "maintain an adequate system of control and accountability". Article (11)(1)(d) to (f) impose three requirements in respect of the samples themselves : they must be "identical with the smallest presentation on the market", must be marked "free medical sample - not for resale or bear another legend of analogous meaning", and must be accompanied by a copy of the summary of product characteristics. Article 11(1)(g) prohibits the supply of samples of "medicinal products containing psychotropic or narcotic substances within the meaning of international conventions". That final prohibition is unexplained and did not appear in the original Commission proposal. It is presumably contrary to general social policy for free samples of such products to be supplied, and there must also be some fear of abuse (whether commercial or personal) should such products be supplied free to doctors.

Article 11(2) permits the Member States to "place further restrictions on the distribution of samples of certain medicinal products". That apparently allows restrictions of any kind to be imposed, but requires that such restrictions should not be generally applicable but should specify particular categories of products to which the additional restrictions apply. It would not apparently allow stricter general rules.

16.5   Monitoring of advertising : Chapter IV, articles 12 to 16

The principal articles of Chapter IV of the Directive, articles 12 and 13, deal with two distinct but related matters : article 12, which is closely modelled on articles 4 and 5 of Directive (EEC) 84/450 on the control of misleading advertising (the "monitoring mechanisms set up by Directive (EEC) 84/450" are expressly referred to in recital 11 to Directive (EEC) 92/28); and article 13, which requires the holder of a marketing authorisation to establish a scientific information service charged with the responsibility of providing information to the national monitoring authorities and compliance with their decisions. Articles 14 to 16 deal with the implementation of the Directive in the Member States by 1 January 1993, article 14 in particular requiring full application of the Directive's provisions and determination by the Member States of the penalties to be imposed for infringement of the national implementing provisions.

Article 12(1) imposes a general obligation on the Member States to ensure that "there are adequate and effective methods to monitor the advertising of medicinal products". The remainder of the paragraph, and of article 12, sets out specific minimum requirements for the fulfilment of that obligation and also permits certain other steps to be taken.

The minimum requirements are :

(1) The Member States must enact : "legal provisions under which persons or organisations regarded under national law as having a legitimate interest in prohibiting any advertisement inconsistent with this Directive may take legal action against such advertisement, or bring such advertisement before an administrative authority competent either to decide on complaints or to initiate appropriate legal proceedings" (article 12(1)).

Given the nature of the interests protected by the Directive and the prohibitions contained in article 5 in particular in respect of advertising to the general public, it would seem appropriate that the concept of "legitimate interest" should be widely construed, though the Directive clearly leaves the matter to national administrative law to determine (members of the general public would not have so obvious a legitimate interest in advertising to health professionals). Article 12(1) naturally differs from the equivalent provision of Directive (EEC) 84/450 in referring to "any advertisement inconsistent with this Directive" rather than to "misleading advertising".

(2) The Member States must confer powers on such courts or administrative authorities, "in cases where they deem such measures to be necessary taking into account all the interests involved and in particular the public interest", either

(a) (i) to order the cessation of "misleading advertising" or (in the case of administrative authorities) (ii) to commence legal proceedings for its cessation, or

(b) (i) to order the prohibition of publication of such advertising if it "has not yet been published but publication is imminent" or (ii) to commence legal proceedings for such a prohibition;

in each case "even without proof of actual loss or damage or of intention or negligence on the part of the advertiser" (article 12(2), first sub-paragraph).

The courts and administrative authorities thus are required to be given a wide discretion in the monitoring and control of "misleading advertising". In the context of Directive (EEC) 92/28, the use of the expression "misleading advertising" in article 12(2) appears to be a drafting error rather than a limitation on the powers of the relevant authorities : a "purposive" interpretation would take that expression to be equivalent in context to the expression "any advertisement inconsistent with this Directive" in article 12(1). The reference to the "advertiser" is also unexplained : it could refer to the holder of the marketing authorisation or to the person actually responsible for the creation or placing of the advertisement; whatever it means, the authorities are not obliged to take account of "the advertiser's" state of mind, so that the legal position is unaltered.

(3) Provision must be made for "an accelerated procedure" with either (i) interim effect or (ii) definitive effect, "on the understanding that it is for each Member State to decide which of the two options to select" (article 12(2), second sub-paragraph).

The effect of that provision is to compel the Member States to specify a single accelerated procedure, rather than leaving it to the court or administrative authority to exercise a further discretion.

(4) Article 12(3) does not correspond to anything in Directive (EEC) 84/450. It contains the standard provision originally found in article 12 of Directive (EEC) 65/65, that an administrative decision taken under the Community pharmaceutical rules must : (i) state in detail the reasons on which it is based; (ii) be communicated to the person concerned; and (iii) mention the redress available at law and the time limits allowed for access to that redress.

In addition to those four requirements, the Member States are empowered :

(1) to introduce "a system of prior vetting" of advertising of medicinal products (article 12(1));

(2) to confer a power on the relevant courts or authorities, "with a view to eliminating the continuing effects of misleading advertising the cessation of which has been ordered by a final decision", to require : (i) publication of their decision "in full or in part and in such form as they deem adequate; and (ii) "publication of a corrective statement" (article 12(2), third sub-paragraph);

(3) "voluntary control of advertising of medicinal products by self-regulatory bodies and recourse to such bodies"; that possibility is conditional on such control being "in addition" to the compulsory measures set out above.

Article 13(1) requires a holder of a marketing authorisation (as to which see Chapter 3) to establish "within his undertaking a scientific service in charge of information about the medicinal products which he places on the market". Article 13(2) imposes five obligations on "the person responsible for placing the product on the market" (once a product is authorised, the persons referred to in article 14(1) and (2), will be the same person, so the significance in the variation of the wording seems to be limited to cases where advertising relates either to medicinal products which are unauthorised (contrary to article 2(1) of the Directive) or to products the authorisation of which has been revoked). That ensures that the obligations imposed by article 13 do not lapse where a product is not currently authorised. The five obligations are :

(1) to "keep available for, or communicate to, the authorities or bodies responsible for monitoring advertising of medicinal products a sample of all advertisements emanating from his undertaking together with a statement indicating the persons to whom it is addressed, the method of dissemination and the date of first dissemination" (article 13(2), first indent)[1];

(2) to ensure conformity by its advertising to the requirements of the Directive (article 13(2), second indent);

(3) to verify that article 8 has been observed in respect of its medical sales representatives (article 13(2), third indent);

(4) to supply the relevant authorities or bodies with "the information and assistance they require to carry out their responsibilities" (article 13(2), fourth indent); and

(5) to ensure that the decisions of such authorities are "immediately and fully complied with" (article 13(2), fifth indent).

As stated above, the Member States are required by article 14 of the Directive to specify penalties to be imposed "should the provisions adopted in the execution of this Directive be infringed". Directive (EEC) 92/28 thus imposes a considerable further constraint on the commercial conduct of pharmaceutical companies.

---

1. In effect, the company must be in a position to provide full information to the relevant external or self-regulatory body for either prospective or retrospective control over its advertising.

APPENDICES

APPENDIX 1

COUNCIL DIRECTIVE (EEC) 65/65
of 26 January 1965

on the approximation of provisions laid down by law, regulation or administrative action relating to medicinal products[1]

THE COUNCIL OF THE EUROPEAN ECONOMIC COMMUNITY,

Having regard to the Treaty establishing the European Economic Community, and in particular Article 100 thereof;

Having regard to the proposal from the Commission;

Having regard to the Opinion of the European Parliament[2];

Having regard to the Opinion of the Economic and Social Committee[3];

Whereas the primary purpose of any rules concerning the production and distribution of medicinal products must be to safeguard public health;

Whereas, however, this objective must be attained by means which will not hinder the development of the pharmaceutical industry or trade in medicinal products within the Community;

Whereas trade in medicinal products within the Community is hindered by disparities between certain national provisions, in particular between provisions relating to medicinal products (excluding substances or combinations of substances which are foods, animal feeding-stuffs or toilet preparations); and whereas such disparities directly affect the establishment and functioning of the common market;

Whereas such hindrances must accordingly be removed; and whereas this entails approximation of the relevant provisions;

Whereas, however, such approximation can only be achieved progressively; and whereas priority must be given to eliminating the disparities liable to have the greatest effect on the functioning of the common market;

HAS ADOPTED THIS DIRECTIVE:

CHAPTER I

DEFINITIONS AND SCOPE

Article 1
For the purposes of this Directive, the following shall have the meanings hereby assigned to them;

---

1.   OJ No 22 9.2.65 p369/65. Note that Council Directive (EEC) 89/341, OJ L142 25.5.89 p11, replaces all references in the title, preamble and Chapters II to V to "proprietary medicinal product" by "medicinal product". For reasons of consistency, references to "proprietary products" have also been altered in the text to "products" or "medicinal products" as appropriate.
2.   OJ No 84 4.6.1963 p1571/63.
3.   OJ No 158 16.10.1964 p2508/64.

1.   *Proprietary medicinal product :*

Any ready-prepared medicinal product placed on the market under a special name and in a special pack.

2.   *Medicinal product :*

Any substance or combination of substances presented for treating or preventing disease in human beings or animals.

Any substance or combination of substances which may be administered to human beings or animals with a view to making a medical diagnosis or to restoring, correcting or modifying physiological functions in human beings or in animals is likewise considered a medicinal product.

3.   *Substance :*

Any matter irrespective of origin which may be :

— human, e.g.
     human blood and human blood products;
— animal, e.g.
     micro-organisms, whole animals, parts of organs, animal secretions, toxins, extracts, blood products, etc;
— vegetable, e.g.
     micro-organisms, plants, parts of plants, vegetable secretions, extracts, etc;
— chemical, e.g.
     elements, naturally occurring chemical materials and chemical products obtained by chemical change or synthesis.

[4.   *Magistral formula :*

Any medicinal product prepared in a pharmacy in accordance with a prescription for an individual patient.

5.   *Official formula :*

Any medicinal product which is prepared in a pharmacy in accordance with the prescriptions of a pharmacopoeia and is intended to be supplied directly to the patients served by the pharmacy in question.][1]

Article 2
[1.   Chapters II to V shall apply to proprietary medicinal products for human use intended to be placed on the market in Member States.

2.   Where a Member State authorises the placing on the market of industrially produced medicinal products which do not comply with the definition of a proprietary medicinal product, it shall also apply Chapters II to V to them.

3.   Chapters II to V shall not apply to :

— medicinal products prepared on the basis of a magistral or official formula,
— medicinal products intended for research and development trials,

---

1.   Inserted by Council Directive (EEC) 89/341, OJ L142 25.5.89 p11.

—   intermediate products intended for further processing by an authorised manufacturer.

4.   A Member State may, in accordance with legislation in force and to fulfil special needs, exclude from Chapters II to V medicinal products supplied in response to a bona fide unsolicited order, formulated in accordance with the specifications of an authorised health care professional and for use by his individual patients on his direct personal responsibility.][1]

CHAPTER II

AUTHORISATION TO PLACE MEDICINAL PRODUCTS ON THE MARKET

Article 3

[No medicinal product may be placed on the market of a Member State unless a marketing authorisation has been issued by the competent authorities of that Member State in accordance with this Directive or an authorisation has been granted in accordance with Regulation (EEC) No 2309/93 of 22 July 1993 laying down Community procedures for the authorisation and supervision of medicinal products for human and veterinary use and establishing a European Agency for the Evaluation of Medicinal Products[2].

The provisions of this Directive shall not affect the powers of the Member States' authorities either as regards the setting of prices for medicinal products or their inclusion in the scope of national health insurance schemes, on the basis of health, economic and social conditions.][3]

Article 4

In order to obtain an authorisation to place a medicinal product on the market as provided for in Article 3, the person responsible for placing that product on the market shall make application to the competent authority of the Member State concerned.

[The person responsible for placing medicinal products on the market shall be established in the Community. In respect of medicinal products authorised on the date of implementation of this Directive, the Member State shall if necessary apply this provision at the time of the five-yearly renewal of the marketing authorisation provided for in Article 10.][4]

The application shall be accompanied by the following particulars and documents :

1.   Name or corporate name and permanent address of the person responsible for placing the product on the market and, where applicable, of the manufacturer.

---

1.   Replaced by Council Directive (EEC) 89/341, OJ L14 25.5.89 p12-13.
2.   OJ L214 14.8.93 p1.
3.   Replaced by Council Directive (EEC) 93/39, OJ L214 24.8.93 p23 with effect from 1 January 1995.
      Pre-1993 Text read as follows :
          "No medicinal product may be placed on the market in a Member State unless an authorisation has been issued by the competent authority of that Member State."
4.   Added by Council Directive (EEC) 93/39, OJ L214 24.8.93 p23 with effect from 1 January 1995.
      Pre 1993 Text to be read without insertion at second sub-paragraph.

2. Name of the product (brand name, or common name together with a trade mark or name of the manufacturer, or scientific name together with a trade mark or name of the manufacturer).

3. Qualitative and quantitative particulars of all the constituents of the product in usual terminology, but excluding empirical chemical formulae, with mention of the international non-proprietary name recommended by the World Health Organisation where such name exists.

4. Brief description of the method of preparation.

5. Therapeutic indications, contra-indications and side-effects.

[6. Posology, pharmaceutical form, method and route of administration and expected shelf life.

If applicable, reasons for any precautionary and safety measures to be taken for the storage of the medicinal product, its administration to patients and for the disposal of waste products, together with an indication of any potential risks presented by the medicinal product for the environment.][1]

[7. Description of the control methods employed by the manufacturer (qualitative and quantitative analysis of the constituents and of the finished product, special tests, e.g. sterility tests, tests for the presence of pyrogenic substances, the presence of heavy metals, stability tests, biological and toxicity tests, controls carried out at an intermediate stage of the manufacturing process).][2]

[8. Results of :

— physico-chemical, biological or microbiological tests;
— pharmacological and toxicological tests;
— clinical trials.

However, and without prejudice to the law relating to the protection of industrial and commercial property :

(a) The applicant shall not be required to provide the results of pharmacological and toxicological tests or the results of clinical trials if he can demonstrate :

(i) either that the medicinal product is essentially similar to a product authorised in the country concerned by the application and that the person responsible for the marketing of the original medicinal product has consented to the pharmacological, toxicological or clinical references contained in the file on the original medicinal product being used for the purpose of examining the application in question;

(ii) or by detailed references to published scientific literature presented in accordance with the second paragraph of Article 1 of Directive 75/318/EEC that the constituent or constituents of the medicinal product have a well established medicinal use, with recognised efficacy and an acceptable level of safety;

---

1. Replaced by Council Directive (EEC) 93/39, OJ L214 24.8.93 p23 with effect from 1 January 1995.
   Pre 1993 Text read as follows :
   "Posology, pharmaceutical form, method and route of administration and expected shelf life."
2. Replaced by Council Directive (EEC) 75/319, OJ L147 9.6.75 p21.

(iii)   or that the medicinal product is essentially similar to a product which has been authorised within the Community, in accordance with Community provisions in force, for not less than six years and is marketed in the Member State for which the application is made; this period shall be extended to 10 years in the case of high-technology medicinal products within the meaning of Part A in the Annex to Directive 87/22/EEC[1] or of a medicinal product within the meaning of Part B in the Annex to that Directive for which the procedure laid down in Article 2 thereof has been followed; furthermore, a Member State may also extend this period to 10 years by a single Decision covering all the products marketed on its territory where it considers this necessary in the interest of public health. Member States are at liberty not to apply the abovementioned six-year period beyond the date of expiry of a patent protecting the original product.

However, where the medicinal product is intended for a different therapeutic use from that of the other medicinal products marketed or is to be administered by different routes or in different doses, the results of appropriate pharmacological and toxicological tests and/or of appropriate clinical trials must be provided.

(b)   In the case of new medicinal products containing known constituents not hitherto used in combination for therapeutic purposes, the results of pharmacological and toxicological tests and of clinical trials relating to that combination must be provided, but it shall not be necessary to provide references relating to each individual constituent.][2]

[9.   A summary, in accordance with Article 4a, of the product characteristics, one or more specimens or mock-ups of the sales presentation of the product, together with a package leaflet where one is to be enclosed.][3]

10.   A document showing that the manufacturer is authorised in his own country to produce medicinal products.

[11.   Copies of any authorisation obtained in another Member State or in a third country to place the relevant medicinal product on the market, together with a list of those Member States in which an application for authorisation submitted in accordance with this Directive is under examination. Copies of the summary of the product characteristics proposed by the applicant in accordance with Article 4a or approved by the competent authorities of the Member State in accordance with Article 4b. Copies of the package leaflet proposed in accordance with Article 6 of Directive 92/27/EEC or approved by the competent authorities of the Member State in accordance with Article 10 of the same Directive. Details of any decision to refuse authorisation, whether in the Community or in a third country, and the reasons for such decision.

This information shall be updated on a regular basis.][4]

---

1.   OJ L15 17.1.87 p38.
2.   Amended by Council Directive (EEC) 87/21, OJ L15 17.1.87 p37.
3.   Replaced by Council Directive (EEC) 83/570, OJ L332 28.11.83 p2.
4.   Replaced by Council Directive (EEC) 93/39, OJ L214 24.8.93 p23 with effect from 1 January 1995.
       Pre 1993 Text read as follows :
       "Any authorisation obtained in another Member State or in a third country to place the relevant product on the market."

Article 4a

[The summary of the product characteristics referred to in point 9 of the second paragraph of Article 4 shall contain the following information :

1.   Name of the medicinal product.

2.   Qualitative and quantitative composition in terms of the active ingredients and constituents of the excipient, knowledge of which is essential for proper administration of the medicinal product; the international non-proprietary names recommended by the World Health Organisation shall be used, where such names exist, or failing this, the usual common name or chemical description.

3.   Pharmaceutical form.

4.   Pharmacological properties and, in so far as this information is useful for therapeutic purposes, pharmacokinetic particulars.

5.   Clinical particulars :
    5.1.   therapeutic indications,
    5.2.   contra-indications,
    5.3.   undesirable effects (frequency and seriousness),
    5.4.   special precautions for use,
    5.5.   use during pregnancy and lactation,
    5.6.   interaction with other medicaments and other forms of interaction,
    5.7.   posology and method of administration for adults and, where necessary, for children,
    5.8.   overdose (symptoms, emergency procedures, antidotes),
    5.9.   special warnings,
    5.10. effects on ability to drive and to use machines.

6   Pharmaceutical particulars :
    6.1.   incompatibilities (major),
    6.2.   shelf life, when necessary after reconstitution of the product or when the container is opened for the first time,
    6.3.   special precautions for storage,
    6.4.   nature and contents of container,
    6.5.   name or style and permanent address or registered place of business of the holder of the marketing authorisation,][1]
    [6.6.   special precautions for disposal of unused products or waste materials derived from such products, if appropriate.][2]

[Article 4b

When the marketing authorisation referred to in Article 3 is issued, the person responsible for placing that product on the market shall be informed, by the competent authorities of the Member State concerned, of the summary of the product characteristics as approved by it. The competent authorities shall take all necessary measures to ensure that the information given in the summary is in conformity with that accepted when the marketing authorisation is issued or subsequently. The competent authorities shall forward to the European Agency for the Evaluation of Medicinal Products a copy of the authorisation together with the summary of the product characteristics referred to in Article 4a.

Furthermore, the competent authorities shall draw up an assessment report and comments on the dossier as regards the results of the analytical and

1.   Inserted by Council Directive (EEC) 83/570, OJ L332 28.11.83 p2.
2.   Added by Council Directive (EEC) 89/341, OJ L142 25.5.89 p12.

pharmacotoxicological tests and the clinical trials of the medicinal product concerned. The assessment report shall be updated whenever new information becomes available which is of importance for the evaluation of the quality, safety or efficacy of the medicinal product concerned.][1]

Article 5

The authorisation provided for in Article 3 shall be refused if, after verification of the particulars and documents listed in Article 4, it proves that the medicinal product is harmful in the normal conditions of use, or that its therapeutic efficacy is lacking or is insufficiently substantiated by the applicant, or that its qualitative and quantitative composition is not as declared.

Authorisation shall likewise be refused if the particulars and documents submitted in support of the application do not comply with Article 4.

Article 6

[This Directive shall not affect the application of national legislation prohibiting or restricting the sale, supply or use of medicinal products as contraceptives or abortifacients. The Member States shall communicate the national legislation concerned to the Commission.][2]

Article 7

[1.   Member States shall take all appropriate measures to ensure that the procedure for granting an authorisation to place a medicinal product on the market is completed within 210 days of the submission of a valid application.

2   Where a Member State notes that an application for authorisation submitted after 1 January 1995 is already under active examination in another Member State in respect of that medicinal product, the Member State concerned may decide to suspend the detailed examination of the application in order to await the assessment report prepared by the other Member State in accordance with Article 4b.

The Member State concerned shall inform the other Member State and the applicant of its decision to suspend detailed examination of the application in question. As soon as it has completed the examination of the application and

---

1.   Originally inserted by Council Directed 83/570, OJ L332 28.11.83, subsequently replaced by Council Directive (EEC) 93/39, OJ L214 24.8.93 p23 with effect from 1 January 1995.
       Pre 1993 Text read as follows :
            "When the marketing authorisation referred to in Article 3 is issued, the person responsible for placing the product on the market shall be informed, by the competent authorities of the Member State concerned, of the summary of the product characteristics as approved by them. The competent authorities shall take all necessary measures to ensure that the information given in the summary is in conformity with that accepted when the marketing authorisation is issued or subsequently."
2.   Replaced by Council Directive (EEC) 93/39, OJ L214 24.8.93 p24 with effect from 1 January 1995.
       Pre 1993 Text read as follows :
            "The competent authorities of Member States may refuse to authorise the placing on the market of a medicinal product for use as a contraceptive where the sale of proprietary products intended principally for such purposes is prohibited under their laws."

reached a decision, the other Member State shall forward a copy of its assessment report to the Member State concerned.

Within 90 days of the receipt of the assessment report, the Member State concerned shall either recognise the decision of the other Member State and the summary of the product characteristics as approved by it, or, if it considers that there are grounds for supposing that the authorisation of the medicinal product concerned may present a risk to public health[1], it shall apply the procedures set out in Articles 10 to 14 of Directive 75/319/EEC.][2]

[*Article 7a*

With effect from 1 January 1998, where a Member State is informed in accordance with point 11 of the second paragraph of Article 4 that another Member State has authorised a medicinal product which is the subject of an application for authorisation in the Member State concerned, that Member State shall forthwith request the authorities of the Member State which has granted the authorisation to forward to it the assessment report referred to in the second paragraph of Article 4b. Within 90 days of the receipt of the assessment report, the Member State concerned shall either recognise the decision of the first Member State and the summary of the product characteristics as approved by it or, if it considers that there are grounds for supposing that the authorisation of the medicinal product concerned may present a risk to public health[3], it shall apply the procedures set out in Articles 10 to 14 of Directive 75/319/EEC.][4]

Article 8

Member States shall take all appropriate measures to ensure that the holder of an authorisation furnishes proof that the controls have been carried out on the finished product in accordance with the methods described by the applicant pursuant to item 7 of the second paragraph of Article 4.

Article 9

Authorisation shall not affect the civil and criminal liability of the manufacturer and, where applicable, of the person responsible for placing the medicinal product on the market.

[*Article 9a*

After an authorisation has been issued, the person responsible for placing the product on the market must, in respect of the methods of preparation and control

---

1. "The expression 'risk to public health' refers to the quality, safety and efficacy of the medicinal product."
2. Replaced by Council Directive (EEC) 93/39, OJ L214 24.8.93 p24 with effect from 1 January 1995.
   Pre 1993 Text read as follows :
   "Member States shall take all appropriate measures to ensure that the procedure for granting an authorisation to place a medicinal product on the market is completed within 120 days of the date of submitting the application.

   In exceptional cases this time limit may be extended for a further 90 days. The applicant shall be notified of such extension before the expiry of the initial time limit."
3. See footnote 1 above.
4. Inserted by Council Directive (EEC) 93/39, OJ L214 24.8.93 p24 with effect from 1 January 1998.
   Pre 1993 Text to be read without insertion of article 7a.

provided for in points 4 and 7 of the second paragraph of Article 4, take account of technical and scientific progress and introduce any changes that may be required to enable that medicinal product to be manufactured and checked by means of generally accepted scientific methods. These changes shall be subject to the approval of the competent authority of the Member State concerned.][1]

Article 10

[1.   Authorisation shall be valid for five years and shall be renewable for five-year periods, on application by the holder at least three months before the expiry date and after consideration by the competent authority of a dossier containing in particular details of the data on pharmacovigilance and other information relevant to the monitoring of the medicinal product.

2.   In exceptional circumstances, and following consultation with the applicant, an authorisation may be granted subject to certain specific obligations, including :

— the carrying out of further studies following the granting of authorisation;
— the notification of adverse reactions to the medicinal product.

These exceptional decisions may be adopted only for objective and verifiable reasons and shall be based on one of the causes referred to in Part 4(G) of the Annex to Directive 75/318/EEC.][2]

CHAPTER III

SUSPENSION AND REVOCATION OF AUTHORISATION TO MARKET MEDICINAL PRODUCTS

Article 11

The competent authorities of the Member States shall suspend or revoke an authorisation to place a medicinal product on the market where that product proves to be harmful in the normal conditions of use, or where its therapeutic efficacy is lacking, or where its qualitative and quantitative composition is not as declared. Therapeutic efficacy is lacking when it is established that therapeutic results cannot be obtained with the product.

[An authorisation shall also be suspended or revoked where the particulars supporting the application as provided for in Articles 4 and 4a are incorrect or have not been amended in accordance with Article 9a, or when the controls referred to in Article 8 of this Directive or in Article 27 of Second Council Directive

---

1.   Replaced by Council Directive (EEC) 93/39, OJ L214 24.8.93 p24 with effect from 1 January 1995.
      Pre 1993 Text read as follows :
      "When an authorisation has been issued, the person responsible for placing the product on the market must, in respect of the control methods provided for in Article 4(7), take account of technical and scientific progress and introduce any changes that may be required to enable the medicinal product to be checked by means of generally accepted scientific methods. These changes must be accepted by the competent authorities of the Member States concerned."
2.   Originally amended by Council Directive (EEC) 83/570, OJ L332 28.11.83 p3, subsequently replaced by Council Directive (EEC) 93/39, OJ L214 24.8.93 p24 with effect from 1 January 1995.
      Pre 1993 Text read as follows :
      "An authorisation shall be valid for five years and be renewable for five-year periods on application by the holder at least three months before expiry."

75/319/EEC of 20 May 1975 on the approximation of provisions laid down by law, regulation or administrative action relating to medicinal products[1] have not been carried out.][2]

Article 12

All decisions taken pursuant to Articles 5, 6 or 11 shall state in detail the reasons on which they are based. A decision shall be notified to the party concerned, who shall at the same time be informed of the remedies available to him under the laws in force and of the time limit allowed for the exercise of such remedies.

Authorisations to place a medicinal product on the market and decisions to revoke authorisations shall be published by each Member State in the appropriate official publication.

CHAPTER IV

LABELLING OF MEDICINAL PRODUCTS

[*Article 13*][3]

[*Article 14*][4]

[*Article 15*][5]

[*Article 16*][6]

[*Article 17*][7]

[*Article 18*][8]

[*Article 19*][9]

[*Article 20*][10]

---

1.   OJ L147 9.6.75 p13.
2.   Amended by Council Directive (EEC) 83/570, OJ L332 28.11.83 p3.
3.   Repealed by Council Directive (EEC) 92/27, OJ L113 30.4.92 p8.
4.   Repealed by ibid.
5.   Repealed by ibid.
6.   Repealed by Council Directive (EEC) 87/21, OJ L15 17.1.87 p37.
7.   Repealed by Council Directive (EEC) 92/27, OJ L113 30.4.92 p8.
8.   Repealed by ibid.
9.   Repealed by ibid.
10.   Repealed by ibid.

CHAPTER V

GENERAL AND FINAL PROVISIONS

Article 21

An authorisation to market a medicinal product shall not be refused, suspended or revoked except on the grounds set out in this Directive.

Article 22

Member States shall put into force the measures needed in order to comply with this Directive [not later than 31 December 1966][1] and shall inform the Commission forthwith.

Article 23

Member States shall ensure that they communicate to the Commission the text of the main provisions of national law which they adopt in the field covered by this Directive.

Article 24

[Within the time limits and under the conditions laid down in Article 39(2) and (3) of second Directive 75/319/EEC the rules laid down in this Directive shall be applied progressively to medicinal products covered by an authorisation to place on the market by virtue of previous provisions.][2]

Article 25

This Directive is addressed to the Member States.

Done at Brussels, 26 January 1965.

For the Council

The President

M. COUVE DE MURVILLE

---

1.   Amended by Council Directive 66/454, OJ No 144 5.8.66 p2658/66.
2.   Amended by Council Directive (EEC) 75/319, OJ L147 9.6.75 p21.

APPENDIX 2

COUNCIL DIRECTIVE (EEC) 75/318
of 20 May 1975

on the approximation of the laws of Member States relating to analytical, pharmacotoxicological and clinical standards and protocols in respect of the testing of medicinal products[1]

THE COUNCIL OF THE EUROPEAN COMMUNITIES,

Having regard to the Treaty establishing the European Economic Community, and in particular Article 100 thereof;

Having regard to the proposal from the Commission;

Whereas the approximation begun by Council Directive 65/65/EEC[2] of 26 January 1965 on the approximation of provisions laid down by law, regulation or administrative action relating to medicinal products should be continued and the implementation of the principles laid down in that Directive should be ensured;

Whereas among existing disparities those relating to the control of medicinal products are of fundamental importance and point 8 of Article 4, second paragraph of the said Directive requires that applications for authorisation to place a medicinal product on the market should be accompanied by particulars and documents relating to the results of tests and trials carried out on the product concerned;

Whereas standards and protocols for the performance of tests and trials on medicinal products are an effective means of control of these products and hence of protecting public health and can facilitate the movement of these products by laying down uniform rules applicable to tests and trials, the compilation of dossiers and the examination of applications;

Whereas the adoption of the same standards and protocols by all the Member States will enable the competent authorities to arrive at their decisions on the basis of uniform tests and by reference to uniform criteria and will therefore help to avoid differences in evaluation;

Whereas the physico-chemical, biological or microbiological tests provided for in point 8 of Article 4, second paragraph, of Directive 65/65/EEC are closely related to points 3, 4, 6 and 7 of the same paragraph and it is therefore necessary to specify the data to be provided pursuant to these points;

Whereas the quality of the tests is the essential consideration; whereas therefore tests carried out in accordance with these provisions must be taken into consideration irrespective of the nationality of the experts who perform them or the country in which they are carried out;

Whereas the concepts of "harmfulness" and "therapeutic efficacy" referred to in Article 5 of Directive 65/65/EEC can only be examined in relation to each other and have only a relative significance depending on the progress of scientific

---

1.   OJ L147 9.6.75 p1. Note that Council Directive (EEC) 89/341 replaces all references to "proprietary medicinal product" or to "proprietary product" by "medicinal product".
2.   OJ No 22 2.9.65 p369/65.

knowledge and the use for which the medicinal product is intended; whereas the particulars and documents which must accompany an application for authorisation to place a medicinal product on the market demonstrate that potential risks are outweighed by the therapeutic efficacy of the product; whereas failing such demonstration, the application must be rejected;

Whereas the evaluation of "harmfulness" and "therapeutic efficacy" may be modified in the light of new discoveries and standards and protocols must be amended periodically to take account of scientific progress,

HAS ADOPTED THIS DIRECTIVE :

Article 1
Member States shall take all appropriate measures to ensure that the particulars and documents which must accompany applications for authorisation to place a medicinal product on the market (marketing authorisation), pursuant to points 3, 4, 6, 7 and 8 of Article 4, second paragraph, of Directive 65/65/EEC, are submitted by the persons concerned in accordance with the Annex to this Directive.

Where, pursuant to point 8(a) and (b) of Article 4, second paragraph, of the abovementioned Directive, references to published data are submitted, the provisions of this Directive shall apply in like manner.

Article 2
Notwithstanding the provisions of other Directives on medicinal products, Member States shall take all appropriate measures to ensure that the competent authorities examine the particulars and documents submitted in support of applications for marketing authorisation in accordance with the criteria of the Annex to this Directive.

[Article 2a
Any changes which are necessary in order to adapt the Annex to take account of technical progress shall be adopted in accordance with the procedure laid down in Article 2c.

If appropriate, the Commission shall propose to the Council that the procedure in Article 2c be reviewed in connection with the detailed rules set for the exercise of the powers of implementation granted to the Commission.

Article 2b
1.   A [Standing Committee on Medicinal Products for Human Use][1], hereinafter called "the Committee", is hereby set up; it shall consist of representatives of the Member States with a representative of the Commission as chairman.

2.   The Committee shall adopt its own rules of procedure.

Article 2c

---

1.   Amended by Council Directive (EEC) 93/39, OJ L214 24.8.93 p25 with effect from 1 January 1995.
       Pre 1993 Text read as follows :
          "A Committee on the Adaptation to Technical Progress of the Directives on the Removal of Technical Barriers to Trade in the Medicinal Products Sector".

1.   Where the procedure laid down in this Article is to be followed, matters shall be referred to the Committee by the chairman either on his own initiative or at the request of the representative of a Member State.

2.   The representative of the Commission shall submit to the Committee a draft of the measures to be adopted. The Committee shall deliver its opinion on the draft within a time limit set by the chairman, having regard to the urgency of the matter. It shall act by a qualified majority, the votes of the Member States being weighted as provided in Article 148(2) of the Treaty. The chairman shall not vote.

3. (a)   The Commission shall adopt the measures envisaged where they are in accordance with the opinion of the Committee.
   (b)   Where the measures envisaged are not in accordance with the opinion of the Committee, or if no opinion is adopted, the Commission shall without delay propose to the Council the measures to be adopted. The Council shall act by a qualified majority.
   (c)   If, within three months of the proposal being submitted to it, the Council has not acted, the proposed measures shall be adopted by the Commission.][1]

Article 3

Member States shall bring into force the provisions needed in order to comply with this Directive within 18 months of its notification and shall forthwith inform the Commission thereof.

Member States shall ensure that they communicate to the Commission the text of the main provisions of national law which they adopt in the field covered by this Directive.

Article 4

This Directive is addressed to the Member States.

Done at Brussels, 20 May 1975.

For the Council

The President

R. RYAN

---

1.   Inserted by Council Directive (EEC) 87/19, OJ L15 17.1.87 pp31-32.

ANNEX[1]

INTRODUCTION

The particulars and documents accompanying an application for marketing authorisation pursuant to Article 4 of Council Directive 65/65/EEC[2] shall be presented in four parts, in accordance with the requirements set out in this Annex and taking account of the guidance published by the Commission in *The rules governing medicinal products in the European Community,* Volume 11 : *Notice to applicants for marketing authorisations for medicinal products for human use in the Member States of the European Community.*

In assembling the dossier for application for marketing authorisation, applicants shall take into account the Community guidelines relating to the quality, safety and efficacy of medicinal products published by the Commission in *The rules governing medicinal products in the European Community,* Volume III and its supplements: *Guidelines on the quality, safety and efficacy of medicinal products for human use.*

All information which is relevant to the evaluation of the medicinal product concerned shall be included in the application, whether favourable or unfavourable to the product. In particular, all relevant details shall be given of any incomplete or abandoned pharmacotoxicological or clinical test or trial relating to the medicinal product. Moreover, in order to monitor the benefit/risk assessment after marketing authorisation has been granted, any change to the data in the dossier, any new information not in the original application and all pharmacovigilance reports, shall be submitted to the competent authorities.

The general sections of this Annex give the requirements for all categories of medicinal products; they are supplemented by sections containing additional special requirements for radiopharmaceuticals and for biological medicinal products, such as vaccines, serums, toxins, allergen products, medicinal products derived from human blood or plasma. The additional special requirements for biological medicinal products are also applicable to medicinal products obtained through processes mentioned in List A and the first indent of List B of the Annex to Directive 87/22/EEC.

Member States shall also ensure that all tests on animals are conducted in accordance with Council Directive 86/609/EEC[3].

PART 1

SUMMARY OF THE DOSSIER

A.   Administrative data

The medicinal product which is the subject of the application shall be identified by name and name of the active ingredient(s), together with the pharmaceutical form, the method of administration, the strength and the final presentation, including packaging.

The name and address of the applicant shall be given, together with the name and address of the manufacturers and the sites involved in the different stages of the

---

1.   Text of the Annex as replaced by Commission Directive (EEC) 91/507, OJ L270 26.9.91 p32.
2.   OJ No 22, 9.2.65 p369/65.
3.   OJ L358 18.12.86 p1.

manufacture (including the manufacturer of the finished product and the manufacturer(s) of the active ingredient(s)), and where relevant the name and address of the importer.

The applicant shall identify the number of volumes of documentation submitted in support of the application and indicate what samples, if any, are also provided.

Annexed to the administrative data shall be copies of the manufacturing authorisation as defined in Article 16 of Council Directive 75/319/EEC[1], together with a list of countries in which authorisation has been granted, copies of all the summaries of product characteristics in accordance with Article 4a of Directive 65/65/EEC as approved by Member States and a list of countries in which an application has been submitted.

B.   Summary of product characteristics

The applicant shall propose a summary of the product characteristics, in accordance with Article 4a of Directive 65/65/EEC.

In addition the applicant shall provide samples or mock-ups of the packaging, labels and package leaflets for the medicinal product concerned.

C.   Expert reports

In accordance with Article 2 of Directive 75/319/EEC, expert reports must be provided on the chemical, pharmaceutical and biological documentation, the pharmacotoxicological documentation and the clinical documentation respectively.

The expert report shall consist of a critical evaluation of the quality of the product and the investigations carried out on animals and human beings and bring out all the data relevant for evaluation. It shall be worded so as to enable the reader to obtain a good understanding of the properties, quality, the proposed specifications and control methods, the safety, the efficacy, the advantages and disadvantages of the product.

All important data shall be summarised in an appendix to the expert report, whenever possible including report formats in tabular or in graphic form. The expert report and the summaries shall contain precise cross references to the information contained in the main documentation.

Each expert report shall be prepared by a suitably qualified and experienced person. It shall be signed and dated by the expert, and attached to the report shall be brief information about the educational background, training and occupational experience of the expert. The professional relationship of the expert to the applicant shall be declared.

PART 2

CHEMICAL, PHARMACEUTICAL AND BIOLOGICAL TESTING OF MEDICINAL
PRODUCTS

All the test procedures shall correspond to the state of scientific progress at the time and shall be validated procedures; results of the validation studies shall be provided.

---

1.   OJ L147 9.6.75 p13.

All the test procedure(s) shall be described in sufficiently precise detail so as to be reproducible in control tests, carried out at the request of the competent authority; any special apparatus and equipment which may be used shall be described in adequate detail, possibly accompanied by a diagram. The formulae of the laboratory reagents shall be supplemented, if necessary, by the method of preparation. In the case of test procedures included in the *European Pharmacopoeia* or the pharmacopoeia of a Member State, this description may be replaced by a detailed reference to the pharmacopoeia in question.

A.   Qualitative and quantitative particulars of the constituents

The particulars and documents which must accompany applications for marketing authorisation, pursuant to point 3 of Article 4 (2) of Directive 65/65/EEC shall be submitted in accordance with the following requirements.

1.   *Qualitative particulars*

1.1   "Qualitative particulars" of all the constituents of the medicinal product shall mean the designation or description of:

—   the active ingredient(s),
—   the constituent(s) of the excipients, whatever their nature or the quantity used, including colouring matter, preservatives, adjuvants, stabilisers, thickeners, emulsifiers, flavouring and aromatic substances, etc.,
—   the constituents, intended to be ingested or otherwise administered to the patient, of the outer covering of the medicinal products - capsules, gelatine capsules, rectal capsules, etc.

These particulars shall be supplemented by any relevant data concerning the container and, where appropriate, its manner of closure, together with details of devices with which the medicinal product will be used or administered and which will be delivered with the product.

1.2.   In the context of a radiopharmaceutical kit, which is to be radiolabelled after supply by the manufacturer, the active ingredient is considered to be that part of the formulation which is intended to carry or bind the radionuclide. Details of the source of the radionuclide shall be stated. In addition, any compounds essential for the radiolabelling shall be stated.

In a generator, both mother and daughter radionuclides are to be considered as active ingredients.

2.   The "usual terminology", to be used in describing the constituents of medicinal products, shall mean, notwithstanding the application of the other provisions of point 3 of Article 4(2) of Directive 65/65/EEC:

—   in respect of substances which appear in the *European Pharmacopoeia* or, failing this, in the national pharmacopoeia of one of the Member States, the main title at the head of the monograph in question, with reference to the pharmacopoeia concerned,
—   in respect of other substances, the international non-proprietary name recommended by the World Health Organisation, which may be accompanied by another non-proprietary name, or, failing these, the exact scientific designation; substances not having an international non-proprietary name or an exact scientific designation shall be

described by a statement of how and from what they were prepared, supplemented, where appropriate, by any other relevant details,

— in respect of colouring matter, designation by the "E" code assigned to them in Council Directive 78/25/EEC[1] of 12 December 1977 on the approximation of the rules of the Member States concerning the colouring matters authorised for use in medicinal products.

3.   *Quantitative particulars*

3.1   In order to give "quantitative particulars" of the active ingredients of the medicinal products, it is necessary, depending on the pharmaceutical form concerned, to specify the mass, or the number of units of biological activity, either per dosage-unit or per unit of mass or volume, of each active ingredient.

Units of biological activity shall be used for substances which cannot be defined chemically. Where an International Unit of biological activity has been defined by the World Health Organisation, this shall be used. Where no International Unit has been defined, the units of biological activity shall be expressed in such a way as to provide unambiguous information on the activity of the substances.

Whenever possible, biological activity per units of mass shall be indicated.

This information shall be supplemented :

— in respect of injectable preparations, by the mass or units of biological activity of each active ingredient in the unit container, taking into account the usable volume of the product, after reconstitution, where appropriate,

— in respect of medicinal products to be administered by drops, by the mass or units of biological activity of each active ingredient contained in the number of drops corresponding to l ml or l g of the preparation,

— in respect of syrups, emulsions, granular preparations and other pharmaceutical forms to be administered in measured quantities, by the mass or units of biological activity of each active ingredient per measured quantity.

3.2   Active ingredients present in the form of compounds or derivatives shall be described quantitatively by their total mass, and if necessary or relevant, by the mass of the active entity or entities of the molecule.

3.3   For medicinal products containing an active ingredient which is the subject of an application for marketing authorisation in any Member State for the first time, the quantitative statement of an active ingredient which is a salt or hydrate shall be systematically expressed in terms of the mass of the active entity or entities in the molecule. All subsequently authorised medicinal products in the Member States shall have their quantitative composition stated in the same way for the same active ingredient.

3.4   For allergen products, the quantitative particulars shall be expressed by units of biological activity, except for well defined allergen products for which the concentration may be expressed by mass/unit of volume.

3.5   The requirement to express the content of active ingredients in terms of the mass of active entities, as in point 3.3. above, may not apply to

---

1.   OJ L11 14.1.78 p18.

radiopharmaceuticals. For radionuclides, radioactivity shall be expressed in becquerels at a given date and, if necessary, time with reference to time zone. The type of radiation shall be indicated.

4.   *Development pharmaceutics*

4.1   An explanation should be provided with regard to the choice of composition, constituents and container and the intended function of the excipients in the finished product. This explanation shall be supported by scientific data on development pharmaceutics. The overage, with justification thereof, should be stated.

4.2   For radiopharmaceuticals this should include a consideration of chemical/radiochemical purity and its relationship to biodistribution.

B.   Description of method of preparation

1.   The description of the method of preparation accompanying the application for marketing authorisation pursuant to point 4 of Article 4(2) of Directive 65/65/EEC, shall be drafted in such a way as to give an adequate synopsis of the nature of the operations employed.

For this purpose it shall include at least :

—   mention of the various stages of manufacture, so that an assessment can be made of whether the processes employed in producing the pharmaceutical form might have produced an adverse change in the constituents,

—   in the case of continuous manufacture, full details concerning precautions taken to ensure the homogeneity of the finished product,

—   the actual manufacturing formula, with the quantitative particulars of all the substances used, the quantities of excipients, however, being given in approximate terms in so far as the pharmaceutical form makes this necessary; mention shall be made of any substances that may disappear in the course of manufacture; any overage shall be indicated and justified,

—   a statement of the stages of manufacture at which sampling is carried out for in-process control tests, where other data in the documents supporting the application show such tests to be necessary for the quality control of the finished product,

—   experimental studies validating the manufacturing process, where a non-standard method of manufacture is used or where it is critical for the product,

—   for sterile products, details of the sterilisation processes and/or aseptic procedures used.

2.   For radiopharmaceutical kits, the description of the method of preparation shall also include details of the manufacture of the kit and details of its recommended final processing to produce the radioactive medicinal product.

For radionuclides, the nuclear reactions involved shall be discussed.

C.   Controls of starting materials

1.   For the purposes of this paragraph, "starting materials" shall mean all the constituents of the medicinal product and, if necessary, of its container, as referred to in paragraph A, point 1, above.

In the case of :

—   an active ingredient not described in the *European Pharmacopoeia* or in the pharmacopoeia of a Member State, or
—   an active ingredient described in the *European Pharmacopoeia* or in the pharmacopoeia of a Member State when prepared by a method liable to leave impurities not mentioned in the pharmacopoeia monograph and for which the monograph is inappropriate to adequately control its quality,

which is manufactured by a person different from the applicant, the latter may arrange for the detailed description of the manufacturing method, quality control during manufacture and process validation to be supplied directly to the competent authorities by the manufacturer of the active ingredient. In this case, the manufacturer shall however provide the applicant with all the data which may be necessary for the latter to take responsibility for the medicinal product. The manufacturer shall confirm in writing to the applicant that he shall ensure batch to batch consistency and not modify the manufacturing process or specifications without informing the applicant. Documents and particulars supporting the application for such a change shall be supplied to the competent authorities.

The particulars and documents accompanying the application for marketing authorisation pursuant to points 7 and 8 of Article 4(2) of Directive 65/65/EEC shall include the results of the tests, including batch analyses particularly for active ingredients, relating to quality control of all the constituents used. These shall be submitted in accordance with the following provisions.

1.1.   *Starting materials listed in pharmacopoeias*

The monographs of the *European Pharmacopoeia* shall be applicable to all substances appearing in it.

In respect of other substances, each Member State may require observance of its own national pharmacopoeia with regard to products manufactured in its territory.

Constituents fulfilling the requirements of the *European Pharmacopoeia* or the pharmacopoeia of one of the Member States shall be deemed to comply sufficiently with point 7 of Article 4(2) of Directive 65/65/EEC. In this case the description of the analytical methods may be replaced by a detailed reference to the pharmacopoeia in question.

However, where a starting material in the *European Pharmacopoeia* or in the pharmacopoeia of a Member State has been prepared by a method liable to leave impurities not controlled in the pharmacopoeia monograph, these impurities and their maximum tolerance limits must be declared and a suitable test procedure must be described.

Colouring matter shall, in all cases, satisfy the requirements of Directive 78/25/EEC.

The routine tests carried out on each batch of starting materials must be as stated in the application for marketing authorisation. If tests other than those mentioned in the pharmacopoeia are used, proof must be supplied that the starting materials meet the quality requirements of that pharmacopoeia.

In cases where a specification contained in a monograph of the *European Pharmacopoeia* or in the national pharmacopoeia of a Member State might be insufficient to ensure the quality of the substance, the competent authorities may request more appropriate specifications from the person responsible for placing the product on the market.

The competent authorities shall inform the authorities responsible for the pharmacopoeia in question. The person responsible for placing the product on the market shall provide the authorities of that pharmacopoeia with the details of the alleged insufficiency and the additional specifications applied.

In cases where a starting material is described neither in the *European Pharmacopoeia* nor in the pharmacopoeia of a Member State, compliance with the monograph of a third country pharmacopoeia can be accepted; in such cases, the applicant shall submit a copy of the monograph accompanied where necessary by the validation of the test procedures contained in the monograph and by a translation where appropriate.

1.2. *Starting materials not in a pharmacopoeia*

Constituents which are not given in any pharmacopoeia shall be described in the form of a monograph under the following headings :

(a) The name of the substance, meeting the requirements of paragraph A, point 2, shall be supplemented by any trade or scientific synonyms;

(b) the definition of the substance, set down in a form similar to that used in the *European Pharmacopoeia,* shall be accompanied by any necessary explanatory evidence, especially concerning the molecular structure where appropriate; it must be accompanied by an appropriate description of the method of synthesis. Where substances can only be described by their method of preparation, the description should be sufficiently detailed to characterise a substance which is constant both in its composition and in its effects;

(c) methods of identification may be described in the form of complete techniques as used for production of the substance, and in the form of tests which ought to be carried out as a routine matter;

(d) purity tests shall be described in relation to the sum total of predictable impurities, especially those which may have a harmful effect, and, if necessary, those which, having regard to the combination of substances to which the application refers, might adversely affect the stability of the medicinal product or distort analytical results;

(e) with regard to complex substances of plant or animal/human origin, a distinction must be made between the case where multiple pharmacological effects render chemical, physical or biological control of the principal constitutents necessary, and the case of substances containing one or more groups of principles having similar activity, in respect of which an overall method of assay may be accepted;

(f) when materials of animal/human origin are used, measures to ensure freedom from potentially pathogenic agents shall be described;

(g) for radionuclides, the nature of the radionuclide, the identity of the isotope, likely impurities, the carrier, the use and the specific activity shall be given;

(h)   any special precautions that may be necessary during storage of the starting material and, if necessary, the maximum period of storage before retesting shall be given.

1.3.   *Physico-chemical characteristics liable to effect bio-availability*

The following items of information concerning active ingredients, whether or not listed in the pharmacopoeias, shall be provided as part of the general description of the active ingredients if the bio-availability of the medicinal product depends on them :

— crystalline form and solubility coefficients,
— particle size, where appropriate after pulverisation,
— state of solvation,
— oil/water coefficient of partition[1]

The first three indents are not applicable to substances used solely in solution.

2.   For biological medicinal products, such as vaccines, serums, toxins, allergen products and medicinal products derived from human blood or plasma, the requirements of this paragraph shall apply.

For the purposes of this paragraph, starting materials shall mean any substance used in the manufacture of the medicinal product; this includes the constituents of the medicinal product, and, if necessary, of its container, as referred to in paragraph A, point I above, as well as source materials such as micro-organisms, tissues of either plant or animal origin, cells or fluits (including blood) of human or animal origin, and biotechnological cell constructs. The origin and history of starting materials shall be described and documented.

The description of the starting material shall include the manufacturing strategy, purification/inactivation procedures with their validation and all in-process control procedures designed to ensure the quality, safety and batch to batch consistency of the finished product.

2.1   When cell banks are used, the cell characteristics shall be shown to have remained unchanged at the passage level used for the production and beyond.

2.2   Seed materials, cell banks, pools of serum or plasma and other materials of biological origin and, whenever possible, the source materials from which they are derived shall be tested for adventitious agents.

If the presence of potentially pathogenic adventitious agents is inevitable, the material shall be used only when further processing ensures their elimination and/or inactivation, and this shall be validated.

2.3   Whenever possible, vaccine production shall be based on a seed lot system and on established cell banks; for serums, defined pools of starting materials shall be used.
For bacterial and viral vaccines, the characteristics of the infectious agent shall be demonstrated on the seed. In addition, for live vaccines, the stability of the attenuation characteristics shall be demonstrated on the seed;

---

1.   The competent authorities may also request the pK and pH values if they think this information is essential.

if this proof is not sufficient, the attenuation characteristics shall also be demonstrated at the production stage.

2.4   For allergen products, the specifications and control methods for the source materials shall be described. The description shall include particulars concerning collection, pretreatment and storage.

2.5   For medicinal products derived from human blood or plasma, the origin and the criteria and procedures for collection, transportation and storage of the source material shall be described and documented.

Defined pools of source material shall be used.

3.   For radiopharmaceuticals, starting materials include irradiation target materials.

D.   Control tests carried out at intermediate stages of the manufacturing process

1.   The particulars and documents accompanying an application for marketing authorisation, pursuant to points 7 and 8 of Article 4(2) of Directive 65/65/EEC, shall include particulars relating to the product control tests that may be carried out at an intermediate stage of the manufacturing process, with a view to ensuring the consistency of the technical characteristics and the production process.

These tests are essential for checking the conformity of the medicinal product with the formula when, exceptionally, an applicant proposes an analytical method for testing the finished product which does not include the assay of all the same requirements as the active ingredients).

The same applies where the quality control of the finished product depends on in-process control tests, particularly if the substance is essentially defined by its method or preparation.

For biological medicinal products, such as vaccines, serums, toxins, allergen products and medicinal products derived from human blood or plasma, the procedures and the criteria of acceptability published as recommendations of the WHO *(Requirements for Biological Substances)* shall serve as guidelines for all controls of production stages which are not specified in the *European Pharmacopoeia,* or falling this, in the national pharmacopoeia of a Member State.

For inactivated or detoxified vaccines, effective inactivation or detoxification shall be verified during each production run, unless this control is dependent upon a test for which the availability of susceptible animals is limited. In this case, the test shall be carried out until consistency of production and correlation with appropriate in process controls have been established and thereafter compensated by appropriate in-process controls.

For modified or adsorbed allergens, the allergen products shall be qualitatively and quantitatively characterised at an intermediate stage, as late as possible in the manufacturing process.

E.   Control tests on the finished product

1.   For the control of the finished product, a batch of a finished product comprises all the units of a pharmaceutical form which are made from the same initial quantity of material and have undergone the same series of manufacturing and/or sterilisation operations or, in the case of a continuous production process, all the units manufactured in a given period of time.

The application for marketing authorisation shall list those tests which are carried out routinely on each batch of finished product. The frequency of the tests which are not carried out routinely shall be stated. Release limits shall be indicated.

The particulars and documents accompanying the application for marketing authorisation pursuant to points 7 and 8 of Article 4 (2) of Directive 65/65/EEC, shall include particulars relating to control tests on the finished product at release. They shall be submitted in accordance with the following requirements.

The provisions of the monographs for pharmaceutical forms, immunosera, vaccines and radiopharmaceutical preparations of the *European Pharmacopoeia* or failing that, of a Member State, shall be applicable to all products such as vaccines, serums, toxins, allergen products and medicinal products derived from human blood or plasma which are not specified in the European *Pharmacopoeia* or falling this, in the pharmacopoeia of a Member State, the procedures and the criteria of acceptability published as recommendations in the WHO *(Requirements for biological Substances)* shall serve as guidelines.

If test procedures and limits other than those mentioned in the monographs of the *European Pharmacopoeia* or falling this, in the national pharmacopoeia of a Member State, are used, proof shall be supplied that the finished product would, if tested in accordance with those monographs, meet the quality requirements of that pharmacopoeia for the pharmaceutical form concerned.

1.1   *General characteristics of the finished product*

Certain tests of the general characteristics of a product shall always be included among the tests on the finished product. These tests shall, wherever applicable, relate to the control of average masses and maximum deviations, to mechanical, physical or microbiological tests, organoleptic characteristics, physical characteristics such as density, pH, refractive index, etc. For each of these characteristics, standards and tolerance limits shall be specified by the applicant in each particular case.

The conditions of the tests, where appropriate, the equipment/apparatus employed and the standards shall be described in precise details whenever they are not given in the *European Pharmacopoeia* or the pharmacopoeia of the Member States; the same shall apply in cases where the methods prescribed by such pharmacopoeias are not applicable.

Furthermore, solid pharmaceutical forms having to be administered orally shall be subjected to *in vitro* studies on the liberation and dissolution rate of the active ingredient or ingredients; these studies shall also be carried out where administration is by another means if the competent authorities of the Member State concerned consider this necessary.

1.2   *Identification and assay of active ingredient(s)*

Identification and assay of the active ingredient(s) shall be carried out either in a representative sample from the production batch or in a number of dosage-units analysed individually.

Unless there is appropriate justification, the maximum acceptable deviation in the active-ingredient content of the finished product shall not exceed + 5 % at the time of manufacture.

On the basis of the stability tests, the manufacturer must propose and justify maximum acceptable tolerance limits in the active-ingredient content of the finished product up to the end of the proposed shelf-life.

In certain exceptional cases of particularly complex mixtures, where assay of active ingredients which are very numerous or present in very low amounts would necessitate an intricate investigation difficult to carry out in respect of each production batch, the assay of one or more active ingredients in the finished product may be omitted, on the express condition that such assays are made at intermediate stages in the production process. This relaxation may not be extended to the characterisation of the substances concerned. This simplified technique shall be supplemented by a method of quantitative evaluation, enabling the competent authority to have the conformity of the medicinal product with its specification verified after it has been placed on the market.

An *in vivo* or *in vitro* biological assay shall be obligatory when physico-chemical methods cannot provide adequate information on the quality of the product. Such an assay shall, whenever possible, include reference materials and statistical analysis allowing calculation of confidence limits. Where these tests cannot be carried out on the finished product, they may be performed at an intermediate stage, as late as possible in the manufacturing process.

Where the particulars given in section B show that a significant overage of an active ingredient is employed in the manufacture of the medicinal product, the description of the control tests on the finished product shall include, where appropriate, the chemical and, if necessary, the toxico-pharmacological investigation of the changes that this substance has undergone, and possibly the characterisation and/or assay of the degradation products.

1.3   *Identification and assay of excipient constituents*

In so far as is necessary, the excipient(s) shall be subject at least to identification tests.

The test procedure proposed for identifying colouring matters must enable a verification to be made that such matters appear in the list annexed to Directive 78/25/EEC.

An upper and lower limit test shall be obligatory in respect of preserving agents and an upper limit test for any other excipient constituent liable to affect adversely physiological functions; an upper and lower limit test shall be obligatory in respect of the excipient if it is liable to affect the bio-availability of an active substance, unless bio-availability is guaranteed by other appropriate tests.

1.4   *Safety tests*

Apart from the toxico-pharmacological tests submitted with the application for marketing authorisation, particulars of safety tests, such as sterility, bacterial endotoxin, pyrogenicity and local tolerance in animals shall be included in the analytical particulars wherever such tests must be undertaken as a matter of routine in order to verify the quality of the product.

For all controls of biological medicinal products, such as vaccines, serums, toxins, allergen products and medicinal products derived from human blood or plasma, which are not specified in the European Pharmacopoeia, or failing this, in the national pharmacopoeia of a Member State, the procedures and the criteria of acceptability published as recommendations in the WHO *(Requirements for Biological Substances)* shall serve as guidelines.

For radiopharmaceuticals, radionuclidic purity, radiochemical purity and specific activity shall be described For content of radioactivity, the deviation from that stated on the label should not exceed + 10%.

For generators, details on the testing for mother and daughter radionuclides are required For generator-eluates, tests for mother radionuclides and for other components of the generator system shall be provided.

For kits, the specifications of the finished product shall include tests on performance of products after radiolabelling. Appropriate controls on radiochemical and radionuclidic purity of the radiolabelled compound shall be included. Any material essential for radiolabelling shall be identified and assayed.

F.   **Stability tests**

1.   The particulars and documents accompanying the application for marketing authorisation pursuant to points 6 and 7 of Article 4(2) of Directive 65/65/EEC shall be submitted in accordance with the following requirements.

A description shall be given of the investigations by which the shelf life, the recommended storage conditions and the specifications at the end of the shelf-life proposed by the applicant have been determined.

Where a finished product is liable to give rise to degradation products, the applicant must declare these and indicate characterisation methods and test procedures.

The conclusions shall contain the results of analyses, justifying the proposed shelf life under the recommended storage conditions and the specifications of the finished product at the end of the shelf-life under these recommended storage conditions.

The maximum acceptable level of degradation products at the end of shelf-life shall be indicated.

A study of the interaction between product and container shall be submitted wherever the risk of such interaction is regarded as possible, especially where injectable preparations or aerosols for internal use are concerned.

2.   Where for biological medicinal products, such as vaccines, serums, toxins, allergen products and medicinal products derived from human blood or plasma, stability tests cannot be carried out on the finished products, it is acceptable to carry out stability indicating tests at an intermediate stage of production as late as possible in the manufacturing process. In addition, there should be an evaluation of the stability of the finished product using other secondary tests.

3.   For radiopharmaceuticals, information on stability shall be given for generators, kits and radiolabelled products. The stability during use of radiopharmaceuticals in multi-dose vials shall be documented.

PART 3

TOXICOLOGICAL AND PHARMACOLOGICAL TESTS

1.   Introduction

1.   The particulars and documents accompanying the application for marketing authorisation pursuant to point 8 of Article 4, second paragraph, Directive 65/65/EEC shall he given in accordance with the requirements below.

Member States shall ensure that the safety tests are carried out in conformity with the provisions relating to good laboratory practice laid down by Directives 87/18/EEC[1] and 88/320/EEC[2].

The toxicological and pharmacological tests must show :

(a)   the potential toxicity of the product and any dangerous or undesirable toxic effects that may occur under the proposed conditions of use in human beings; these should be evaluated in relation to the pathological condition concerned;

(b)   the pharmacological properties of the product, in both qualitative and quantitative relationship to the proposed use in human beings. All results must be reliable and of general applicability. Whenever appropriate, mathematical and statistical procedures shall be used in designing the experimental methods and in evaluating the results.

Additionally, it is necessary for clinicians to be given information about the therapeutic potential of the product.

2.   Where a medicinal product is intended for topical use, systemic absorption must be investigated, due account also being taken of the possible use of the product on broken skin and absorption through other relevant surfaces. Only if it is proved that systematic absorption under these conditions is negligible may repeated dose systematic toxicity tests, foetal toxicity tests and studies of reproductive function be omitted.

If, however, systematic absorption is demonstrated during therapeutic experimentation, toxicity tests shall be carried out on animals, including where necessary, foetal toxicity tests.

In all cases, tests of local tolerance after repeated application shall be carried out with particular care and include histological examinations; the

---

1.   OJ L15 17.9.187 p29.
2.   OJ L145 11.6.88 p35.

possibility of sensitisation shall be investigated and any carcinogenic potential investigated in the cases referred to in paragraph II E of this Part.

3. For biological medicinal products such as vaccines, serums, toxins, allergen products and medicinal products derived from human blood or plasma, the requirements of this Part may have to be adapted for individual products; therefore the testing programme carried out shall be justified by the applicant.

    In establishing the testing programme, the following shall be taken into consideration :

    — all tests requiring repeated administration of the product shall be designed to take account of the possible induction of, and interference by, antibodies;
    — examination of reproductive function, of embryo/foetal and perinatal toxicity, of mutagenic potential and of carcinogenic potential shall be considered. Where components other than the active ingredient(s) are incriminated, validation of their removal may replace the study.

4. For radiopharmaceuticals, it is appreciated that toxicity may be associated with a radiation dose. In diagnosis, this is a consequence of the use of radiopharmaceuticals; in therapy, it is the wanted property. The evaluation of safety and efficacy of radiopharmaceuticals shall, therefore, address requirements for medicinal products and radiation dosimetry aspects. Organ/tissue exposure to radiation shall be documented. Absorbed radiation dose estimates shall be calculated according to a specified, internationally recognised system by a particular route of administration.

5. The toxicology and pharmacokinetics of an excipient used for the first time in the pharmaceutical field shall be investigated.

6. Where there is a possibility of significant degradation during storage of the medicinal product, the toxicology of degradation products must be considered.

II.   Performance of tests

A.   *Toxicity*

1.   Single dose toxicity

An acute test is a qualitative and quantitative study of the toxic reactions which may result from a single administration of the active substance or substances contained in the medicinal product, in the proportions and physico-chemical state in which they are present in the actual product.

The acute toxicity test must be carried out in two or more mammalian species of known strain unless a single species can be justified. At least two different routes of administration shall normally be used, one being identical with or similar to that proposed for use in human beings and the other ensuring systemic exposure to the substance.

This study will cover the signs observed, including local reactions. The period during which the test animals are observed shall be fixed by the investigator as being adequate to reveal tissue or organ damage or recovery, usually for a period of 14 days but not less than seven days, but without exposing the animals to prolonged suffering. Animals dying during the observation period should be subject to autopsy as also should all animals surviving to the end of the observation period. Histopathological examinations should be considered on any organ showing macroscopic changes at autopsy. The maximum amount of information should be obtained from the animals used in the study.

The single dose toxicity tests should be conducted in such a way that signs of acute toxicity are revealed and the mode of death assessed as far as reasonably possible. In suitable species a quantitative evaluation of the approximate lethal dose and information on the dose effect relationship should be obtained, but a high level of precision is not required.

These studies may give some indication of the likely effects of acute overdosage in man and may be useful for the design of toxicity studies requiring repeated dosing on the suitable animal species.

In the case of active substances in combination, the study must be carried out in such a way as to check whether or not there is enhancement of toxicity or if novel toxic effects occur.

2.   Repeated dose toxicity (sub-acute or chronic toxicity)

Repeated dose toxicity tests are intended to reveal any physiological and/or pathological changes induced by repeated administration of the active substance or combination of active substances under examination, and to determine how these changes are related to dosage.

Generally, it is desirable that two tests be performed: one short-term, lasting two to four weeks, the other long-term. The duration of the latter shall depend on the conditions of clinical use. Its purpose shall be to determine by experiment the non-toxic dose range of the product and normally it shall last three to six months.

In respect of medicinal products to be administered once only to humans, a single test lasting two to four weeks shall be performed.

If, however, having regard to the proposed duration of use in human beings, the investigator sees fit to carry out experiments of greater or lesser duration than indicated above, he must give adequate reasons for doing so.

Reasons should also be given for the dosages chosen.

Repeated dose toxicity tests shall be carried out on two species of mammals one of which must be a non-rodent. The choice of route(s) of administration employed shall depend on the intended therapeutic use and the possibilities of systemic absorption. The method and frequency of dosage shall be clearly stated.

The maximum dose should be chosen so as to bring harmful effects to light. The lower doses will then enable the animal's tolerance of the product to be determined.

Wherever possible, and always in experiments on small rodents, the design of the experiment and the control procedures must be suited to the scale of the problem being tackled and enable fiducial limits to be determined.

The evaluation of the toxic effects shall be based on observation of behaviour, growth, haematological and biochemical tests, especially those relating to the excretory mechanism, and also on autopsy reports and accompanying histological data. The choice and range of each group of tests will depend on the species of animal used and the state of scientific knowledge at the time.

In the case of new combinations of known substances that have been investigated in accordance with the provisions of this Directive, the long-term tests may, except where acute and sub-acute toxicity tests have demonstrated potentiation or novel toxic effects, be suitable modified by the investigator who shall submit his reasons for such modification.

B.   *Examination of reproductive function*

If the results of other tests reveal anything suggesting harmful effects on progeny or impairment of male or female reproductive function, this shall be investigated by appropriate tests.

C.   *Embryo/foetal and perinatal toxicity*

This investigation comprises a demonstration of the toxic and especially the teratogenic effects observed in the issue of conception when the substance under investigation has been administered to the female during pregnancy.

Although up to the present these tests have had only a limited predictive value in regard to the application of the results to human beings, they are thought to provide important information where the results show effects such as resorptions and other anomalies.

Omission of these tests, either because the medicinal product will not normally be used by women capable of child-bearing or for other reasons, must be adequately justified.

Embryo/foetal toxicity studies shall normally be conducted on two mammalian species, one of which should be other than a rodent. Peri- and postnatal studies shall be conducted in at least one species. Where metabolism of a medicinal product in a particular species is known to be similar to that in man, it is desirable to include this species. Also, it is desirable that one of the species is the same as in the repeated dose toxicity studies.

The details of the test (number of animals, amounts administered, timing of administration and criteria for evaluation of results) shall depend on the state of scientific knowledge at the time when the application is lodged, and the level of statistical significance that the results must attain.

D.   *Mutagenic potential*

The purpose of the study of mutagenic potential is to reveal the changes which a substance may cause in the genetic material of individuals or cells and which have the effect of making successors permanently and hereditarily different from their predecessors. This study is obligatory for any new substance.

The number and types of results and the criteria for their evaluation shall depend on the state of scientific knowledge at the time when the application is lodged.

E.   *Carcinogenic potential*

Tests to reveal carcinogenic effects shall normally be required :

(a)   in respect of substances having a close chemical analogy with known carcinogenic or cocarcinogenic compounds;

(b)   in respect of substances which have given rise to suspicious changes during the long-term toxicological tests;

(c)   in respect of substances which have given rise to suspicious results in the mutagenicpotential tests or in other short-term carcinogenicity tests.

Such tests may also be required in respect of substances to be included in medicinal products likely to be administered regularly over a prolonged period of a patient's life.

The state of scientific knowledge at the time when the application is lodged shall be taken into account when determining the details of the tests.

F.   *Pharmacodynamies*

This heading covers the variations caused by the substance in the functions of the physiological systems, whether these functions are normal or experimentally modified.

This study shall follow two distinct lines of approach :

Firstly, the actions on which the recommended application in therapeutic practice is based shall be adequately described. The results shall be expressed in quantitative terms using, for example, dose-effect curves, time-effect curves etc., and wherever possible, compared with data relating to a substance whose activity is known. Where a higher therapeutic potency is being claimed for a substance, the difference shall be demonstrated and shown to be statistically significant.

Secondly, the investigator shall provide a general pharmacological characterisation of the substance, with special reference to collateral effects. In general, the main functions of the physiological systems should be investigated. The depth of this investigation must be increased as the doses liable to produce side-effects approach those producing the main effect for which the substance is being proposed.

The experimental techniques, unless they are standard procedures, must be described in such detail as to allow them to be reproduced, and the investigator must establish their validity. The experimental results shall be set out clearly and, when relevant to the test, their statistical significance quoted.

Unless good reasons are given to the contrary, any quantitative modification of responses resulting from repeated administration of the substance shall be investigated.

Tests on combinations of active substances may be prompted either by pharmacological premisses or by indications of therapeutic effect.

In the first case, the pharmacodynamic study shall demonstrate those interactions which might make the combination of value in therapeutic use.

In the second case, where scientific justification for the combination is sought through therapeutic experimentation, the investigation shall determine whether the effects expected from the combination can be demonstrated in animals, and the importance of any collateral effects shall at least be investigated.

If a combination includes a novel active substance, the latter must previously have been studied in depth.

G.   *Pharmacokinetics*

Pharmacokinetics means the study of the fate of the active substance within the organism, and covers the study of the absorption, distribution, biotransformation and excretion of the substance.

The study of these different phases may be carried out both by means of physical, chemical or biological methods, and by observation of the actual pharmacodynamic activity of the substance itself.

Information on distribution and elimination (i.e. biotransformation and excretion) shall be necessary in all cases where such data are indispensable to determine the dosage for humans, and in respect of chemotherapeutic substances (antibiotics, etc.) and substances whose use depends on their non-pharmacodynamic effects (e.g. numerous diagnostic agents, etc.).

Pharmacokinetic investigation of pharmacologically active substances is necessary.

In the case of new combinations of known substances which have been investigated in accordance with the provisions of this Directive pharmacokinetic studies may not be required, if the toxicity tests and therapeutic experimentation justify their omission.

H.   *Local tolerance*

The purpose of local tolerance studies is to ascertain whether medicinal products (both active ingredients and excipients) are tolerated at sites in the body which may come into contact with the products as a result of its administration in clinical use The testing strategy shall be such that any mechanical effects of administration or purely physico-chemical actions of the product can be distinguished from toxicological or pharmacodynamic ones.

PART 4

CLINICAL DOCUMENTATION

The particulars and documents accompanying applications for marketing authorisations pursuant to point 8 of Article 4(2) of Directive 65/65/EEC shall be submitted in accordance with the provisions below.

A clinical trial is any systematic study of medicinal products in human subjects whether in patients or non-patient volunteers in order to discover or verify the effects of and/or identify any adverse reaction to investigational products, and/or study their absorption, distribution, metabolism and excretion in order to ascertain the efficacy and safety of the products.

Evaluation of the application for marketing authorisation shall be based on clinical trials including clinical pharmacological trials designed to determine the efficacy and safety of the product under normal conditions of use, having regard to the therapeutic indications for use in human beings. Therapeutic advantages must outweigh potential risks.

A.   General requirements

The clinical particulars to be provided pursuant to point 8 of Article 4 (2) of Directive 65/65/EEC must enable a sufficiently well-founded and scientifically valid opinion to be formed as to whether the medicinal product satisfies the criteria governing the granting of a marketing authorisation. Consequently, an essential requirement is that the results of all clinical trials should be communicated, both favourable and unfavourable.

Clinical trials must always be preceded by adequate pharmacological and toxicological tests, carried out on animals in accordance with the requirements of Part 3 of this Annex. The investigator must acquaint himself with the conclusions drawn from the pharmacological and toxicological studies and hence the applicant must provide him at least with the investigator's brochure, consisting of all the relevant information known prior to the onset of a clinical trial including chemical, pharmaceutical and biological data, toxicological, pharmacokinetic and pharmacodynamic data in animals and the results of earlier clinical trials, with adequate data to justify the nature, scale and duration of the proposed trial; the complete pharmacological and toxicological reports shall be provided on request. For materials of human or animal origin, all available means shall be employed to ensure safety from transmission of infectious agents prior to the commencement of the trial.

B.   Conduct of trials

1.   *Good clinical practice*

1.1.   All phases of clinical investigation, including bio-availability and bio-equivalence studies, shall be designed, implemented and reported in accordance with good clinical practice.

1.2.   All clinical trials shall be carried out in accordance with the ethical principles laid down in the current revision of the Declaration of Helsinki. In principle, the freely given informed consent of each trial subject shall be obtained and documented.

The trial protocol, procedures (including statistical design) and documentation shall be submitted by the sponsor and/or investigator for an opinion to the relevant ethics committee. The trials shall not begin before the opinion of this committee has been received in writing.

1.3.   Pre-established, systematic written procedures for the organisation, conduct, data collection, documentation and verification of clinical trials shall be required.

1.4. In the case of radiopharmaceuticals, clinical trials shall be carried out under the responsibility of a medical doctor authorised to use radionuclides for medical purposes.

2. *Archiving*

The person responsible for placing the medicinal product on the market shall make arrangements for archiving of documentation.

(a) The investigator shall arrange for the retention of the patient identification codes for at least 15 years after the completion or discontinuation of the trial.

(b) Patient files and other source data shall be kept for the maximum period of time permitted by the hospital, institution or private practice.

(c) The sponsor or other owner of the data shall retain all other documentation pertaining to the trial as long as the product is authorised. These procedures shall include :

— the protocol including the rationale, objectives and statistical design and methodology of the trial, with conditions under which it is performed and managed, and details of the investigational product, the reference medicinal product and/or the placebo used,
— standard operating procedures,
— all written opinions on the protocol and procedures,
— the investigator's brochure,
— case report forms on each trial subject,
— final report,
— audit certificate(s), if available.

(d) The final report shall be retained by the sponsor or subsequent owner, for five years after the product is no longer authorised.

Any change of ownership of the data shall be documented. All data and documents shall be made available if requested by relevant authorities.

C. Presentation of results

1. The particulars of each clinical trial must contain sufficient detail to allow an objective judgement to be made :

— the protocol, including the rationale, objectives and statistical design and methodology of the trial, with conditions under which it is performed and managed, and details of the investigational product used,
— audit certificate(s), if available,
— the list of investigator(s), and each investigator shall give his name, address, appointments, qualifications and clinical duties, state where the trial was carried out and assemble the information in respect of each patient individually, including case report forms on each trial subject,
— final report signed by the investigator and for multicentre trials, by all the investigators or the coordinating (principal) investigator.

2. The particulars of clinical trials referred to above shall be forwarded to the competent authorities. However, in agreement with the competent authorities, the applicant may omit part of this information. Complete documentation shall be provided forthwith upon request.

3. The clinical observations shall be summarised for each trial indicating :

    (a) the number and sex of patients treated;
    (b) the selection and age-distribution of the groups of patients being investigated and the control groups;
    (c) the number of patients withdrawn prematurely from the trials and the reasons for such withdrawal;
    (d) where controlled trials were carried out under the above conditions, whether the control group :
         — received no treatment,
         — received a placebo,
         — received another medicinal product of known effect,
         — received treatment other than therapy using medicinal products;
    (e) the frequency of observed side-effects;
    (f) details concerning patients who may be at increased risk, e.g. elderly people, children, women during pregnancy or menstruation, or whose physiological or pathological condition requires special consideration;
    (g) parameters or evaluation criteria of efficacy and the results in terms of these parameters;
    (h) a statistical evaluation of the results when this is called for by the design of the trials and the variable factors involved.

4. The investigator shall, in his conclusions on the experimental evidence, express an opinion on the safety of the product under normal conditions of use, its compatibility, its efficacy and any useful information relating to indications and contra-indications, dosage and average duration of treatment as well as any special precautions to be taken during treatment and the clinical symptoms of overdosage. In reporting the results of a multi-centre study, the principal investigator shall, in his conclusions, express an opinion on the safety and efficacy of the investigational product on behalf of all centres.

5. In addition, the investigator shall always indicate his observations on :

    (a) any signs of habituation, addiction or difficulty in weaning patients from the medicinal product;
    (b) any interactions that have been observed with other medicinal products administered concomitantly;
    (c) the criteria determining exclusion of certain patients from the trials;
    (d) any deaths which occurred during the trial or within the follow-up period.

6. Particulars concerning a new combination of medicinal substances must be identical to those required for new medicinal products and must substantiate the safety and efficacy of the combination.

7. Total or partial omission of data must be explained. Should unexpected results occur during the course of the trials, further preclinical toxicological and pharmacological tests must be undertaken and reviewed.

If the medicinal product is intended for long-term administration, particulars shall be given of any modification of the pharmacological action following repeated administration, as well as the establishment of long-term dosage.

D.   Clinical pharmacology

1.   *Pharmacodynamics*

The pharmacodynamic action correlated to the efficacy shall be demonstrated including :

— the dose-response relationship and its time course,
— justification for the dosage and conditions of administration,
— the mode of action, if possible.

The pharmacodynamic action not related to efficacy shall be described.

The demonstration of pharmacodynamic effects in human beings shall not in itself be sufficient to justify conclusions regarding any particular potential therapeutic effect.

2.   *Pharmacokinetics*

The following pharmacokinetic characteristics shall be described :

— absorption (rate and extent),
— distribution,
— metabolism,
— excretion.

Clinically significant features including the implication of the kinetic data for the dosage regimen especially for patients at risk, and differences between man and animal species used in the preclinical studies, shall be described.

3.   *Interactions*

If the product is normally to be administered concomitantly with other medicinal products, particulars shall be given of joint administration tests performed to demonstrate possible modification of the pharmacological action.

If pharmacodynamic/pharmacokinetic interactions exist between the substance and other medical products or substances like alcohol, caffeine, tobacco or nicotine, likely to be taken simultaneously, or if such interactions are likely, they should be described and discussed; particularly from the point of view of clinical relevance and the relationship to the statement concerning interactions in the summary of product characteristics presented in accordance with Article 4a, point 5.6 of Directive 65/65/EEC.

E.   Bio-availability/bio-equivalence

The assessment of bio-availability must be undertaken in all cases where it is necessary, e.g. where the therapeutic dose is near the toxic dose or where the previous tests have revealed anomalies which may be related to pharmacokinetic properties, such as variable absorption.

In addition, an assessment of bio-availability shall be undertaken where necessary to demonstrate bio-equivalence for the medicinal products referred to in Article 4(2) point 8(i) (ii) and (iii) of Directive 65/65/EEC.

F. Clinical efficacy and safety

1. In general, clinical trials shall be done as "controlled clinical trials" and if possible, randomised; any other design shall be justified. The control treatment of the trials will vary from case to case and also will depend on ethical considerations; thus it may, in some instances, be more pertinent to compare the efficacy of a new medicinal product with that of an established medicinal product of proven therapeutic value rather than with the effect of a placebo.

    As far as possible, and particularly in trials where the effect of the product cannot be objectively measured, steps shall be taken to avoid bias, including methods of randomisation and blinding.

2. The protocol of the trial must include a thorough description of the statistical methods to be employed, the number and reasons for inclusion of patients (including calculations of the power of the trial), the level of significance to be used and a description of the statistical unit. Measures taken to avoid bias, particularly methods of randomisation, shall be documented. Inclusion of a large number of subjects in a trial must not be regarded as an adequate substitute for a properly controlled trial.

3. Clinical statements concerning the efficacy or safety of a medicinal product under normal conditions of use which are not scientifically substantiated cannot be accepted as valid evidence.

4. The value of data on the efficacy and safety of a medicinal product under normal conditions of use will be very greatly enhanced if such data come from several competent investigators working independently.

5. For vaccines and serums, the immunological status and age of the trial population and the local epidemiology are of critical importance and shall be monitored during the trial and fully described.

    For live attenuated vaccines, clinical trials shall be so designed as to reveal potential transmission of the immunising agent from vaccinated to non-vaccinated subjects. If transmission is possible, the genotypic and phenotypic stability of the immunising agent shall be studied.

    For vaccines and allergen products, follow-up studies shall include appropriate immunological tests, and where applicable, antibody assays.

6. The pertinence of the different trials to the assessment of safety and the validity of methods of evaluation shall be discussed in the expert report.

7. All adverse events including abnormal laboratory values shall be presented individually and discussed, especially :

    — in terms of overall adverse experience and
    — as a function of the nature, seriousness and causality of effects.

8. A critical assessment of relative safety, taking into account adverse reactions, shall be made in relation to :

—   the disease to be treated,
—   other therapeutic approaches,
—   particular characteristics in sub-groups of patients,
—   preclinical data on toxicology and pharmacology.

9.   Recommendations shall be made for the conditions of use, with the intention of reducing the incidence of adverse reactions.

G.   Documentation for applications in exceptional circumstances

When, in respect of particular therapeutic indications, the applicant can show that he is unable to provide comprehensive data on the quality, efficacy and safety under normal conditions of use, because :

—   the indications for which the product in question is intended are encountered so rarely that the applicant cannot reasonably be expected to provide comprehensive evidence, or
—   in the present state of scientific knowledge comprehensive information cannot be provided, or
—   it would be contrary to generally accepted principles of medical ethics to collect such information,

marketing authorisation may be granted on the following conditions :

(a)   the applicant completed an identified programme of studies within a time period specified by the competent authority, the results of which shall form the basis of a reassessment of the benefit/risk profile,
(b)   the medicinal product in question may be supplied on medical prescription only and may in certain cases be administered only under strict medical supervision, possibly in a hospital and for a radiopharmaceutical, by an authorised person,
(c)   the package leaflet and any medical information shall draw the attention of the medical practitioner to the fact that the particulars available concerning the medicinal product in question are as yet inadequate in certain specified respects.

H.   Post-marketing experience

1.   If the medicinal product is already authorised in other countries, information shall be given in respect of adverse drug reactions of the medicinal product concerned and medicinal products containing the same active ingredient(s), in relation to the usage rates if possible. Information from world-wide studies relevant to the safety of the medicinal product shall be included.

For this purpose, an adverse drug reaction is a reaction which is noxious and unintended and which occurs at doses normally used in man for prophylaxis, diagnosis or therapy of disease or for the modification of physiological function.

2.   In the case of vaccines already authorised in other countries, information on the monitoring of vaccinated subjects to evaluate the prevalence of the disease in question as compared to nonvaccinated subjects shall be submitted, when available.

3.   For allergen products, response in periods of increased antigen exposure shall be identified.

APPENDIX 3[1]

COUNCIL DIRECTIVE (EEC) 75/319
of 20 May 1975

on the approximation of provisions laid down by law, regulation or administrative action relating to proprietary medicinal products[2]

THE COUNCIL OF THE EUROPEAN COMMUNITIES,

Having regard to the Treaty establishing the European Economic Community, and in particular Article 100 thereof;

Having regard to the proposal from the Commission;

Having regard to the Opinion of the European Parliament[3];

Having regard to the Opinion of the Economic and Social Committee[4];

Whereas the approximation begun by Council Directive 65/65/EEC[5] of 26 January 1965 on the approximation of provisions laid down by law, regulation or administrative action relating to proprietary medicinal products should be continued and the implementation of the principles laid down in that Directive should be ensured;

Whereas in order to reduce the disparities which remain, rules should be laid down on the control of proprietary medicinal products and the duties incumbent upon the Member States' competent authorities should be specified with a view to ensuring compliance with legal requirements;

Whereas, in order to progress towards free movement of proprietary medicinal products, the issue of authorisations to place one and the same proprietary medicinal product on the market in two or more Member States should be facilitated;

Whereas, for this purpose, a Committee for Proprietary Medicinal Products should be set up, consisting of representatives of the Member States and of the Commission, responsible for giving an opinion as to whether a particular proprietary medicinal product complies with the requirements set out in Directive 65/65/EEC;

Whereas this Directive represents merely one step towards achievement of the objective of the free movement of proprietary medicinal products; whereas, therefore, further measures with a view to abolishing any remaining barriers to the free movement of proprietary medicinal products will be necessary in the light of experience gained, particularly in the abovementioned Committee;

Whereas in order to facilitate the movement of proprietary medicinal products and to prevent the controls carried out in one Member State from being repeated in

---

1.   *Author's note* : It should be borne in mind that the references in Directive (EEC) 75/319 to "proprietary" medicinal products are anachronistic since the coming into force of Directive (EEC) 89/341 (OJ L142 25.5.89 p11) and should be disregarded.
2.   OJ L147 9.6.75 p13.
3.   OJ No 96 2.6.65 p1677/65.
4.   OJ No 107 19.6.75 p1825/65.
5.   OJ No 22 9.2.65 p369/65.

another, minimum requirements should be laid down for manufacture and imports coming from third countries and for the grant of the authorisation relating thereto; Whereas it should be ensured that, in the Member States, the supervision and control of the manufacture of proprietary medicinal products is carried out by a person who fulfils minimum conditions of qualification;

Whereas, moreover, the provisions of this Directive and of that of Directive 65/65/EEC which relate to proprietary medicinal products, although appropriate, are inadequate for vaccines, toxins and serums, proprietary medicinal products based on human blood or blood constituents, proprietary medicinal products based on radio-active isotopes and homeopathic proprietary medicinal products whereas the application thereof should consequently not be imposed at the present time in respect of such proprietary medicinal products;

Whereas certain rules in this Directive entail amendments to various provisions of Directive, 65/65/EEC,

HAS ADOPTED THIS DIRECTIVE :

CHAPTER I

Application for authorisation to place proprietary medicinal products on the market

Article 1

Member States shall take all appropriate measures to ensure that the documents and particulars listed in points 7 and 8 of Article 4, second paragraph, of Directive 65/65/EEC are drawn up by experts with the necessary technical or professional qualifications before they are submitted to the competent authorities. These documents and particulars shall be signed by the experts.

Article 2

The duties of the experts according to their respective qualifications shall be :

(a) to perform tasks falling within their respective disciplines (analysis, pharmacology and similar experimental sciences, clinical trials) and to describe objectively the results obtained (qualitatively and quantitatively);

(b) to describe their observations in accordance with Council Directive 75/318/EEC[1] of 20 May 1975, on the approximation of the laws of the Member States relating to analytical, pharmacotoxicological and clinical standards and protocols in respect of the testing of proprietary medicinal products, and to state, in particular :

— in the case of the analyst, whether the product is consistent with the declared composition, giving any substantiation of the control methods employed by the manufacturer;

— in the case of the pharmacologist or the specialist with similar experimental competence, the toxicity of the product and the pharmacological properties observed;

— in the case of the clinician, whether he has been able to ascertain effects on persons treated with the product which correspond to the particulars given by the applicant in accordance with Article 4 of Directive 65/65/EEC, whether the patient tolerates the product well, the posology the clinician advises and any contra-indications and side-effects;

---

1. See OJ L147 9.6.75 p1.

(c)   where applicable, to state the grounds for using the published references mentioned in point 8(a) and (b) of Article 4, second paragraph, of Directive 65/65/EEC under the conditions set out in Directive 75/318/EEC.

Detailed reports by the experts shall form part of the particulars accompanying the application which the applicant submits to the competent authorities.

Article 3

In the event of Article 2 of this Directive not being complied with, Article 5, second paragraph, of Directive 65/65/EEC shall apply.

CHAPTER II

Examination of the application for authorisation to place proprietary medical products on the market

Article 4

In order to examine the application submitted in accordance with Article 4 of Directive 65/65/EEC, the competent authorities of the Member States :

(a)   must verify whether the particulars submitted in support of the application comply with the said Article 4 and examine whether the conditions for issuing an authorisation to place proprietary medicinal products on the market (marketing authorisation) are complied with;

[(b)   may submit the medicinal product, its starting materials and, if need be, its intermediate products or other constituent materials for testing by a State laboratory or by a laboratory designated for that purpose in order to ensure that the control methods employed by the manufacturer and described in the particulars accompanying the application in accordance with the second subparagraph of point 7 of Article 4 of Directive 65/65/EEC are satisfactory;][1]

(c)   may, where appropriate, require the applicant to supplement the particulars accompanying the application in respect of the items listed in the second paragraph of Article 4 of Directive 65/65/EEC. Where the competent authorities avail themselves of this option, the time limits laid down in Article 7 of the said Directive shall be suspended until such time as the supplementary information required has been provided. Likewise, these time limits shall be suspended for the time allowed the applicant, where appropriate, for giving oral or written explanation.

Article 5

Member States shall take all appropriate measures to ensure that :

(a)   the competent authorities verify that manufacturers and importers of products coming from third countries are able to carry out manufacture in compliance with the particulars supplied pursuant to point 4 of Article 4, second paragraph, of Directive 65/65/EEC and/or to carry out controls according to the methods described in the particulars accompanying the application in accordance with point 7 of Article 4, second paragraph, of that Directive;

(b)   the competent authorities may allow manufacturers and importers of products coming from third countries, in exceptional and justifiable cases, to have certain stages of manufacture and/or certain of the controls referred

---

1.   Article 4(b) is replaced by Council Directive (EEC) 89/341, OJ L142 25.5.89 p11.

to in (a) carried out by third parties; in such cases, the verifications by the competent authorities shall also be made in the establishment designated.

[*Articles 6*]¹

[*Article 7*]²

[CHAPTER III]³

Committee for Proprietary Medicinal Products

Article 8

1.   In order to facilitate the adoption of common decisions by Member States on the authorisation of medicinal products for human use on the basis of the scientific criteria of quality, safety and efficacy, and to achieve thereby the free movement of medicinal products within the Community, a Committee for Proprietary Medicinal Products, hereinafter referred to as "the Committee", is hereby set up. The Committee shall be part of the European Agency for the Evaluation of Medicinal Products established by Council Regulation (EEC) No 2309/93 of 22 July 1993 laying down Community procedures for the authorisation and supervision of medicinal products for human and veterinary use and establishing a European Agency for the Evaluation of Medicinal Products⁴, hereinafter referred to as "the Agency".

2.   In addition to the other responsibilities conferred upon it by Community law, the Committee shall examine any question relating to the granting, variation, suspension or withdrawal of marketing authorisation for a medicinal product which is submitted to it in accordance with this Directive.

Article 9

1.   In order to obtain the recognition according to the procedures laid down in this Chapter in one or more of the Member States of an authorisation issued by a Member State in accordance with Article 3 of Directive 65/65/EEC, the holder of the authorisation shall submit an application to the competent authorities of the Member State or Member States concerned, together with the information and particulars referred to in Articles 4, 4a and 4b of Directive 65/65/EEC. He shall testify that the dossier is identical to that accepted by the first Member State, or shall identify any additions or amendments it may contain. In the latter case, he shall certify that the summary of the product characteristics proposed by him in accordance with Article 4a of Directive 65/65/EEC is identical to that accepted by the first Member State in accordance with Article 4b of Directive 65/65/EEC. Moreover he shall certify that all the dossiers filed as part of the procedure are identical.

2.   The holder of the marketing authorisation shall notify the Committee of this application, inform it of the Member States concerned and of the dates of submission of the application and send it a copy of the authorisation granted by the

---

1.   Repealed by Council Directive (EEC) 92/27, OJ L113 30.4.92 p8.
2.   Repealed by ibid.
3.   Chapter III (Articles 8 to 15c) is replaced by Council Directive (EEC) 93/39, OJ L214 24.8.93 p25, with effect from 1 January 1995. For the position prior to that date see italicised text at the end of this Appendix at pp310-312.
4.   OJ L214 24.8.93 p1.

first Member State. He shall also send the Committee copies of any such authorisation which may have been granted by the other Member States in respect of the medicinal product concerned, and shall indicate whether any application for authorisation is currently under consideration in any Member State.

3.   Except in cases referred to in Article 7a of Directive 65/65/EEC, before submitting the application, the holder of the authorisation shall inform the Member State which granted the authorisation on which the application is based that an application is to be made in accordance with this Directive and shall notify it of any additions to the original dossier; that Member State may require the applicant to provide it with all the particulars and documents necessary to enable it to check that the dossiers filed are identical.

In addition the holder of the authorisation shall request the Member State which granted the initial authorisation to prepare an assessment report in respect of the medicinal product concerned, or, if necessary, to update any existing assessment report. That Member State shall prepare the assessment report, or update it, within 90 days of the receipt of the request.

At the same time as the application is submitted in accordance with paragraph 1 the Member State which granted the initial authorisation shall forward the assessment report to the Member State or Member States concerned by the application.

4.   Save in the exceptional case provided for in Article 10(1), each Member State shall recognise the marketing authorisation granted by the first Member State within 90 days of receipt of the application and the assessment report. It shall inform the Member State which granted the initial authorisation, the other Member States concerned by the application, the Committee, and the person responsible for placing the medicinal product on the market.

Article 10

1.   Notwithstanding Article 9(4), where a Member State considers that there are grounds for supposing that the authorisation of the medicinal product concerned may present a risk to public health[1], it shall forthwith inform the applicant, the Member State which granted the initial authorisation, any other Member States concerned by the application and the Committee. The Member State shall state its reasons in detail and shall indicate what action may be necessary to correct any defect in the application.

2.   All the Member States concerned shall use their best endeavours to reach agreement on the action to be taken in respect of the application. They shall provide the applicant with the opportunity to make his point of view known orally or in writing. However, if the Member States have not reached agreement within the time limit referred to in Article 9(4) they shall forthwith refer the matter to the Committee for the application of the procedure laid down in Article 13.

3.   Within the time limit referred to in paragraph 2, the Member States concerned shall provide the Committee with a detailed statement of the matters on which they have been unable to reach agreement and the reasons for their disagreement. The applicant shall be provided with a copy of this information.

---

1.   "The expression 'risk to public health' refers to the quality, safety and efficacy of the medicinal product."

4.   As soon as he is informed that the matter has been referred to the Committee, the applicant shall forthwith forward to the Committee a copy of the information and particulars referred to in Article 9(1).

Article 11

If several applications submitted in accordance with Article 4 and 4a of Directive 65/65/EEC have been made for marketing authorisation for a particular medicinal product, and Member States have adopted divergent decisions concerning the authorisation of the medicinal product or its suspension or withdrawal from the market, a Member State, or the Commission, or the person responsible for placing the medicinal product on the market may refer the matter to the Committee for application of the procedure laid down in Article 13.

The Member State concerned, the person responsible for placing the medicinal product on the market or the Commission shall clearly identify the question which is referred to the Committee for consideration and, where appropriate, shall inform the aforementioned person thereof.

The Member State and the person responsible for placing the medicinal product on the market shall forward to the Committee all available information relating to the matter in question.

Article 12

The Member States or the Commission or the applicant or holder of the marketing authorisation may, in specific cases where the interests of the Community are involved, refer the matter to the Committee for the application of the procedure laid down in Article 13 before reaching a decision on a request for a marketing authorisation or on the suspension or withdrawal of an authorisation, or on any other variation to the terms of a marketing authorisation which appears necessary, in particular to take account of the information collected in accordance with Chapter Va.

The Member State concerned or the Commission shall clearly identify the question which is referred to the Committee for consideration and shall inform the person responsible for placing the medicinal product on the market.

The Member States and the aforementioned person shall forward to the Committee all available information relating to the matter in question.

Article 13

1.   When reference is made to the procedure described in this Article, the Committee shall consider the matter concerned and issue a reasoned opinion within 90 days of the date on which the matter was referred to it.

However, in cases submitted to the Committee in accordance with Articles 11 and 12, this period may be extended by 90 days.

In case of urgency, on a proposal from its Chairman, the Committee may agree to impose a shorter deadline.

2.   In order to consider the matter, the Committee may appoint one of its members to act as rapporteur. The Committee may also appoint individual experts to advise it on specific questions. When appointing experts, the Committee shall define their tasks and specify the time limit for the completion of these tasks.

3.   In the cases referred to in Articles 10 and 11, before issuing its opinion, the Committee shall provide the person responsible for placing the medicinal product on the market with an opportunity to present written or oral explanations.

In the case referred to in Article 12, the person responsible for placing the medicinal product on the market may be asked to explain himself orally or in writing.

If it considers it appropriate, the Committee may invite any other person to provide information relating to the matter before it.

The Committee may suspend the time limit referred to in paragraph 1 in order to allow the person responsible for placing the medicinal product on the market to prepare explanations.

4.   Where the opinion of the Committee is that :

—   the application does not satisfy the criteria for authorisation, or
—   the summary of the product characteristics proposed by the applicant in accordance with Article 4a of Directive 65/65/EEC should be amended, or
—   the authorisation should be granted subject to conditions, with regard to conditions considered essential for the safe and effective use of the medicinal product including pharmacovigilance, or
—   a marketing authorisation should be suspended, varied or withdrawn,

the Agency shall forthwith inform the person responsible for placing the medicinal product on the market. Within 15 days of the receipt of the opinion, the aforementioned person may notify the Agency in writing of his intention to appeal. In that case, he shall forward the detailed grounds for appeal to the Agency within 60 days of receipt of the opinion. Within 60 days of receipt of the grounds for appeal, the Committee shall consider whether its opinion should be revised, and the conclusions reached on the appeal shall be annexed to the assessment report referred to in paragraph 5.

5.   Within 30 days of its adoption, the Agency shall forward the final opinion of the Committee to the Member States, the Commission and the person responsible for placing the medicinal product on the market together with a report describing the assessment of the medicinal product and stating the reasons for its conclusions.

In the event of an opinion in favour of granting or maintaining an authorisation to place the medicinal product concerned on the market, the following documents shall be annexed to the opinion.

(a)   a draft summary of the product characteristics, as referred to in Article 4a of Directive 65/65/EEC;
(b)   any conditions affecting the authorisation within the meaning of paragraph 4.

Article 14

1.   Within 30 days of the receipt of the opinion, the Commission shall prepare a draft of the decision to be taken in respect of the application, taking into account Community law.

In the event of a draft decision which envisages the granting of marketing authorisation, the documents referred to in Article 13(5)(a) and (b) shall be annexed.

Where, exceptionally, the draft decision is not in accordance with the opinion of the Agency, the Commission shall also annex a detailed explanation of the reasons for the differences.

The draft decision shall be forwarded to the Member States and the applicant.

2.   A final decision on the application shall be adopted in accordance with the procedure laid down in Article 37b.

3.   The rules of procedure of the Committee referred to in Article 37b shall be adjusted to take account of the tasks incumbent upon it in accordance with this Directive.

These adjustments shall involve the following :

—   except in cases referred to in the third subparagraph of paragraph 1, the opinion of the Standing Committee shall be obtained in writing,
—   each Member State is allowed at least 28 days to forward written observations on the draft decision to the Commission,
—   each Member State is able to require in writing that the draft decision be discussed by the Standing Committee, giving its reasons in detail.

Where, in the opinion of the Commission, the written observations of a Member State raise important new questions of a scientific or technical nature which have not been addressed in the opinion of the Agency, the Chairman shall suspend the procedure and refer the application back to the Agency for further consideration.

The provisions necessary for the implementation of this paragraph shall be adopted by the Commission in accordance with the procedure laid down in Article 37a.

4.   A decision adopted in accordance with this Article shall be addressed to the Member States concerned by the matter and to the person responsible for placing the medicinal product on the market. The Member States shall either grant or withdraw marketing authorisation, or vary the terms of a marketing authorisation as necessary to comply with the decision within 30 days of its notification. They shall inform the Commission and the Committee thereof.

5.   The procedure referred to in Articles 8 to 14 shall not apply in the cases provided for in Article 9(2) of Council Directive 92/73/EEC of 22 September 1992[1] widening the scope of Directive 65/65/EEC and 75/319/EEC on the approximation of the laws of the Member States on medicinal products and laying down additional provisions on homeopathic medicinal products.

Article 15

Any application by the person responsible for placing the medicinal product on the market to vary a marketing authorisation which has been granted in accordance with the provisions of this Chapter shall be submitted to all the Member States which have previously authorised the medicinal product concerned.

The Commission shall, in consultation with the Agency, adopt appropriate arrangements for the examination of variations to the terms of a marketing authorisation.

---

1.   OJ L297 13.10.92 p8.

These arrangements shall include a notification system or administration procedures concerning minor variations and define precisely the concept of "a minor variation".

These arrangements shall be adopted by the Commission in the form of an Implementing Regulation in accordance with the procedure laid down in Article 37a.

The procedure laid down in Articles 13 and 14 shall apply by analogy to variations made to marketing authorisations for products subject to the Commission's arbitration.

Article 15a

1.   Where a Member State considers that the variation of the terms of a marketing authorisation which has been granted in accordance with the provisions of this Chapter or its suspension or withdrawal is necessary for the protection of public health, the Member State concerned shall forthwith refer the matter to the Committee for the application of the products laid down in Articles 13 and 14.

2.   Without prejudice to the provisions of Article 12, in exceptional cases, where urgent action is essential to protect public health, until a definitive decision is adopted a Member State may suspend the marketing and the use of the medicinal product concerned on its territory. It shall inform the Commission and the other Member States no later than the following working day of the reasons for its action.

Article 15b

Articles 15 and 15a shall apply by analogy to medicinal products authorised by Member States following an opinion of the Committee given in accordance with Article 4 of Directive 87/22/EEC before 1 January 1995.

Article 15c

1.   The Agency shall publish an annual report on the operation of the procedures laid down in this chapter and shall forward that report to the European Parliament and the Council for information.

2.   By 1 January 2001, the Commission shall publish a detailed review of the operation of the procedures laid down in this chapter and shall propose any amendments which may be necessary to improve these procedures.

The Council shall decide, under the conditions provided for in the Treaty, on the Commission proposal within one year of its submission.

CHAPTER IV

Manufacture and imports coming from third countries

Article 16

[1.   Member States shall take all appropriate measures to ensure that the manufacture of medicinal products is subject to the holding of an authorisation. This manufacturing authorisation shall be required notwithstanding that the medicinal products manufactured are intended for export.][1]

---

1.   Article 16(1) is replaced by Council Directive (EEC) 89/341, OJ L142 25.5.89 p11.

2.   The authorisation referred to in paragraph 1 shall be required for both total and partial manufacture, and for the various processes of dividing up, packaging or presentation.

However, such authorisation shall not be required for preparation, dividing up, changes in packaging or presentation where these processes are carried out, solely for retail supply, by pharmacists in dispensing pharmacies or by persons legally authorised in the Member States to carry out such processes.

3.   Authorisation referred to in paragraph 1 shall also be required for imports coming from third countries into a Member State; this Chapter and Article 29 shall have corresponding application to such imports as they have to manufacture.

Article 17

In order to obtain the authorisation referred to in Article 16, the applicant must meet at least the following requirements :

(a)   specify the proprietary medicinal products and pharmaceutical forms which are to be manufactured or imported and also the place where they are to be manufactured and/or controlled;

(b)   have at his disposal, for the manufacture or import of the above, suitable and sufficient premises, technical equipment and control facilities complying with the legal requirements which the Member State concerned lays down as regards both manufacture and control and the storage of products, in accordance with Article 5(a).

(c)   have at his disposal the services of at least one qualified person within the meaning of Article 21.

The applicant must provide particulars in support of the above in his application.

Article 18

1.   The competent authority of the Member State shall issue the authorisation referred to in Article 16 only after having made sure of the accuracy of the particulars supplied pursuant to Article 17, by means of an inquiry carried out by its agents.

2.   In order to ensure that the requirements referred to in Article 17 are complied with, authorisation may be made conditional on the carrying out of certain obligations imposed either when authorisation is granted or at a later date.

3.   The authorisation shall apply only to the premises specified in the application and to the proprietary medicinal products and pharmaceutical forms specified in that same application.

Article 19

The holder of an authorisation referred to in Article 16 shall at least be obliged :

(a)   to have at his disposal the services of staff who comply with the legal requirements existing in the Member State concerned both as regards manufacture and controls;

(b)   to dispose of the authorised proprietary medicinal products only in accordance with the legislation of the Member States concerned;

(c)   to give prior notice to the competent authority of any changes he may wish to make to any of the particulars supplied pursuant to Article 17; the competent authority shall in any event be immediately informed if the qualified person referred to in Article 21 is replaced unexpectedly;

(d) to allow the agents of the competent authority of the Member State concerned access to his premises at any time;

(e) to enable the qualified person referred to in Article 21 to carry out his duties, for example by placing at his disposal all the necessary facilities.

[(f) to comply with the principles and guidelines of good manufacturing practice for medicinal products as laid down by Community law.]¹

[*Article 19a*

The principles and guidelines of good manufacturing practices for medicinal products referred to in Article 19(f) shall be adopted in the form of a directive addressed to the Member States, in accordance with the procedure laid down in Article 37a of Directive 75/318/EEC. Detailed guidelines in line with those principles will be published by the Commission and revised as necessary to take account of technical and scientific progress.]²

Article 20

1. The Member States shall take all appropriate measures to ensure that the time taken for the procedure for granting the authorisation referred to in Article 16 does not exceed 90 days from the day on which the competent authority receives the application.

2. If the holder of the authorisation requests a change in any of the particulars referred to in Article 17 (a) and (b), the time taken for the procedure relating to this request shall not exceed 30 days. In exceptional cases this period of time may be extended to 90 days.

3. Member States may require from the applicant further information concerning the particulars supplied pursuant to Article 17 and concerning the qualified person referred to in Article 21; where the competent authority concerned exercises this right, application of the time limits referred to in paragraphs 1 and 2 shall be suspended until the additional data required have been supplied.

Article 21

1. Member States shall take all appropriate measures to ensure that the holder of the authorisation referred to in Article 16 has permanently and continuously at his disposal the services of at least one qualified person, in accordance with the conditions laid down in Article 23, responsible in particular for carrying out the duties specified in Article 22.

2. If he personally fulfils the conditions laid down in Article 23, the holder of the authorisation may himself assume the responsibility referred to in paragraph 1.

Article 22

1. Member States shall take all appropriate measures to ensure that the qualified person referred to in Article 21, without prejudice to his relationship with the holder of the authorisation referred to in Article 16, is responsible, in the context of the procedures referred to in Article 25, for securing :

---

1. Article 19, point (f), is added by Council Directive (EEC) 89/341, OJ L142 25.5.89 p11.
2. Article 19a is inserted by Council Directive (EEC) 89/341, OJ L142 25.5.89 p11.

(a)   in the case of proprietary medicinal products manufactured within the Member States concerned that each batch of proprietary medicinal products has been manufactured and checked in compliance with the laws in force in that Member State and in accordance with the requirements of the marketing authorisation;

(b)   in the case of proprietary medicinal products coming from third countries, that each production batch has undergone in the importing country a full qualitative analysis, a quantitative analysis of at least all the active constituents and all the other tests or checks necessary to ensure the quality of proprietary medicinal products in accordance with the requirements of the marketing authorisation.

The batches of products which have undergone such controls in a Member State shall be exempt from the above controls if they are imported into another Member State, accompanied by the control reports signed by the qualified person.

[In the case of medicinal products imported from a third country, where appropriate arrangements have been made by the Community with the exporting country to ensure that the manufacturer of the medicinal product applies standards of good manufacturing practice at least equivalent to those laid down by the Community and to ensure that the controls referred to under (b) have been carried out in the exporting country, the qualified person may be relieved of responsibility for carrying out those controls.][1]

2. In all cases and particularly where the proprietary medicinal products are released for sale the qualified person must certify in a register or equivalent document provided for that purpose that each production batch satisfies the provisions of this Article; the said register or equivalent document must be kept up to date as operations are carried out and must remain at the disposal of the agents of the competent authority for the period specified in the provisions of the Member State concerned and in any event for at least five years.

Article 23

Member States shall ensure that the qualified person referred to in Article 21 fulfils the following minimum conditions of qualification :

(a)   Possession of a diploma, certificate or other evidence of formal qualifications awarded on completion of a university course of study, or a course recognised as equivalent by the Member State concerned, extending over a period of at least four years of theoretical and practical study in one of the following scientific disciplines: pharmacy, medicine, veterinary medicine, chemistry, pharmaceutical chemistry and technology, biology. However :

—   the minimum duration of the university course may be three and a half years where the course is followed by a period of theoretical and practical training of a minimum duration of one year and including a

---

1.   Article 22(1), third subparagraph, is replaced by Council Directive (EEC) 93/39, OJ L214 24.8.93 p22.
        Pre-1993 Text read as follows :
        "A Member States may relive the qualified person of responsibility for the controls prescribed under (b) for imported proprietary medicinal products which are to remain in that Member State, if appropriate arrangements have been made with the exporting country to ensure that those controls have been carried out in the exporting country. Where these products are imported in the packaging in which they are to be sold by retail, Member States may allow exceptions to the requirements laid down in Article 17."

              training period of at least six months in a pharmacy open to the public, corroborated by an examination at university level;

—   where two university courses or two courses recognised by the State as equivalent co-exist in a Member State and where one of these extends over four years and the other over three years, the three-year course leading to a diploma, certificate or other evidence of formal qualifications awarded on completion of a university course or its recognised equivalent shall be considered to fulfil the condition of duration referred to in (a) in so far as the diplomas, certificates or other evidence of formal qualifications awarded on completion of both courses are recognised as equivalent by the State in question.

The course shall include theoretical and practical study bearing upon at least the following basic subjects :

Applied physics
General and inorganic chemistry
Organic chemistry
Analytical chemistry
Pharmaceutical chemistry, including analysis of medicinal products
General and applied biochemistry (medical)
Physiology
Microbiology
Pharmacology
Pharmaceutical technology
Toxicology
Pharmacognosy (medical aspects) (study of the composition and effects of the active principles of natural substances of plant and animal origin).

Studies in these subjects should be so balanced as to enable the person concerned to fulfil the obligations specified in Article 22.

In so far as certain diplomas, certificates or other evidence of formal qualifications mentioned in (a) do not fulfil the criteria laid down above, the competent authority of the Member State shall ensure that the person concerned provides evidence of adequate knowledge of the subjects involved.

(b)   Practical experience for at least two years, in one or more undertakings which are authorised to manufacture proprietary medicinal products, in the activities of qualitative analysis of medicinal products, of quantitative analysis of active substances and of the testing and checking necessary to ensure the quality of proprietary medicinal products.

The duration of practical experience may be reduced by one year where a university course lasts for at least five years and by a year and a half where the course lasts for at least six years.

Article 24

1.   A person engaging in the activities of the person referred to in Article 21 in a Member State at the time when this Directive is brought into force in that State but without complying with the provisions of Article 23 shall be eligible to continue to engage in those activities in the State concerned.

2.   The holder of a diploma, certificate or other evidence of formal qualifications awarded on completion of a university course - or a course recognised as equivalent by the Member State concerned - in a scientific discipline

allowing him to engage in the activities of the person referred to in Article 21 in accordance with the laws of that State may - if he began his course prior to the notification of this Directive - be considered as qualified to carry out in that State the duties of the person referred to in Article 21 provided that he has previously engaged in the following activities for at least two years before the end of the tenth year following notification of this Directive in one or more undertakings authorised pursuant to Article 16 : production supervision and/or qualitative analysis, quantitative analysis of active substances, and the necessary testing and checking under the direct authority of the person referred to in Article 21 to ensure the quality of the proprietary medicinal products.

If the person concerned has acquired the practical experience referred to in the first subparagraph more than 10 years prior to the notification of this Directive, a further one year's practical experience in accordance with the conditions referred to in the first subparagraph will be required to be completed immediately before he engages in such activities.

3.   A person who, at the time when this Directive is brought into force, is engaged in direct collaboration with a person referred to in Article 21 in production supervision activities and/or in qualitative and quantitative analysis of active substances and the testing and checking necessary to ensure the quality of proprietary medicinal products may, for a period of five years after this Directive has been brought into force, be considered as qualified to take up in that State the duties of the person referred to in Article 21 provided that that Member State ensures that the person shows evidence of adequate theoretical and practical knowledge and has engaged in the activities mentioned for at least five years.

Article 25

Member States shall ensure that the duties of qualified persons referred to in Article 21 are fulfilled, either by means of appropriate administrative measures or by making such persons subject to a professional code of conduct.

Member States may provide for the temporary suspension of such a person upon the commencement of administrative or disciplinary procedures against him for failure to fulfil his obligations.

CHAPTER V

Supervision and sanctions

Article 26

[The competent authority of the Member State concerned shall ensure, by means of repeated inspections, that the legal requirements governing medicinal products are complied with.

After every inspection as referred to in the first subparagraph, the officials representing the competent authority shall report on whether the manufacturer complies with the principles and guidelines of good manufacturing practice laid down by Community law. The content of such reports shall be communicated to the manufacturer who has to undergo the inspection.][1]

Such inspections shall be carried out by officials representing the competent authority who must be empowered to :

---

1.   Article 26, first subparagraph is replaced and the second subparagraph is inserted by Council Directive (EEC) 89/341, OJ L142 25.5.89 p11.

(a)   inspect manufacturing or commercial establishments and any laboratories entrusted by the holder of the authorisation referred to in Article 16 with the task of carrying out checks pursuant to Article 5(b);

(b)   take samples;

(c)   examine any documents relating to the object of the inspection, subject to the provisions in force in the Member States at the time of notification of this Directive and which place restrictions on these powers with regard to the descriptions of the method of preparation.

Article 27

Member States shall take all appropriate measures to ensure that the person responsible for marketing a proprietary medicinal product and, where appropriate, the holder of the authorisation referred to in Article 16, furnish proof of the controls carried out on the finished product and/or the ingredients and of the controls carried out at an intermediate stage of the manufacturing process, in accordance with the methods laid down for the purposes of the marketing authorisation.

Article 28

1.   Notwithstanding the measures provided for in Article 11 of Directive 65/65/EEC, Member States shall take all appropriate measures to ensure that the supply of the proprietary medicinal product shall be prohibited and the proprietary medicinal product withdrawn from the market if :

(a)   the proprietary medicinal product proves to be harmful under normal conditions of use;

(b)   it is lacking in therapeutic efficacy;

(c)   its qualitative and quantitative composition is not as declared;

(d)   the controls on the finished product and/or on the ingredients and the controls at an intermediate stage of the manufacturing process have not been carried out or if some other requirement or obligation relating to the grant of the authorisation referred to in Article 16 has not been fulfilled.

2.   The competent authority may limit the prohibition to supply the product, or its withdrawal from the market, to those batches which are the subject of dispute.

[Article 28a

At the request of the manufacturer, the exporter or the authorities of an importing third country, Member States shall certify that a manufacturer of medicinal products is in possession of the authorisation referred to in Article 16(1). When issuing such certificates they shall comply with the following conditions :

1.   Member States shall have regard to the prevailing administrative arrangements of the World Health Organisation.

2.   For medicinal products intended for export which are already authorised on their territory, they shall supply the summary of the product characteristics as approved in accordance with Article 4(b) of Directive 65/65/EEC.

3.   When the manufacturer is not in possession of a marketing authorisation he shall provide the authorities responsible for establishing the certificate referred to above with a declaration explaining why no marketing authorisation is available.][1]

---

1.   Article 28a is inserted by Council Directive (EEC) 89/341, OJ L142 25.5.89 p11.

Article 29

1.   The competent authority of a Member State shall suspend or revoke the authorisation referred to in Article 16 for a category of preparations or all preparations where any one of the requirements laid down in Article 17 is no longer met.

2.   In addition to the measures specified in Article 28, the competent authority of a Member State may suspend manufacture or imports of proprietary medicinal products coming from third countries or suspend or revoke the authorisation referred to in Article 16 for a category of preparations or all preparations where Articles 18, 19, 22 and 27 are not complied with.

[CHAPTER Va][1]

Pharmacovigilance

Article 29a

In order to ensure the adoption of appropriate regulatory decisions concerning the medicinal products authorised within the Community, having regard to information obtained about adverse reactions to medicinal products under normal conditions of use, the Member States shall establish a pharmacovigilance system. This system shall be used to collect information useful in the surveillance of medicinal products, with particular reference to adverse reactions in human beings, and to evaluate such information scientifically.

Such information shall be collated with data on consumption of medicinal products.

This system shall also collate information on frequently observed misuse and serious abuse of medicinal products.

Article 29b

For the purpose of this Directive, the following definitions shall apply :

—   "adverse reaction" means a reaction which is harmful and unintended and which occurs at doses normally used in man for the prophylaxis, diagnosis or treatment of disease or the modification of physiological function,
—   "serious adverse reaction" means an adverse reaction which is fatal, life-threatening, disabling, incapacitating, or which results in or prolongs hospitalisation,
—   "unexpected adverse reaction" means an adverse reaction which is not mentioned in the summary of product characteristics,
—   "serious unexpected adverse reaction" means an adverse reaction which is both serious and unexpected.

Article 29c

The person responsible for placing the medicinal product on the market shall have permanently and continuously at his disposal an appropriately qualified person responsible for pharmacovigilance.

That qualified person shall be responsible for the following :

---

1.   Chapter Va (Articles 29a to 29i) is added by Council Directive (EEC) 93/39, OJ L214 24.8.93 p22.

(a) the establishment and maintenance of a system which ensures that information about all suspected adverse reactions which are reported to the personnel of the company, and to medical representatives, is collected and collated at a single point within the Community;

(b) the preparation for the competent authorities of the reports referred to in Article 29d, in such form as may be laid down by those authorities, in accordance with the relevant national or Community guidelines;

(c) ensuring that any request from the competent authorities for the provision of additional information necessary for the evaluation of the benefits and risks afforded by a medicinal product is answered fully and promptly, including the provision of information about the volume of sales or prescriptions of the medicinal product concerned.

Article 29d

1. The person responsible for placing the medicinal product on the market shall be required to record and to report all suspected serious adverse reactions which are brought to his attention by a health care professional to the competent authorities immediately, and in any case within 15 days of their receipt at the latest.

2. In addition, the person responsible for placing the medicinal product on the market shall be required to maintain detailed records of all other suspected adverse reactions which are reported to him by a health care professional.

Unless other requirements have been laid down as a condition of the granting of authorisation, these records shall be submitted to the competent authorities immediately upon request or at least every six months during the first two years following authorisation, and once a year for the following three years. Thereafter, the records shall be submitted at five-yearly intervals together with the application for renewal of the authorisation, or immediately upon request. These records shall be accompanied by a scientific evaluation.

Article 29e

The Member States shall take all appropriate measures to encourage doctors and other health care professionals to report suspected adverse reactions to the competent authorities.

The Member States may impose specific requirements on medical practitioners, in respect of the reporting of suspected serious or unexpected adverse reactions, in particular where such reporting is a condition of the authorisation.

Article 29f

The Member States shall ensure that reports of suspected serious adverse reactions are immediately brought to the attention of the Agency and the person responsible for placing the medicinal product on the market, and in any case within 15 days of their notification, at the latest.

Article 29g

In order to facilitate the exchange of information about pharmacovigilance within the Community, the Commission, in consultation with the Agency, Member States and interested parties, shall draw up guidance on the collection, verification and presentation of adverse reaction reports.

This guidance shall take account of international harmonisation work carried out with regard to terminology and classification in the field of pharmacovigilance.

Article 29h

Where as a result of the evaluation of adverse reaction reports a Member State considers that a marketing authorisation should be varied, suspended or withdrawn, it shall forthwith inform the Agency and the person responsible for placing the medicinal product on the market.

In case of urgency, the Member State concerned may suspend the marketing of a medicinal product, provided the Agency is informed at the latest on the following working day.

Article 29i

Any amendments which may be necessary to update provisions of this Chapter to take account of scientific and technical progress shall be adopted in accordance with the procedure laid down in Article 37a.

CHAPTER VI

Miscellaneous provisions

Article 30

Member States shall take all appropriate measures to ensure that the competent authorities concerned communicate to each other such information as is appropriate to guarantee that the requirements for the authorisations referred to in Article 16 or marketing authorisations are fulfilled.

[Upon reasoned request, Member States shall forthwith communicate the reports referred to in the third subparagraph of Article 26 to the competent authorities of another Member State. If, after considering the reports, the Member State receiving the reports considers that it cannot accept the conclusions reached by the competent authorities of the Member State in which the report was established, it shall inform the competent authorities concerned of its reasons and may request further information. The Member States concerned shall use their best endeavours to reach agreement. If necessary, in the case of serious differences of opinion, the Commission shall be informed by one of the Member States concerned.][1]

Article 31

All decisions taken pursuant to Articles 18, 28 and 29 and all negative decisions taken pursuant to Articles 5(b) and 11(3) shall state in detail the reasons on which they are based. Such decisions shall be notified to the party concerned, who shall at the same time be informed of the remedies available to him under the laws in force and of the time limit allowed for applying for such remedies.

Article 32

No decision concerning suspension of manufacture or of importation of proprietary medicinal products coming from third countries, prohibition of supply or withdrawal from the market of a proprietary medicinal product may be taken except on the ground set out in Articles 28 and 29.

---

1.   Article 30, second subparagraph, is inserted by Council Directive (EEC) 89/341, OJ L142 25.5.89 p11.

Article 33

1.   Each Member State shall take all the appropriate measures to ensure that decisions authorising marketing, refusing or revoking a marketing authorisation, cancelling a decision refusing or revoking a marketing authorisation, prohibiting supply, or withdrawing a product from the market, together with the reasons on which such decisions are based, are brought to the attention of the Committee forthwith.

[2.   The person responsible for the marketing of a medicinal product shall be obliged to notify the Member States concerned forthwith of any action taken by him to suspend the marketing of a product or to withdraw a product from the market, together with the reasons for such action if the latter concerns the efficacy of the medicinal product or the protection of public health. Member States shall ensure that this information is brought to the attention of the committee.

3.   Member States shall ensure that appropriate information about action taken pursuant to paragraphs 1 and 2 which may affect the protection of public health in third countries is forthwith brought to the attention of the World Health Organisation, with a copy to the committee.

4.   The Commission shall publish annually a list of the medicinal products which are prohibited in the Community.][1]

Article 34

[This Directive shall apply to medicinal products for human use within the limits referred to in Article 2 of Directive 65/65/EEC.][2]

Chapters II to V of Directive 65/65/EEC and this Directive shall not apply to proprietary medicinal products consisting of vaccines, toxins or serums, to proprietary medicinal products based on human blood or blood constituents or radioactive isotopes, or to homeopathic proprietary medicinal products. A list, for information purposes, of these vaccines, toxins and serums is given in the Annex.

[Articles 35 to 37 amend Directive 65/65 and are not reproduced here]

[CHAPTER VIa][3]

Standing Committee procedures

Article 37a

Where the procedure laid down in this Article is to be followed the Commission shall be assisted by the Standing Committee on Medicinal Products for Human Use.

The representative of the Commission shall submit to the Committee a draft of the measures to be taken. The Committee shall deliver its opinion on the draft within a time limit which the Chairman may lay down according to the urgency of the matter. The opinion shall be delivered by the majority laid down in Article 148(2) of the Treaty in the case of decisions which the Council is required to adopt on a

---

1.   Article 33, paragraphs 2, 3 and 4 are added by Council Directive (EEC) 89/341, OJ L142 25.5.89 p11.
2.   Article 34, first paragraph is amended by Council Directive (EEC) 89/341, OJ L142 25.5.89 p11.
3.   Chapter VIa (Articles 37a and 37b) is inserted by Council Directive (EEC) 93/39, OJ L214 24.8.93 p22.

proposal from the Commission. The votes of the representatives of the Member States within the Committee shall be weighted in the manner set out in that Article. The Chairman shall not vote.

The Commission shall adopt the measures envisaged if they are in accordance with the opinion of the Committee.

If the measures envisaged are not in accordance with the opinion of the Committee, or if no opinion is delivered, the Commission shall, without delay, submit to the Council a proposal relating to the measures to be taken. The Council shall act by a qualified majority.

If on the expiry of a period of three months from the date of referral to the Council, the Council has not acted, the proposed measures shall be adopted by the Commission.

Article 37b

Where the procedure laid down in this Article is to be followed the Commission shall be assisted by the Standing Committee on Medicinal Products for Human Use.

The representative of the Commission shall submit to the Committee a draft of the measures to be taken. The Committee shall deliver its opinion on the draft within a time limit which the Chairman may lay down according to the urgency of the matter. The opinion shall be delivered by the majority laid down in Article 148(2) of the Treaty in the case of decisions which the Council is required to adopt on a proposal from the Commission. The votes of the representatives of the Member States within the Committee shall be weighted in the manner set out in that Article. The Chairman shall not vote.

The Commission shall adopt the measures envisaged if they are in accordance with the opinion of the Committee.

If the measures envisaged are not in accordance with the opinion of the Committee, or if no opinion is delivered, the Commission shall, without delay submit to the Council a proposal relating to the measures to be taken. The Council shall act by a qualified majority.

If on the expiry of a period of three months from the date of referral to the Council, the Council has not acted, the proposed measures shall be adopted by the Commission, save where the Council has decided against the said measures by a simple majority[1].]

CHAPTER VII

Implementing provisions and transitional measures

Article 38

Member States shall bring into force the laws, regulations and administrative provisions needed in order to comply with this Directive within 18 months of its notification and shall forthwith inform the Commission thereof.

1.　Chapter VIa (Articles 37a and 37b) is inserted by Council Directive (EEC) 93/39, OJ L214 24.8.93 p22.
　　Pre 1993 Text to be read without insertion of Chapter VIa.

Member States shall communicate to the Commission the text of the main provisions of national law which they adopt in the field covered by this Directive.

Article 39

1.   As regards the authorisations referred to in Article 16 issued before the expiry of the time limit laid down in Article 38, Member States may grant an additional period of one year to the undertakings concerned to enable them to comply with the provisions of Chapter IV.

2.   Within 15 years of the notification referred to in Article 38, the other provisions of this Directive shall be applied progressively to proprietary medicinal products placed on the market by virtue of previous provisions.

3.   Member States shall notify the Commission, within three years following the notification of this Directive, of the number of proprietary medicinal products covered by paragraph 2, and, each subsequent year, of the number of these products for which a marketing authorisation referred to in Article 3 of Directive 65/65/EEC, has not yet been issued.

Article 40

This Directive is addressed to the Member States.

Done at Brussels, 20 May 1975.

For the Council

The President

R. RYAN

ANNEX

The expression "vaccines, toxins or serums" used in Article 34 shall cover in particular :

— *agents used to produce active immunity*
 (such as cholera vaccine, BCG, polio vaccine, smallpox vaccine);

— *agents used to diagnose the state of immunity*
 including in particular tuberculin and tuberculin PPD, toxins for the Schick and Dick Tests, brucellin;

— *agents used to produce passive immunity*
 (such as diphtheria antitoxin, anti-smallpox globulin, antilymphocytic globulin).

CHAPTER III[1]

Committee for Proprietary Medicinal Products

Article 8

1. In order to facilitate the adoption of a common position by the Member States with regard to decisions on the issuing of marketing authorisations and to promote thereby the free movement of proprietary medicinal products, a Committee for Proprietary Medicinal Products, hereinafter referred to as "the Committee", is hereby set up. The Committee shall consist of representatives of the Member States and of the Commission.

2. The Committee's task shall be to examine, at the request of a Member State or the Commission and in accordance with Articles 9 to 14, questions concerning the application of Articles 5, 11 or 20 of Directive 65/65/EEC.

3. The Committee shall draw up its own rules of procedure.

Article 9

1. In order to make it easier to obtain a marketing authorisation in at least two other Member States taking into due consideration an authorisation issued in one Member State in accordance with Article 3 of Directive 65/65/EEC, the holder of the latter authorisation may submit an application to the competent authorities of the Member States concerned together with the information and documents referred to in Articles 4, 4a and 4b of Directive 65/65/EEC. He shall testify to its identity with the dossier accepted by the first Member State, specifying any additions it may contain, and shall certify that all the dossiers filed as part of this procedure are identical.

2. The holder of the marketing authorisation shall notify the Committee of this application, inform it of the Member States concerned and send it a copy of his authorisation. He shall also inform the Member State which granted him the initial authorisation and notify it of any additions to the original dossier; that State may require the applicant to provide it with all the particulars and documents necessary to enable it to check the identity of the dossiers filed with the dossier on which it took its decision.

3. The holder of the marketing authorisation shall notify the dates on which the dossiers were sent to the Member States concerned. As soon as the Committee has noted that all the Member States concerned are in possession of the dossier, it shall forthwith inform all the Member States and the applicant of the date on which the last Member State concerned received the dossier. The Member State(s) concerned shall either grant the authorisation valid for their markets within a period of 120 days of the aforementioned date, taking into due consideration the authorisation issued within the meaning of paragraph 1, or put forward a reasoned objection.

Article 10

1. Where a Member State considers that it is unable to grant a marketing authorisation, it shall forward to the Committee and to the person responsible for placing the proprietary medicinal product on the market its reasoned objection in

---

1.   Text of 75/319 as replaced by Directive 83/570. Please note this text has now been replaced by Directive 93/39 and is included here to indicate the position until 1 January 1995 when the amendments made by Directive 93/39 are to be implemented in the Member States.

accordance with Article 5 of Directive 65/65/EEC, within the time limits stipulated in Article 9 (3).

2. Upon the expiry of this period, the matter shall be referred to the Committee and the procedure referred to in Article 14 shall be applied.

3. On receipt of the reasoned objection referred to in paragraph 1, the person responsible for placing the product on the market shall immediately send the Committee a copy of the particulars and documents enumerated in Article 9 (1).

Article 11

If several applications submitted in accordance with Articles 4 and 4a of Directive 65/65/EEC have been made for a marketing authorisation for a particular proprietary medicinal product, and one or more Member States have granted an authorisation while one or more of the other Member States have refused it, one of the Member States concerned or the Commission may refer the matter to the Committee for application of the procedure referred to in Article 14 of this Directive.

The same shall apply where one or more Member States have suspended or revoked a marketing authorisation while one or more other Member States have not done so.

In both cases, the person responsible for placing the proprietary medicinal product on the market shall be informed of any decision of the Committee to apply the procedure laid down in Article 14.

Article 12

The competent authorities of Member States may, in specific cases where the interests of the Community are involved, refer the matter to the Committee before reaching a decision on a request for a marketing authorisation or on the suspension or revocation of an authorisation.

Article 13

1. The competent authorities shall draw up an assessment report and comments on the dossier as regards the results of the analytical and toxico-pharmacological tests on, and clinical trials of, any proprietary products containing a new active substance which are the subject of a request for a marketing authorisation in the Member States concerned for the first time.

2. As soon as the notification referred to in Article 9 is received, the competent authorities shall immediately communicate to the Member States concerned any assessment report accompanied by a summary of the dossier relating to a particular proprietary product. This report shall also be communicated to the Committee where a matter is referred to the Committee pursuant to Article 10.

The assessment report shall also be forwarded to the other Member States concerned and to the Committee as soon as a matter is referred to the Committee under the procedure laid down in Article 11. Any assessment report so forwarded shall remain confidential.

The competent authorities shall bring the assessment report up to date as soon as it is in possession of information which is of importance for the evaluation of the balance between effectiveness and risk.

Article 14

1. When reference is made to the procedure described in this Article, the Committee shall consider the matter concerned and issue a reasoned opinion within 60 days of the date on which the matter was referred to it.

In the cases referred to in Article 10 the person responsible for placing the product on the market may, at his request, explain himself orally or in writing before the Committee issues its opinion. The Committee may extend the time limit referred to in the preceding paragraph to give the applicant time to explain himself orally or in writing.

In the case referred to in Article 11, the person responsible for placing the product on the market may be asked to explain himself orally or in writing.

2. The Committee's opinion shall concern the grounds for the objection provided for in Article 10 (1) and the grounds on which the marketing authorisation has been refused, suspended or withdrawn in the cases described in Article 11.

The Committee shall immediately inform the Member State(s) concerned and the person responsible for placing the product on the market of its opinion or of those of its members in the case of divergent opinions.

3. The Member State(s) concerned shall decide what action to take on the Committee's opinion within 60 days of receipt of the information referred to in paragraph 2. They shall immediately inform the Committee of their decision.

Article 15

1. The Commission shall report to the Council every two years on the operation of the procedure laid down in this chapter and its effects on the development of intra-Community trade.

2. In the light of experience, the Commission shall, not later than four years after the entry into force of this Directive, submit to the Council a proposal containing appropriate measures leading towards the abolition of any remaining barriers to the free movement of proprietary medicinal products.

3. The Council shall decide on the Commission proposal no later than one year after its submission.

APPENDIX 4

COUNCIL DIRECTIVE (EEC) 87/22
of 22 December 1986

on the approximation of national measures relating to the placing on the market of high-technology medicinal products, particularly those derived from biotechnology[1]

THE COUNCIL OF THE EUROPEAN COMMUNITIES,

Having regard to the Treaty establishing the European Economic Community, and in particular Article 100 thereof,

Having regard to the proposal from the Commission[2],

Having regard to the opinion of the European Parliament[3],

Having regard to the opinion of the Economic and Social Committee[4],

Whereas the essential aim of any rules governing the production and distribution of medicinal products must be to safeguard public health;

Whereas high-technology medicinal products requiring lengthy periods of costly research will continue to be developed in Europe only if they benefit from a favourable regulatory environment, particularly identical conditions governing their placing on the market throughout the Community;

Whereas Council Directive 75/319/EEC of 20 May 1975 on the approximation of provisions laid down by law, regulation or administrative action relating to proprietary medicinal products[5], as last amended by Directive 83/570/EEC[6], makes provision for certain procedures for co-ordinating national decisions relating to the placing on the market of proprietary medicinal products for human use; whereas pharmaceutical undertakings may, according to these provisions, request a Member State to take due account of an authorisation already issued by another Member State;

Whereas Council Directive 81/851/EEC of 28 September 1981 on the approximation of the laws of the Member States relating to veterinary medicinal products[7] makes provision for a procedure for co-ordinating national decisions relating to veterinary medicinal products;

Whereas, however, these procedures are not sufficient to open up to high-technology medicinal products the large Community-wide single market they require;

Whereas, in this technically advanced sector, the scientific expertise available to each of the national authorities is not always sufficient to resolve problems posed by high-technology medicinal products;

1.   OJ L15 17.1.87 p38.
2.   OJ C293 5.11.84 p1.
3.   OJ C36 17.2.86 p152.
4.   OJ C160 1.7.85 p18.
5.   OJ L147 9.6.75 p13.
6.   OJ L332 28.11.83 p1.
7.   OJ L317 6.11.81 p1.

Whereas it is consequently important to provide for a Community mechanism for concertation, prior to any national decision relating to a high-technology medicinal product, with a view to arriving at uniform decisions throughout the Community;

Whereas it is desirable to extend this Community concertation to immunological products and substitutes for blood constituents developed by means of new biotechnological processes, and to new products based on radio-isotopes, the development of which in Europe can only take place if a sufficiently large and homogeneous market exists;

Whereas the need for the adoption of new technical rules applying to high-technology medicinal products or for the amendment of existing rules must be examined during a preliminary concertation between the Member States and the Commission within the competent Committees so as not to endanger the advance of pharmaceutical research whilst at the same time ensuring optimum protection of public health within the Community,

HAS ADOPTED THIS DIRECTIVE :

Article 1

Before taking a decision on a marketing authorisation or on the withdrawal or, subject to Article 4(2), suspension of a marketing authorisation in respect of the medicinal products listed in the Annex, Member States' authorities shall, in accordance with Articles 2, 3 and 4, refer the matter for an opinion to the Committees referred to in Article 8 of Directive 75/319/EEC and Article 16 of Directive 81/851/EEC.

Article 2

1. As soon as they receive an application for marketing authorisation relating to a medicinal product referred to in the Annex (Lists A and B), the competent authorities shall, at the request of the person responsible for placing the product on the market, bring the matter before either the Committee for Proprietary Medicinal Products or the Committee for Veterinary Medicinal Products, in accordance with their competence, for an opinion. Any such request shall be submitted in writing to the competent authorities concerned at the same time as the application for marketing authorisation and a copy shall be sent to the Committee concerned.

2. As soon as they receive an application for marketing authorisation relating to a medicinal product developed by means of new biotechnological processes and referred to in List A in the Annex, the competent authorities shall be required to bring the matter before the Committee for Proprietary Medicinal Products or the Committee for Veterinary Medicinal Products, in accordance with their competence, for an opinion.

3. Paragraph 2 shall not apply if, when submitting the application for marketing authorisation, the applicant certifies to the competent authorities of the Member State concerned that :

(i)   neither he nor any other natural or legal person with whom he is connected has, during the preceding five years, applied for authorisation to place a product containing the same active principle(s) on the market of another Member State; and

(ii)   neither he nor any other natural or legal person with whom he is connected intends, within the five years following the date of the application, to seek authorisation to place a product containing the same active principle(s) on the market of another Member State.

In this case, the competent authorities shall notify the appropriate Committee of the application and forward to it a summary of product characteristics as described in Article 4a of Directive 65/65/EEC[1], as last amended by Directive 87/21/EEC[2] or an equivalent document provided by the applicant if a proprietary medicinal product referred to in the second paragraph of Article 34 of Directive 75/319/EEC or a veterinary medicinal product is involved.

If, within five years of the first application, one or more subsequent applications for authorisation to place a product containing the same active principle derived from the same route of synthesis on the market are made to the competent authorities of the other Member States by the person responsible for placing the original product on the market or with his consent, that person shall forthwith inform the competent authorities of the Member State to whom the first application was made and the matter shall be brought before the appropriate Committee for an opinion.

4.   Where the Committee has, in accordance with this Directive, issued a favourable opinion on the placing on the market of a high-technology medicinal product, the competent authorities shall refer the matter to the Committee for a new opinion before deciding on the withdrawal or, subject to Article 4(2), suspension of the marketing authorisation for the medicinal product in question.

5.   The competent authorities or the Commission may also consult the Committee for Proprietary Medicinal Products on any technical question concerning the proprietary medicinal products referred to in the second paragraph of Article 34 of Directive 75/319/EEC.

6.   The competent authorities or the Commission may also consult the Committee for Veterinary Medicinal Products on any technical question concerning the veterinary medicinal products referred to in the second and third indents of Article 2(2) of Directive 81/851/EEC.

Article 3

1.   The representative of the Member State which initiated the procedure referred to in Article 2 shall act as rapporteur and shall provide all information relevant to the evaluation of the medicinal product. Information thus disclosed shall be strictly confidential.

2.   The person responsible for placing the medicinal product in question on the market shall immediately be informed of the referral to the Committee. He may, at his own request, provide the Committee with oral or written explanations.

3.   When placing the matter before the Committee, the Member State concerned shall ensure that the person responsible for placing the medicinal product on the market transmits to all the members of the Committee an identical summary of the dossier consisting of the summary of the product characteristics together with the reports of the analytical, pharmaco-toxicological and clinical experts.

In addition, a complete and updated copy of the dossier for the application for marketing authorisation lodged with the Member State or Member States concerned shall be transmitted to the Committee by the person responsible for placing the product on the market, who shall certify that all the dossiers submitted to the competent authorities and to the Committee in respect of the medicinal product in question are identical.

---

1.   OJ No 22 9.2.65 p369/65.
2.   See OJ L15 17.1.87 p36.

4.   All available evaluation reports and drug-monitoring reports relating to the same medicinal product shall be forwarded to the Committee by the authorities of the Member States and by the person responsible for placing the product in question on the market.

Article 4

1.   When the questions referred to it relate to an application for marketing authorisation, the Committee shall issue its opinion thirty days before the expiry of the time limits provided for in Article 7 of Directive 65/65/EEC and Article 4(c) of Directive 75/319/EEC, or in Articles 8 and 9(3) of Directive 81/851/EEC, as appropriate. To this end, the Member State which referred the matter shall inform the Committee without delay of any extension and of the beginning and end of any suspension of the time limits concerned.

2.   When a proposal to suspend or withdraw a marketing authorisation is referred to it, the Committee shall fix an appropriate time limit for issuing its reasoned opinion, having regard to the requirements for the protection of public health. However, in cases of urgency, the Member States may suspend the marketing authorisation in question without waiting for the opinion of the Committee provided that they forthwith inform the Committee thereof, indicating the reasons for the suspension and justifying the urgency of this measure.

3.   The Committee shall forthwith notify its opinion and, where relevant, any dissenting opinions expressed therein, to the Member State concerned and the person responsible for placing the product on the market.

4.   The Member State concerned shall reach a decision on the action it intends to take following the Committee's opinion not later than 30 days after receipt of the information provided for in paragraph 3. It shall forthwith inform the Committee of its decision.

Article 5

Subject to the application of other Community provisions, Member States shall communicate to the Commission in accordance with Articles 8 and 9 of Council Directive 83/189/EEC of 28 March 1983 laying down a procedure for the provision of information in the field of technical standards regulations[1], draft technical regulations relating to the production and marketing or proprietary medicinal products as defined in Article 1 of Directive 65/65/EEC.

Within one year of adoption of this Directive, the Commission will submit to the Council proposals for Regulations to harmonise, along the lines of Directive 75/319/EEC, the conditions for authorising the manufacture and placing on the market of the proprietary medicinal products excluded by Article 34 of Directive 75/319/EEC and of the veterinary medicinal products referred to in Article 2(2) of Directive 81/851/EEC, in view of in particular of the safety problems arising in production and use.

Article 6

Member States shall take the measures necessary to comply with this Directive not later than 1 July 1987. They shall forthwith inform the Commission thereof.

---

1.   OJ L109 26.4.83 p8.

Article 7

This Directive is addressed to the Member States.

Done at Brussels, 22 December 1986.

For the Council

The President

G. SHAW

ANNEX

LIST OF HIGH-TECHNOLOGY MEDICINAL PRODUCTS

A. **Medicinal products developed by means of the following biotechnological processes :**

-   recombinant DNA technology,
-   controlled expression of genes coding for biologically active proteins in prokaryotes and eukaryotes, including transformed mammalian cells,
-   hybridoma and monoclonal antibody methods.

B. **Other high-technology medicinal products :**

-   other biotechnological processes which, in the opinion of the competent authority concerned constitute a significant innovation,
-   medicinal products administered by means of new delivery systems which, in the opinion of the competent authority concerned, constitute a significant innovation,
-   medicinal products containing a new substance or an entirely new indication which, in the opinion of the competent authority concerned, is of significant therapeutic interest,
-   new medicinal products based on radio-isotopes which, in the opinion of the competent authority concerned, are of significant therapeutic interest,
-   medicinal products the manufacture of which employs processes which, in the opinion of the competent authority concerned, demonstrate a significant technical advance such as two-dimensional electrophoresis under micro-gravity.

APPENDIX 5

COUNCIL REGULATION (EEC) 2309/93
of 22 July 1993

laying down Community procedures for the authorisation and supervision of medicinal products for human and veterinary use and establishing a European Agency for the Evaluation of Medicinal Products[1]

THE COUNCIL OF THE EUROPEAN COMMUNITIES,

Having regard to the Treaty establishing the European Economic Community, and in particular Article 235 thereof,

Having regard to the proposal from the Commission[2],

Having regard to the opinion of the European Parliament[3],

Having regard to the opinion of the Economic and Social Committee[4],

Whereas Council Directive 87/22/EEC of 22 December 1986 on the approximation of national measures relating to the placing on the market of high-technology medicinal products particularly those derived from biotechnology[5] has established a Community mechanism for concertation, prior to any national decision relating to a high-technology medicinal product, with a view to arriving at uniform decisions throughout the Community; whereas this route should be followed, particularly in order to ensure the smooth functioning of the internal market in the pharmaceutical sector;

Whereas the experience acquired as a result of Directive 87/22/EEC has shown that it is necessary to establish a centralised Community authorisation procedure for technologically advanced medicinal products, in particular those derived from biotechnology; whereas this procedure should also be available to persons responsible for placing on the market medicinal products containing new active substances which are intended for use in human beings or in food-producing animals;

Whereas in the interest of public health it is necessary that decisions on the authorisation of such medicinal products should be based on the objective scientific criteria of the quality, the safety and the efficacy of the medicinal product concerned to the exclusion of economic or other considerations; whereas, however, Member States should exceptionally be able to prohibit the use on their territory of medicinal products for human use which infringe objectively defined concepts of public order or public morality; whereas, moreover, a veterinary medicinal product may not be authorised by the Community if its use would contravene the legal measures laid down by the Community within the framework of the common agricultural policy;

Whereas, in the case of medicinal products for human use, the criteria of quality, safety and efficacy have been extensively harmonised by Council Directive

---

1. OJ L214 24.8.93 p1.
2. OJ C330 31.12.90 p1 and OJ C310 30.11.91 p7.
3. OJ C183 15.7.91 p145.
4. OJ C269 14.10.91 p84.
5. OJ L15 17.1.87 p38. See Appendix 4 ante.

65/65/EEC of 26 January 1965 on the approximation of provisions laid down by law, regulation or administrative action relating to medicinal products[1] and the Second Council Directive 75/319/EEC of 20 May 1975 on the approximation of provisions laid down by law, regulation and administrative action relating to proprietary medicinal products[2], and by Council Directive 75/318/EEC of 20 May 1975 on the approximation of the laws of the Member States relating to analytical pharmaco-toxicological and clinical standards and protocols in respect of the testing of medicinal products[3];

Whereas in the case of veterinary medicinal products, the same results have been achieved by Council Directive 81/851/EEC of 28 September 1981 on the approximation of the laws of the Member States relating to veterinary medicinal products[4] and by Council Directive 81/852/EEC of 28 September 1981 on the approximation of the laws of the Member States relating to analytical, pharmaco-toxicological and clinical standards and protocols in respect of the testing of veterinary medicinal products[5];

Whereas the same criteria must be applied to medicinal products which are to be authorised by the Community;

Whereas only after a single scientific evaluation of the highest possible standard of the quality, safety or efficacy of technologically advanced medicinal products, to be undertaken within the European Agency for the Evaluation of Medicinal Products, should a marketing authorisation be granted by the Community by a rapid procedure ensuring close co-operation between the Commission and Member States.

Whereas Council Directive 93/39/EEC of 14 June 1993 amending Directive 65/65/EEC, 75/318/EEC and 75/319/EEC in respect of medicinal products[6] has provided that in the event of a disagreement between Member States about the quality, safety or efficacy of a medicinal product which is the subject of the decentralised Community authorisation procedure, the matter should be resolved by a binding Community decision following a scientific evaluation of the issues involved within a European medicinal product evaluation agency; whereas similar provisions have been laid down in respect of veterinary medicinal products by Council Directive 93/40/EEC of 14 June 1993 amending Directives 81/851/EEC and 81/852/EEC on the approximation of the laws of the Member States relating to veterinary medicinal products[7];

Whereas the Community must be provided with the means to undertake a scientific evaluation of medicinal products which are presented for authorisation in accordance with the centralised Community procedures; whereas, furthermore, in order to achieve the effective harmonisation of the administrative decisions taken by Member States in relation to individual medicinal products which are presented for authorisation in accordance with decentralised procedures, it is necessary to provide the Community with the means of resolving disagreements between Member States about the quality, safety and efficacy of medicinal products;

Whereas it is therefore necessary to establish a European Agency for the Evaluation of Medicinal Products ("the Agency");

1.　　OJ No 22 9.2.65 p369/65. See Appendix 1 ante.
2.　　OJ L147 9.6.75 p13. See Appendix 3 ante.
3.　　OJ L147 9.6.75 p1. See Appendix 2 ante.
4.　　OJ L317 6.11.81 p1.
5.　　OJ L317 6.11.81 p16.
6.　　See OJ L214 24.8.93 p22.
7.　　See OJ L214 24.8.93 p31.

Whereas the primary task of the Agency should be to provide scientific advice of the highest possible quality to the Community institutions and the Member States for the exercise of the powers conferred upon them by Community legislation in the field of medicinal products in relation to the authorisation and supervision of medicinal products;

Whereas it is necessary to ensure close co-operation between the Agency and scientists working within the Member States;

Whereas, therefore, the exclusive responsibility for preparing the opinions of the Agency on all matters relating to medicinal products for human use should be entrusted to the Committee for Proprietary Medicinal Products created by the Second Council Directive 75/319/EEC; whereas in respect of veterinary medicinal products this responsibility should be entrusted to the Committee for Veterinary Medicinal Products created by Directive 81/851/EEC;

Whereas the establishment of the Agency will make it possible to reinforce the scientific role and independence of these two Committees, in particular through the establishment of a permanent technical and administrative secretariat;

Whereas it is also necessary to make provisions for the supervision of medicinal products which have been authorised by the Community and in particular for the intensive monitoring of adverse reactions to those medicinal products through Community pharmacovigilance activities in order to ensure the rapid withdrawal from the market of any medicinal product which presents an unacceptable level of risk under normal conditions of use;

Whereas the Commission, working in close co-operation with the Agency, and after consultation with Member States, should also be entrusted with the task of co-ordinating the discharge of the various supervisory responsibilities of Member States and in particular the provisions of information about medicinal products, monitoring the respect of good manufacturing practices, good laboratory practices and good clinical practices;

Whereas the Agency should also be responsible for co-ordinating the activities of the Member States in the field of the monitoring of adverse reactions to medicinal products (pharmacovigilance);

Whereas it is necessary to provide for the orderly introduction of Community procedures for the authorisation of medicinal products alongside the national procedures of the Member States which have already been extensively harmonised by Directives 65/65/EEC, 75/319/EEC and 81/851/EEC; whereas it is therefore appropriate in the first instance to limit the obligation to use the new Community procedure to certain medicinal products; whereas the scope of the Community procedures should be reviewed in the light of experience at the latest six years after the entry into force of this Regulation;

Whereas risks to the environment may be associated with medicinal products containing or consisting of genetically modified organisms; whereas therefore it is necessary to provide for an environmental risk assessment of such products similar to that provided for by Council Directive 90/220/EEC of 23 April 1990 on the deliberate release into the environment of genetically modified organisms[1] together with the assessment of the quality, safety and efficacy of the product concerned within a single Community procedure;

---

1.   OJ L117 8.5.90 p15.

Whereas the Treaty does not provide, for the adoption of a uniform system at Community level, as provided for by this Regulation, powers other than those of Article 235,

HAS ADOPTED THIS REGULATION :

TITLE I

DEFINITIONS AND SCOPE

Article 1

The purpose of this Regulation is to lay down Community procedures for the authorisation and supervision of medicinal products for human and veterinary use and to establish a European Agency for the Evaluation of Medicinal Products.

The provisions of this Regulation shall not affect the powers of the Member States' authorities as regards the price setting of medicinal products or their inclusion in the scope of the national health system of the Member States' authorities or their inclusion in the scope of the social security schemes on the basis of health, economic and social conditions. For example, the Member States may choose from the marketing authorisation those therapeutic indications and pack sizes which will be covered by their social security organisations.

Article 2

The definitions laid down in Article 1 of Directive 65/65/EEC and those laid down in Article 1(2) of Directive 81/851/EEC shall apply for the purposes of this Regulation.

The person responsible for placing the medicinal products covered by this Regulation on the market must be established in the Community.

Article 3

1.   No medicinal product referred to in Part A of the Annex may be placed on the market within the Community unless a marketing authorisation has been granted by the Community in accordance with the provisions of this Regulation.

2.   The person responsible for placing on the market a medicinal product referred to in Part B of the Annex may request that authorisation to place the medicinal product on the market be granted by the Community in accordance with the provisions of this Regulation.

3.   Before entry into force of this Regulation and after consultation of the Committee for Proprietary Medicinal Products, Parts A and B of the Annex as regards medicinal products for human use shall be re-examined in the light of scientific and technical progress with a view to making any amendments necessary which will be adopted under the procedure laid down in Article 72.

4.   Before entry into force of this Regulation and after consultation of the Committee for Veterinary Medicinal Products, Parts A and B of the Annex as regards veterinary medicinal products shall be re-examined in the light of scientific and technical progress with a view to making any amendments necessary which will be adopted under the procedure laid down in Article 72.

5.   The procedures referred to in paragraphs 3 and 4 shall continue to apply after entry into force of this Regulation.

Article 4

1.   In order to obtain the authorisation referred to in Article 3, the person responsible for placing a medicinal product on the market shall submit an application to the European Agency for the Evaluation of Medicinal Products, hereinafter referred to as "the Agency", set up under Title IV.

2.   The Community shall issue and supervise marketing authorisations for medicinal products for human use in accordance with Title II.

3.   The Community shall issue and supervise marketing authorisations for veterinary medicinal products in accordance with Title III.

TITLE II

AUTHORISATION AND SUPERVISION OF MEDICINAL PRODUCTS FOR HUMAN USE

CHAPTER 1

Submission and examination of applications - authorisations - renewal of authorisation

Article 5

The Committee for Proprietary Medicinal Products established by Article 8 of Directive 75/319/EEC, in this Title referred to as "the Committee", shall be responsible for formulating the opinion of the Agency on any question concerning the admissibility of the files submitted in accordance with the centralised procedure, the granting, variation, suspension or withdrawal of an authorisation to place a medicinal product for human use on the market arising in accordance with the provisions of this Title and pharmacovigilance.

Article 6

1.   An application for authorisation for a medicinal product for human use must be accompanied by the particulars and documents referred to in Articles 4 and 4a of Directive 65/65/EEC, in the Annex to Directive 75/318/EEC and in Article 2 of Directive 75/319/EEC.

2.   In the case of a medicinal product containing or consisting of genetically modified organisms within the meaning of Article 2(1) and (2) of Directive 90/220/EEC, the application must also be accompanied by :

—   a copy of any written consent or consents of the competent authorities to the deliberate release into the environment of the genetically modified organisms for research and development purposes where provided for by Part B of Directive 90/220/EEC,
—   the complete technical dossier supplying the information requested in Annexes II and III to Directive 90/220/EEC and the environmental risk assessment resulting from this information; the results of any investigations performed for the purposes of research or development.

Articles 11 to 18 of Directive 90/220/EEC shall not apply to medicinal products for human use containing or consisting of genetically modified organisms.

3.   The application must also be accompanied by the fee payable to the Agency for the examination of the application.

4.   The Agency shall ensure that the opinion of the Committee is given within 210 days of the receipt of a valid application.

In the case of a medicinal product containing or consisting of genetically modified organisms, the opinion of the Committee shall respect the environmental safety requirements laid down by Directive 90/220/EEC to ensure that all appropriate measures are taken to avoid adverse effects on human health and the environment which might arise from the deliberate release or placing on the market of genetically modified organisms. During the process of evaluating applications for marketing authorisations for products containing or consisting of genetically modified organisms, necessary consultations will be held by the rapporteur with the bodies set up by the Community or the Member States in accordance with Directive 90/220/EEC.

5.   The Commission shall, in consultation with the Agency, the Member States and interested parties, draw up detailed guidance on the form in which applications for authorisation are to be presented.

Article 7
In order to prepare its opinion, the Committee :

(a)   shall verify that the particulars and documents submitted in accordance with Article 6 comply with the requirements of Directives 65/65/EEC, 75/318/EEC and 75/319/EEC, and examine whether the conditions specified in this Regulation for issuing a marketing authorisation for the medicinal product are satisfied;

(b)   may ask for a State laboratory or a laboratory designated for this purpose to test the medicinal product, its starting materials and, if need be, its intermediate products or other constituent materials in order to ensure that the control methods employed by the manufacturer and described in the application documents are satisfactory;

(c)   may, where appropriate, request the applicant to supplement the particulars accompanying the application within a specific time limit. Where the Committee avails itself of this opinion, the time limit laid down in Article 6 shall be suspended until such time as the supplementary information requested has been provided. Likewise, this time limit shall be suspended for the time allowed to the applicant to prepare oral or written explanations.

Article 8
1.   Upon receipt of a written request from the Committee, a Member State shall forward the information establishing that the manufacturer of a medicinal product or the importer from a third country is able to manufacture the medicinal product concerned and/or carry out the necessary control tests in accordance with the particulars and documents supplied pursuant to Article 6.

2.   Where it considers it necessary in order to complete its examination of an application, the Committee may require the applicant to submit to a specific inspection of the manufacturing site of the medicinal product concerned. The inspection, which shall be completed within the time limit referred to in Article 6, shall be undertaken by inspectors from the Member State who possess the appropriate qualifications and who may, if need be, be accompanied by a rapporteur or expert appointed by the Committee.

Article 9

1.   Where the opinion of the Committee is that :

—   the application does not satisfy the criteria for authorisation set out in this
        Regulation, or
—   the summary of the product characteristics proposed by the applicant in
        accordance with Article 6 should be amended, or
—   the labelling or package leaflet of the product is not in compliance with
        Council Directive 92/27/EEC of 31 March 1992 on the labelling of
        medicinal products for human use and on package leaflets[1], or
—   the authorisation should be granted subject to the conditions provided for in
        Article 13(2),

the Agency shall forthwith inform the applicant. Within 15 days of receipt of the
opinion, the applicant may provide written notice to the Agency that he wishes to
appeal. In that case he shall forward the detailed grounds for his appeal to the
Agency within 60 days of receipt of the opinion. Within 60 days of the receipt of
the grounds for appeal, the Committee shall consider whether its opinion should be
revised, and the conclusions reached on the appeal shall be annexed to the
assessment report referred to in paragraph 2.

2.   Within 30 days of its adoption, the Agency shall forward the final opinion of
the Committee to the Commission, the Member States and the applicant together
with a report describing the assessment of the medicinal product by the Committee
and stating the reasons for its conclusions.

3.   In the event of an opinion in favour of granting the relevant authorisation to
place the medicinal product concerned on the market, the following documents
shall be annexed to the opinion :

(a)   a draft summary of the product characteristics, as referred to in Article 4a of
        Directive 65/65/EEC;
(b)   details of any conditions or restrictions which should be imposed on the
        supply or use of the medicinal product concerned, including the conditions
        under which the medicinal product may be made available to patients,
        having regard to the criteria laid down in Council Directive 92/26/EEC of 31
        March 1992 concerning the classification for the supply of medicinal
        products for human use[2] without prejudice to the provisions in Article 3(4)
        of that Directive;
(c)   the draft text of the labelling and package leaflet proposed by the applicant,
        presented in accordance with Directive 92/27/EEC, without prejudice to the
        provisions of Article 7(2) of that Directive;
(d)   the assessment report.

Article 10

1.   Within 30 days of receipt of the opinion, the Commission shall prepare a
draft of the decision to be taken in respect of the application, taking account of
Community law.

In the event of a draft decision which envisages the granting of marketing
authorisation, the documents referred to in Article 9(3)(a), (b) and (c) shall be
annexed.

---

1.   OJ L113 30.4.92 p8. See Appendix 12 post.
2.   OJ L113 30.4.92 p5. See Appendix 11 post.

Where, exceptionally, the draft decision is not in accordance with the opinion of the Agency, the Commission shall also annex a detailed explanation of the reasons for the differences.

The draft decision shall be forwarded to the Member States and the applicant.

2.   A final decision on the application shall be adopted in accordance with the procedure laid down in Article 73.

3.   The rules of procedure of the Committee referred to in Article 73 shall be adjusted to take account of the tasks incumbent upon it in accordance with this Regulation.

These adjustments shall involve the following :

—   except in cases referred to in the third subparagraph of paragraph 1, the opinion of the Standing Committee shall be obtained in writing,
—   each Member State is allowed at least 28 days to forward written observations on the draft decision to the Commission,
—   each Member State is able to require in writing that the draft decision be discussed by the Standing Committee, giving its reasons in detail.

Where, in the opinion of the Commission, the written observations of a Member State raise important new questions of a scientific or technical nature which have not been addressed in the opinion of the Agency, the Chairman shall suspend the procedure and refer the application back to the Agency for further consideration.

The provisions necessary for the implementation of this paragraph shall be adopted by the Commission in accordance with the procedure laid down in Article 72.

4.   The Agency shall, upon request, inform any person concerned of the final decision.

Article 11
Without prejudice to other provisions of Community law, the authorisation provided for in Article 3 shall be refused if, after verification of the information and particulars submitted in accordance with Article 6, it appears that the quality, the safety or the efficacy of the medicinal product have not been adequately or sufficiently demonstrated by the applicant.

Authorisation shall likewise be refused if the particulars and documents provided by the applicant in accordance with Article 6 are incorrect or if the labelling and package leaflets proposed by the applicant are not in accordance with Directive 92/27/EEC.

Article 12
1.   Without prejudice to Article 6 of Directive 65/65/EEC, a marketing authorisation which has been granted in accordance with the procedure laid down in this Regulation shall be valid throughout the Community. It shall confer the same rights and obligations in each of the Member States as a marketing authorisation granted by that Member State in accordance with Article 3 of Directive 65/65/EEC.

The authorised medicinal products shall be entered in the *Community Register of Medicinal Products* and shall be given a number which must appear on the packaging.

2.   The refusal of a Community marketing authorisation shall constitute a prohibition on the placing on the market of the medicinal product concerned throughout the Community.

3.   Notification of marketing authorisation shall be published in the *Official Journal of the European Communities,* quoting in particular the date of authorisation and the number in the Community Register.

4.   Upon request from any interested person, the Agency shall make available the assessment report of the medicinal product by the Committee for Proprietary Medicinal Products and the reasons for its opinion in favour of granting authorisation, after deletion of any information of a commercially confidential nature.

Article 13

1.   Authorisation shall be valid for five years and shall be renewable for five-year periods, on application by the holder at least three months before the expiry date and after consideration by the Agency of a dossier containing up-to-date information on pharmacovigilance.

2.   In exceptional circumstances and following consultation with the applicant, an authorisation may be granted subject to certain specific obligations, to be reviewed annually by the Agency.

Such exceptional decisions may be adopted only for objective and verifiable reasons and must be based on one of the causes mentioned in Part 4G of the Annex to Directive 75/318/EEC.

3.   Some products may be authorised only for use in hospitals or for prescription by some specialists.

4.   Medicinal products which have been authorised by the Community in accordance with the provisions of this Regulation shall benefit from the 10-year period of protection referred to in point 8 of the second paragraph of Article 4 of Directive 65/65/EEC.

Article 14

The granting of authorisation shall not diminish the general civil and criminal liability in the Member States of the manufacturer or, where applicable, of the person responsible for placing the medicinal product on the market.

CHAPTER 2

Supervision and sanctions

Article 15

1.   After an authorisation has been issued in accordance with this Regulation, the person responsible for placing the medicinal product on the market shall, in respect of the methods of production and control provided for in points 4 and 7 of the second paragraph of Article 4 of Directive 65/65/EEC, take account of technical and scientific progress and make any amendments that may be required to enable the medicinal products to be manufactured and checked by means of generally accepted scientific methods. The aforementioned person must apply for approval for these amendments in accordance with this Regulation.

2.   The person responsible for placing the medicinal product on the market shall forthwith inform the Agency, the Commission and the Member States of any new information which might entail the amendment of the particulars and documents referred to in Articles 6 or 9 or in the approved summary of the product characteristics. In particular the aforementioned person shall forthwith inform the Agency, the Commission and the Member States of any prohibition or restriction imposed by the competent authorities of any country in which the medicinal product is placed on the market and of any other new information which might influence the evaluation of the benefits and risks of the medicinal product concerned.

3.   If the person responsible for placing the medicinal product on the market proposes to make any alteration to the information and particulars referred to in Articles 6 and 9, he shall submit an application to the Agency.

4.   The Commission shall, in consultation with the Agency, adopt appropriate arrangements for the examination of variations to the terms of a marketing authorisation.

These arrangements shall include a notification system or administrative procedures concerning minor variations and define precisely the concept of "a minor variation".

These arrangements shall be adopted by the Commission in the form of an implementing Regulation in accordance with the procedure laid down in Article 72.

Article 16

In the case of medicinal products manufactured within the Community, the supervisory authorities shall be the competent authorities of the Member State or Member States which have granted the manufacturing authorisation provided for in Article 16 of Directive 75/319/EEC in respect of the manufacture of the medicinal product concerned.

In the case of medicinal products imported from third countries, the supervisory authorities shall be the competent authorities of the Member States in which the controls referred to in Article 22(1)(b) of Directive 75/319/EEC are carried out unless appropriate arrangements have been made between the Community and the exporting country to ensure that those controls are carried out in the exporting country and that the manufacturer applies standards of good manufacturing practice at least equivalent to those laid down by the Community.

A Member State may request assistance from another Member State or the Agency.

Article 17

1.   The supervisory authorities shall have responsibility for verifying on behalf of the Community that the person responsible for placing the medicinal product on the market or the manufacturer or importer from third countries satisfies the requirements laid down in Chapter IV of Directive 75/319/EEC and for exercising supervision over such persons in accordance with Chapter V of Directive 75/319/EEC.

2.   Where, in accordance with the second paragraph of Article 30 of Directive 75/319/EEC, the Commission is informed of serious differences of opinions between Member States as to whether the person responsible for placing the medicinal product on the market or a manufacturer or importer established within the

Community is satisfying the requirements referred to in paragraph 1, the Commission may, after consultation with the Member States concerned, request an inspector from the supervisory authority to undertake a new inspection of the aforementioned person, the manufacturer or the importer; the inspector in question may be accompanied by an inspector from a Member State which is not party to the dispute and/or by a rapporteur or expert nominated by the Committee.

3.   Subject to any arrangements which may have been concluded between the Community and third countries in accordance with the second subparagraph of Article 16, the Commission may, upon receipt of a reasoned request from a Member State, the Committee for Proprietary Medicinal Products, or on its own initiative, require a manufacturer established in a third country to submit to an inspection. The inspection shall be undertaken by appropriately qualified inspectors from the Member States, who may, if appropriate, be accompanied by a rapporteur or expert nominated by the Committee. The report of the inspectors shall be made available to the Commission, the Member States and the Committee for Proprietary Medicinal Products.

Article 18

1.   Where the supervisory authorities or the competent authorities of any other Member State are of the opinion that the manufacturer or importer from third countries is no longer fulfilling the obligations laid down in Chapter IV of Directive 75/319/EEC, they shall forthwith inform the Committee and the Commission, stating their reasons in detail and indicating the course of action proposed.

The same shall apply where a Member State or the Commission considers that one of the measures envisaged in Chapter V or Va of Directive 75/319/EEC should be applied in respect of the medicinal product concerned or where the Committee for Proprietary Medicinal Products has delivered an opinion to that effect in accordance with Article 20.

2.   The Commission shall in consultation with the Agency forthwith examine the reasons advanced by the Member State concerned. It shall request the opinion of the Committee within a time limit which it shall determine having regard to the urgency of the matter. Whenever practicable, the person responsible for placing the medicinal product on the market shall be invited to provide oral or written explanations.

3.   The Commission shall prepare a draft of the Decision to be taken which shall be adopted in accordance with Article 10.

However, where a Member State has invoked the provisions of paragraph 4, the time limit provided for in Article 73 shall be reduced to 15 calendar days.

4.   Where urgent action is essential to protect human or animal health or the environment, a Member State may suspend the use on its territory of a medicinal product which has been authorised in accordance with this Regulation. It shall inform the Commission and the other Member States no later than the following working day of the reasons for its action. The Commission shall immediately consider the reasons given by the Member State in accordance with paragraph 2 and shall initiate the procedure provided for in paragraph 3.

5.   A Member State which has adopted the suspensive measures referred to in paragraph 4 may maintain them in force until such time as a definitive decision has been reached in accordance with the procedure laid down in paragraph 3.

6.   The Agency shall, upon request, inform any person concerned of the final decision.

CHAPTER 3

Pharmacovigilance

Article 19

For the purpose of this Chapter, the definitions given in Article 29b of Directive 75/319/EEC shall apply.

Article 20

The Agency, acting in close co-operation with the national pharmacovigilance systems established in accordance with Article 29a of Directive 75/319/EEC, shall receive all relevant information about suspected adverse reactions to medicinal products which have been authorised by the Community in accordance with this Regulation. If necessary the Committee may, in accordance with Article 5, formulate opinions on the measures necessary to ensure the safe and effective use of such medicinal products. These measures shall be adopted in accordance with the procedure laid down in Article 18.

The person responsible for placing the medicinal product on the market and the competent authorities of the Member States shall ensure that all relevant information about suspected adverse reactions to medicinal products authorised in accordance with this Regulation are brought to the attention of the Agency in accordance with the provisions of this Regulation.

Article 21

The person responsible for the placing on the market of a medicinal product authorised by the Community in accordance with the provisions of this Regulation shall have permanently and continuously at his disposal an appropriately qualified person responsible for pharmacovigilance.

That qualified person shall be responsible for the following :

(a)   the establishment and maintenance of a system which ensures that information about all suspected adverse reactions which are reported to the personnel of the company and to medical representatives, is collected, evaluated and collated so that it may be accessed at a single point within the Community;

(b)   the preparation of the reports referred to in Article 22 for the competent authorities of the Member States and the Agency in accordance with the requirements of this Regulation;

(c)   ensuring that any request from the competent authorities for the provision of additional information necessary for the evaluation of the benefits and risks of a medicinal product is answered fully and promptly, including the provision of information about the volume of sales or prescriptions for the medicinal product concerned.

Article 22

1.   The person responsible for placing the medicinal product on the market shall ensure that all suspected serious adverse reactions occurring within the Community to a medicinal product authorised in accordance with the provisions of this Regulation which are brought to his attention by a health care professional, are

recorded and reported immediately to the Member States in whose territory the incident occurred, and in no case later than 15 days following the receipt of the information.

The person responsible for placing the medicinal product on the market shall ensure that all suspected serious unexpected adverse reactions occurring in the territory of a third country, are reported immediately to Member States and the Agency and in no case later than 15 days following the receipt of the information.

The arrangements for the reporting of suspected unexpected adverse reactions which are not serious, whether arising in the Community or in a third country, shall be adopted in accordance with Article 26.

2.   In addition, the person responsible for placing the medicinal product on the market shall be required to maintain detailed records of all suspected adverse reactions occurring within or outside the Community which are reported to him by a health care professional. Unless other requirements have been laid down as a condition of the granting of the marketing authorisation by the Community, these records shall be submitted to the Agency and Member States immediately upon request or at least every six months during the first two years following authorisation and once a year for the following three years. Thereafter, the records shall be submitted at five-yearly intervals together with the application of renewal of the authorisation, or immediately upon request. These records shall be accompanied by a scientific evaluation.

Article 23

Each Member State shall ensure that all suspected serious adverse reactions occurring within their territory to a medicinal product authorised in accordance with the provisions of this Regulation which are brought to their attention are recorded and reported immediately to the Agency and the person responsible for placing the medicinal product on the market, and in no case later than 15 days following the receipt of the information.

The Agency shall inform the national pharmacovigilance systems.

Article 24

The Commission in consultation with the Agency, Member States, and interested parties, shall draw up guidance on the collection, verification and presentation of adverse reaction reports.

The Agency, in consultation with the Member States and the Commission, shall set up a data-processing network for the rapid transmission of data between the competent Community authorities in the event of an alert relating to faulty manufacture, serious adverse reactions and other pharmacovigilance data regarding medicinal products marketed in the Community.

Article 25

The Agency shall collaborate with the World Health Organisation on international pharmacovigilance and shall take the necessary steps to submit promptly to the World Health Organisation appropriate and adequate information regarding the measures taken in the Community which may have a bearing on public health protection in third countries and shall send a copy thereof to the Commission and the Member States.

Article 26

Any amendment which may be necessary to update the provisions of this chapter to take account of scientific and technical progress shall be adopted in accordance with the provisions of Article 72.

TITLE III

AUTHORISATION AND SUPERVISION OF VETERINARY MEDICINAL PRODUCTS

CHAPTER 1

Submission and examination of applications - authorisation - renewal of authorisation

Article 27

The Committee for Veterinary Medicinal Products established by Article 16 of Directive 81/851/EEC, in this Title referred to as "the Committee", shall be responsible for formulating the opinion of the Agency on any question concerning the admissibility of the files submitted in accordance with the centralised procedure, the granting, variation, suspension or withdrawal of an authorisation to place a veterinary medicinal product on the market arising in accordance with the provisions of this Title and pharmacovigilance.

Article 28

1.   An application for authorisation for a veterinary medicinal product must be accompanied by the particulars and documents referred to in Articles 5, 5a and 7 of Directive 81/851/EEC.

2.   In the case of a veterinary medicinal product containing or consisting of genetically modified organisms within the meaning of Article 2(1) and (2) of Directive 90/220/EEC, the application must also be accompanied by :

—   a copy of any written consent or consents of the competent authorities to the deliberate release into the environment of the genetically modified organisms for research and development purposes where provided for in Part B of Directive 90/220/EEC,
—   the complete technical dossier supplying the information requested in Annexes II and III to Directive 90/220/EEC and the environmental risk assessment resulting from this information; the results of any investigations performed for the purposes of research or development.

Articles 11 to 18 of Directive 90/220/EEC shall not apply to veterinary medicinal products containing or consisting of genetically modified organisms.

3.   The application shall also be accompanied by the fee payable to the Agency for the examination of the application.

4.   The Agency shall ensure that the opinion of the Committee is given within 210 days of the receipt of a valid application.

In the case of a veterinary medicinal product containing or consisting of genetically modified organisms, the opinion of the Committee shall respect the environmental safety requirements laid down by Directive 90/220/EEC to ensure that all appropriate measures are taken to avoid adverse effects on human health and the environment which might arise from the deliberate release into the environment or placing on the market of genetically modified organisms. During the process of evaluating applications for marketing authorisations for veterinary medicinal products containing or consisting of genetically modified organisms, necessary consultations shall be held by the rapporteur with the bodies set up by the Community or the Member States in accordance with Directive 90/220/EEC.

5.   The Commission shall, in consultation with the Agency, the Member States and interested parties, draw up detailed guidance on the form in which applications for authorisation are to be presented.

Article 29

In order to prepare its opinion, the Committee :

(a)   shall verify that the particulars and documents submitted in accordance with Article 28 comply with the requirements of Directives 81/851/EEC and 81/852/EEC and examine whether the conditions specified in this Regulation for issuing a marketing authorisation are satisfied;

(b)   may ask for a State laboratory or a laboratory designated for this purpose to test the veterinary medicinal product, its starting materials and, if need be, its intermediate products or other constituent materials in order to ensure that the control methods employed by the manufacturer and described in the application documents are satisfactory;

(c)   may request a State laboratory or laboratory designated for this purpose to verify, using samples provided by the applicant, that the analytical detection method proposed by the applicant in accordance with point 8 of the second paragraph of Article 5 of Directive 81/851/EEC is suitable for use in routine checks to reveal the presence of residue levels above the maximum residue level accepted by the Community in accordance with the provisions of Council Regulation (EEC) 2377/90 of 26 June 1990 laying down a Community procedure for the establishment of maximum residue limits of veterinary medicinal products in foodstuffs of animal origin[1];

(d)   may, where appropriate, request the applicant to supplement the particulars accompanying the application within a specific time limit. Where the Committee avails itself of this option, the time limit laid down in Article 28 shall be suspended until such time as the supplementary information requested has been provided. Likewise, this time limit shall be suspended for the time allowed to the applicant to prepare oral or written explanations.

Article 30

1.   Upon receipt of a written request from the Committee, a Member State shall forward the information establishing that the manufacturer of a veterinary medicinal product or the importer from a third country is able to manufacture the veterinary medicinal product concerned and/or carry out the necessary control tests in accordance with the particulars and documents supplied pursuant to Article 28.

2.   Where it considers it necessary in order to complete its examination of an application, the Committee may require the applicant to submit to a specific inspection of the manufacturing site of the veterinary medicinal product concerned. The inspection, which shall be completed within the time limit referred to in Article 28, shall be undertaken by inspectors from the Member State who possess the appropriate qualifications and who may, if need be, be accompanied by a rapporteur or expert appointed by the Committee.

---

1.   OJ L224 18.8.90 p1.

Article 31

1. Where the opinion of the Committee is that :

— the application does not satisfy the criteria for authorisation set out in this Regulation,
or
— the summary of the product characteristics proposed by the applicant in accordance with Article 28 should be amended,
or
— the labelling or package insert of the product is not in compliance with Directive 81/851/EEC,
or
— the authorisation should be granted subject to the conditions provided for in Article 35(2),

the Agency shall forthwith inform the applicant. Within 15 days of receipt of the opinion, the applicant may provide written notice to the Agency that he wishes to appeal. In that case he shall forward the detailed grounds for his appeal to the Agency within 60 days of receipt of the opinion. Within 60 days of the receipt of the grounds for appeal, the Committee shall consider whether its opinion should be revised, and the reasons for the conclusion reached on the appeal shall be annexed to the assessment report referred to in paragraph 2.

2. Within 30 days of its adoption, the Agency shall forward the final opinion of the Committee to the Commission, the Member States and the applicant together with a report describing the assessment of the veterinary medicinal product by the Committee and stating the reasons for its conclusions.

3. In the event of an opinion in favour of granting the relevant authorisation to market the veterinary medicinal product, the following documents shall be annexed to the opinion :

(a) the draft summary of the product characteristics, as referred to in Article 5a of Directive 81/851/EEC; where necessary this will reflect differences in the veterinary conditions pertaining in the Member States;
(b) in the case of a veterinary medicinal product intended for administration to food-producing animals, a statement of the maximum residue level which may be accepted by the Community in accordance with Regulation (EEC) 2377/90;
(c) details of any conditions or restrictions which should be imposed on the supply or use of the veterinary medicinal product concerned, including the conditions under which the veterinary medicinal product may be made available to users, in accordance with the criteria laid down in Directive 81/851/EEC;
(d) the draft text of the labelling and package insert proposed by the applicant, presented in accordance with Directive 81/851/EEC;
(e) the assessment report.

Article 32

1. Within 30 days of receipt of the opinion, the Commission shall prepare a draft of the decision to be taken in respect of the application, taking account of Community law.

In the event of a draft decision which envisages the granting of marketing authorisation, the documents referred to in Article 31(3)(a), (b), (c) and (d) shall be annexed.

Where, exceptionally, the draft decision is not in accordance with the opinion of the Agency, the Commission shall also annex a detailed explanation of the reasons for the differences.

The draft decision shall be forwarded to the Member States and the applicant.

2.   A final decision on the application shall be adopted in accordance with the procedure laid down in Article 73.

3.   The rules of procedure of the Committee referred to in Article 73 shall be adjusted to take account of the tasks incumbent upon it in accordance with this Regulation.

These adjustments shall involve the following :

—   except in the cases referred to in the third subparagraph of paragraph 1, the opinion of the Standing Committee shall be obtained in writing,
—   each Member State is allowed at least 28 days to forward written observations on the draft decision to the Commission,
—   each Member State is able to require in writing that the draft decision be discussed by the Standing Committee giving its reasons in detail.

Where, in the opinion of the Commission, the written observations of a Member State raise important new questions of a scientific or technical nature which have not been addressed in the opinion of the Agency, the Chairman shall suspend the procedure and refer the application back to the Agency for further consideration.

The provisions necessary for the implementation of this paragraph shall be adopted by the Commission in accordance with the procedure laid down in Article 72.

4.   The Agency shall, upon request, inform any person concerned of the final decision.

Article 33

Without prejudice to other provisions of Community law, the authorisation provided for in Article 3 shall be refused if, after verification of the information and particulars submitted in accordance with Article 28, it appears that :

1.   the veterinary medicinal product is harmful under the conditions of use stated at the time of the application for authorisation, has no therapeutic effect or the applicant has not provided sufficient proof of such effect as regards the species of animal which is to be treated, or its qualitative and quantitative composition is not as stated;

2.   the withdrawal period recommended by the applicant is not long enough to ensure that foodstuffs obtained from treated animals do not contain residues which might constitute a health hazard for the consumer or is insufficiently substantiated;

3.   the veterinary medicinal product is offered for sale for a use prohibited under other Community provisions.

Authorisation shall likewise be refused if the particulars and documents provided by the applicant in accordance with Article 28 are incorrect or if the labelling and package inserts proposed by the applicant are not in accordance with Chapter VII of Directive 81/851/EEC.

Article 34

1.   Without prejudice to Article 4 of Council Directive 90/677/EEC of 13 December 1990 extending the scope of Directive 81/851/EEC on the approximation of the laws of the Member States relating to veterinary medicinal products, and laying down additional provisions for immunological veterinary medicinal products[1], a marketing authorisation which has been granted in accordance with the procedure laid down in this Regulation shall apply throughout the Community. It shall confer the same rights and obligations in each of the Member States as a marketing authorisation granted by that Member State in accordance with Article 4 of Directive 81/851/EEC.

The authorised veterinary medicinal products shall be entered in the Community Register of Medicinal Products and shall be given a number which must appear on the packaging.

2.   The refusal of a Community marketing authorisation shall constitute a prohibition on the placing on the market of the veterinary medicinal product concerned throughout the Community.

3.   Notification of marketing authorisation shall be published in the *Official Journal of the European Communities,* quoting in particular the date of authorisation and the number in the Community Register.

4.   Upon request from any interested person, the Agency shall make available the assessment report of the veterinary medicinal product by the Committee for Veterinary Medicinal Products and the reasons for its opinion in favour of granting authorisation, after deletion of any information of a commercially confidential nature.

Article 35

1.   Authorisation shall be valid for five years and shall be renewable for five-year periods, on application by the holder at least three months before the expiry date and after consideration by the Agency of a dossier containing up-to-date information on pharmacovigilance.

2.   In exceptional circumstances and following consultations with the applicant, authorisation may be granted subject to certain specific obligations, to be reviewed annually by the Agency.

Such exceptional decisions may be adopted for objective and verifiable reasons.

3.   Veterinary medicinal products which have been authorised by the Community in accordance with the provisions of this Regulation shall benefit from the 10-year period of protection referred to in point 10 of the second paragraph of Article 5 of Directive 81/851/EEC.

Article 36

The granting of authorisation shall not diminish the general civil and criminal liability in the Member States of the manufacturer or, where applicable, of the person responsible for placing the veterinary medicinal product on the market.

---

1.   OJ L373 31.12.90 p26.

CHAPTER 2

Supervision and sanctions

Article 37

1.   After an authorisation has been issued in accordance with this Regulation, the person responsible for placing the veterinary medicinal product on the market shall, in respect of the methods of production and control provided for in points 4 and 9 of the second paragraph of Article 5 of Directive 81/851/EEC, take account of technical and scientific progress and make changes that may be required to enable the veterinary medicinal product to be manufactured and checked by means of generally accepted scientific methods. The aforementioned person must apply for approval for these changes in accordance with this Regulation.

Upon a request from the Commission, the person responsible for placing the veterinary medicinal product on the market shall also review the analytical detection methods provided for in point 8 of the second paragraph of Article 5 of Directive 81/851/EEC and propose any changes which may be necessary to take account of technical and scientific progress.

2.   The person responsible for placing the veterinary medicinal product on the market shall forthwith inform the Agency, the Commission and the Member States of any new information which might entail the amendment of the particulars and documents referred to in Articles 28 and 31 or in the approved summary of the product characteristics. In particular the aforementioned person shall forthwith inform the Agency, the Commission and the Member States of any prohibition or restriction imposed by the competent authorities of any country in which the veterinary medicinal product is marketed and of any other new information which might influence the evaluation of the benefits and risks of the veterinary medicinal product concerned.

3.   If the person responsible for placing the veterinary medicinal product on the market proposes to make any alteration to the information and particulars referred to in Articles 28 and 31, he shall submit an application to the Agency.

4.   The Commission shall, in consultation with the Agency, adopt appropriate arrangements for the examination of variations to the terms of a marketing authorisation.

These arrangements shall include a notification system or administrative procedures concerning minor variations and define precisely the concept of "a minor variation".

These arrangements shall be adopted by the Commission in the form of an implementing Regulation in accordance with the procedure laid down in Article 72.

Article 38

In the case of veterinary medicinal products manufactured within the Community, the supervisory authorities shall be the competent authorities of the Member State or Member States which have granted the manufacturing authorisation provided for in Article 24 of Directive 85/851/EEC in respect of the manufacture of the veterinary medicinal product concerned.

In the case of veterinary medicinal products imported from third countries, the supervisory authorities shall be the competent authorities of the Member States in which the controls referred to in Article 30(1)(b) of Directive 81/851/EEC are carried out unless appropriate arrangements have been made between the Community and the exporting country to ensure that those controls are carried out in the exporting country and that the manufacturer applies standards of good manufacturing practice at least equivalent to those laid down by the Community.

A Member State may request assistance from another Member State or the Agency.

Article 39

1.   The supervisory authorities shall have responsibility for verifying on behalf of the Community that the person responsible for placing the veterinary medicinal product on the market, or manufacturer or importer from third countries satisfies the requirements laid down in Chapter V of Directive 81/851/EEC and for exercising supervision over such persons in accordance with Chapter VI of Directive 81/851/EEC.

2.   Where, in accordance with the second paragraph of Article 39 of Directive 81/851/EEC, the Commission is informed of serious differences of opinion between Member States as to whether the person responsible for placing the veterinary medicinal product on the market or a manufacturer or importer established within the Community is satisfying the requirements referred to in paragraph 1, the Commission may, after consultation with the Member States concerned, request an inspector from the supervisory authority to undertake a new inspection of the aforementioned person, the manufacturer or the importer; the inspector in question may be accompanied by an inspector from a Member State which is not party to the dispute and/or by a rapporteur or expert nominated by the Committee.

3.   Subject to any arrangements which may have been concluded between the Community and third countries in accordance with the second paragraph of Article 38, the Commission may, upon receipt of a reasoned request from a Member State, the Committee for Veterinary Medicinal Products, or on its own initiative, require a manufacturer established in a third country to submit to an inspection. The inspection shall be undertaken by appropriately qualified inspectors from the Member States, who may, if appropriate, be accompanied by a rapporteur or expert nominated by the Committee. The report of the inspectors shall be made available to the Commission, the Member States and the Committee for Veterinary Medicinal Products.

Article 40

1.   Where the supervisory authorities or the competent authorities of any other Member State are of the opinion that the manufacturer or importer from third countries is no longer fulfilling the obligations laid down in Chapter V of Directive 81/851/EEC, they shall forthwith inform the Committee and the Commission, stating their reasons in detail and indicating the course of action proposed.

The same shall apply where a Member State or the Commission considers that one of the measures envisaged in Chapter VI of Directive 81/851/EEC should be applied in respect of the veterinary medicinal product concerned or where the Committee for Veterinary Medicinal Products has delivered an opinion to that effect in accordance with Article 42.

2.   The Commission shall in consultation with the Agency forthwith examine the reasons advanced by the Member State concerned. It shall request the opinion of the Committee within a time limit to be determined by the Commission having regard to the urgency of the matter. Whenever practicable, the person responsible for placing the veterinary medicinal product on the market shall be invited to provide oral or written explanations.

3.   The Commission shall prepare a draft of the Decision to be taken which shall be adopted in accordance with the procedure laid down in Article 32.

However, where a Member State has invoked the provisions of paragraph 4, the time limit provided for in Article 73 shall be reduced to 15 calendar days.

4.   Where urgent action is essential to protect human or animal health or the environment, a Member State may suspend the use on its territory of a veterinary medicinal product which has been authorised in accordance with this Regulation. It shall inform the Commission and the other Member States no later than the following working day of the reasons for its action. The Commission shall immediately consider the reasons given by the Member State in accordance with paragraph 2 and shall initiate the procedure provided for in paragraph 3.

5.   A Member State which has adopted the suspensive measures referred to in paragraph 4 may maintain them in force until such time as a definitive decision has been reached in accordance with the procedure laid down in paragraph 3.

6.   The Agency shall, upon request, inform any person concerned of the final decision.

CHAPTER 3

Pharmacovigilance

Article 41
For the purpose of this Chapter, the definitions given in Article 42 of Directive 81/851/EEC shall apply.

Article 42
The Agency, acting in close co-operation with the national pharmacovigilance systems established in accordance with Article 42a of Directive 81/851/EEC, shall receive all relevant information about suspected adverse reactions to veterinary medicinal products which have been authorised by the Community in accordance with this Regulation. If necessary the Committee may, in accordance with Article 27, formulate opinions on the measures necessary to ensure the safe and effective use of such veterinary medicinal products. These measures shall be adopted in accordance with the procedure laid down in Article 40.

The person responsible for placing the veterinary medicinal product on the market and the competent authorities of the Member States shall ensure that all relevant information about suspected adverse reactions to veterinary medicinal products authorised in accordance with this Regulation are brought to the attention of the Agency in accordance with the provisions of this Regulation.

Article 43
The person responsible for the placing on the market of a veterinary medicinal product authorised by the Community in accordance with the provisions of this Regulation shall have permanently and continuously at his disposal an appropriately qualified person responsible for pharmacovigilance.

That qualified person shall be responsible for the following :

(a)   the establishment and maintenance of a system which ensures that information about all suspected adverse reactions which are reported to the

(b) personnel of the company and to its representatives is collected, evaluated and collated so that it may be accessed at a single point within the Community;

(b) the preparation of the reports referred to in Article 44 for the competent authorities of the Member States and the Agency in accordance with the requirements of this Regulation;

(c) ensuring that any request from the competent authorities for the provision of additional information necessary for the evaluation of the benefits and risks of a veterinary medicinal product is answered fully and promptly, including the provision of information about the volume of sales or prescriptions for the veterinary medicinal product concerned.

Article 44

1. The person responsible for placing a veterinary medicinal product on the market shall ensure that all suspected serious adverse reactions occurring within the Community to a veterinary medicinal product authorised in accordance with the provisions of this Regulation which are brought to his attention are recorded and reported immediately to the Member States in whose territory the incident occurred, and in no case later than 15 days following the receipt of the information.

The aforementioned person shall ensure that all suspected serious unexpected adverse reactions occurring in the territory of a third country, are reported immediately to the Member States and the Agency and in no case later than 15 days following the receipt of the information.

The arrangements for the reporting of suspected unexpected adverse reactions which are not serious, whether arising in the Community or in a third country, shall be adopted in accordance with Article 48.

2. In addition, the person responsible for placing a veterinary medicinal product on the market shall be required to maintain detailed records of all suspected adverse reactions occurring within or outside the Community which are reported to him. Unless other requirements have been laid down as a condition of the granting of the marketing authorisation by the Community, these records shall be submitted to the Agency and Member States immediately upon request or at least every six months during the first two years following authorisation and once a year for the following three years. Thereafter, the records shall be submitted at five-yearly intervals together with the application of renewal of the authorisation, or immediately upon request. These records shall be accompanied by a scientific evaluation.

Article 45

Each Member State shall ensure that all suspected serious adverse reactions occurring within their territory to a veterinary medicinal product authorised in accordance with the provisions of this Regulation which are brought to their attention are recorded and reported immediately to the Agency and the person responsible for placing the veterinary medicinal product on the market, and in no case later than 15 days following the receipt of the information.

The Agency shall inform the national pharmacovigilance systems.

Article 46

The Commission in consultation with the Agency, Member States, and interested parties, shall draw up guidance on the collection, verification and presentation of adverse reaction reports.

The Agency, in consultation with the Member States and the Commission, shall set up a data-processing network for the rapid transmission of data between the competent Community authorities in the event of an alert relating to faulty manufacture, serious adverse reactions and other pharmacovigilance data regarding veterinary medicinal products marketed in the Community.

Article 47

The Agency shall co-operate with international organisations concerned with veterinary pharmacovigilance.

Article 48

Any amendment which may be necessary to update the provisions of this Chapter to take account of scientific and technical progress shall be adopted in accordance with the provisions of Article 72.

TITLE IV

THE EUROPEAN AGENCY FOR THE EVALUATION OF MEDICINAL PRODUCTS

CHAPTER 1

Tasks of the Agency

Article 49

A European Agency for the Evaluation of Medicinal Products is hereby established.

The Agency shall be responsible for co-ordinating the existing scientific resources put at its disposal by the competent authorities of the Member States for the evaluation and supervision of medicinal products.

Article 50

1.   The Agency shall comprise :

(a)   the Committee for Proprietary Medicinal Products, which shall be responsible for preparing the opinion of the Agency on any question relating to the evaluation of medicinal products for human use;

(b)   the Committee for Veterinary Medicinal Products, which shall be responsible for preparing the opinion of the Agency on any question relating to the evaluation of veterinary medicinal products;

(c)   a Secretariat, which shall provide technical and administrative support for the two Committees and ensure appropriate co-ordination between them;

(d)   an Executive Director, who shall exercise the responsibilities set out in Article 55;

(e)   a Management Board, which shall exercise the responsibilities set out in Articles 56 and 57.

2.   The Committee for Proprietary Medicinal Products and the Committee for Veterinary Medicinal Products may each establish working parties and expert groups.

3.   The Committee for Proprietary Medicinal Products and the Committee for Veterinary Medicinal Products may, if they consider it appropriate, seek guidance on important questions of a general scientific or ethical nature.

Article 51

In order to promote the protection of human and animal health and of consumers of medicinal products throughout the Community, and in order to promote the completion of the internal market through the adoption of uniform regulatory decisions based on scientific criteria concerning the placing on the market and use of medicinal products, the objectives of the Agency shall be to provide the Member States and the institutions of the Community with the best possible scientific advice on any question relating to the evaluation of the quality, the safety, and the efficacy of medicinal products for human or veterinary use, which is referred to it in accordance with the provisions of Community legislation relating to medicinal products.

To this end, the Agency shall undertake the following tasks within its Committees :

(a)   the co-ordination of the scientific evaluation of the quality, safety and efficacy of medicinal products which are subject to Community marketing authorisation procedures;

(b)   the transmission of assessment reports, summaries of product characteristics, labels and package leaflets or inserts for these medicinal products;

(c)   the co-ordination of the supervision, under practical conditions of use, of medicinal products which have been authorised within the Community and the provision of advice on the measures necessary to ensure the safe and effective use of these products, in particular by evaluating and making available through a database information on adverse reactions to the medicinal products in question (pharmacovigilance);

(d)   advising on the maximum limits for residues of veterinary medicinal products which may be accepted in foodstuffs of animal origin in accordance with Regulation (EEC) 2377/90.

(e)   co-ordinating the verification of compliance with the principles of good manufacturing practice, good laboratory practice ant good clinical practice,

(f)   upon request, providing technical and scientific support for steps to improve co-operation between the Community, its Member States, international organisations and third countries on scientific and technical issues relating to the evaluation of medicinal products;

(g)   recording the status of marketing authorisations for medicinal products granted in accordance with Community procedures;

(h)   providing technical assistance for the maintenance of a database on medicinal products which is available for public use;

(i)   assisting the Community and Member States in the provision of information to health care professionals and the general public about medicinal products which have been evaluated within the Agency;

(j)   where necessary, advising companies on the conduct of the various tests and trials necessary to demonstrate the quality, safety and efficacy of medicinal products.

Article 52

1.   The Committee for Proprietary Medicinal Products and the Committee for Veterinary Medicinal Products shall each consist of two members nominated by each Member State for a term of three years which shall be renewable. They shall be chosen by reason of their role and experience in the evaluation of medicinal products for human and veterinary use as appropriate and shall represent their competent authorities.

The Executive Director of the Agency or his representative and representatives of the Commission shall be entitled to attend all meetings of the Committees, their working parties and expert groups.

Members of each Committee may arrange to be accompanied by experts.

2.   In addition to their task of providing objective scientific opinions to the Community and Member States on the questions which are referred to them, the members of each Committee shall ensure that there is appropriate co-ordination between the tasks of the Agency and the work of competent national authorities, including the consultative bodies concerned with the marketing authorisation.

3.   The members of the Committees and the experts responsible for evaluating medicinal products shall rely on the scientific assessment and resources available to the national marketing authorisation bodies. Each Member State shall monitor the scientific level of the evaluation carried out and supervise the activities of members of the Committees and the experts it nominates, but shall refrain from giving them any instruction which is incompatible with the tasks incumbent upon them.

4.   When preparing the opinion, each Committee shall use its best endeavours to reach a scientific consensus. If such a consensus cannot be reached, the opinion shall consist of the position of the majority of members and may, at the request of those concerned, include the divergent positions with their grounds.

Article 53
1.   Where, in accordance with the provisions of this Regulation, the Committee for Proprietary Medicinal Products or the Committee for Veterinary Medicinal Products is required to evaluate a medicinal product, the Committee shall appoint one of its members to act as rapporteur for the co-ordination of the evaluation, taking into consideration any proposal from the applicant for the choice of a rapporteur. The Committee may appoint a second member to act as co-rapporteur.

The Committee shall ensure that all its members undertake the role of rapporteur or co-rapporteur.

2.   Member States shall transmit to the Agency a list of experts with proven experience in the assessment of medicinal products who would be available to serve on working parties or expert groups of the Committee for Proprietary Medicinal Products or the Committee for Veterinary Medicinal Products, together with an indication of their qualifications and specific areas of expertise.

This list shall be updated as necessary.

3.   The provision of services by rapporteurs or experts shall be governed by a written contract between the Agency and the person concerned, or where appropriate between the Agency and his employer. The person concerned, or his employer, shall be remunerated in accordance with a fixed scale of fees to be included in the financial arrangements established by the Management Board.

4.   On a proposal from the Committee for Proprietary Medicinal Products or the Committee for Veterinary Medicinal Products, the Agency may also avail itself of the services of rapporteurs or experts for the discharge of other specific responsibilities of the Agency.

Article 54

1.   The membership of the Committee for Proprietary Medicinal Products and the Committee for Veterinary Medicinal Products shall be made public. When each appointment is published, the professional qualifications of each member shall be specified.

2.   Members of the Management Board, Committee members, rapporteurs and experts shall not have financial or other interests in the pharmaceutical industry which could affect their impartiality. All indirect interests which could relate to this industry shall be entered in a register held by the Agency which the public may consult.

Article 55

1.   The Executive Director shall be appointed by the Management Board, on a proposal from the Commission, for a period of five years, which shall be renewable.

2.   The Executive Director shall be the legal representative of the Agency. He shall be responsible :

—   for the day-to-day administration of the Agency,
—   for the provision of appropriate technical support for the Committee for Proprietary Medicinal Products and the Committee for Veterinary Medicinal Products, and their working parties and expert groups;
—   for ensuring that the time limits laid down in Community legislation for the adoption of opinions by the Agency are respected,
—   for ensuring appropriate co-ordination between the Committee for Proprietary Medicinal Products and the Committee for Veterinary Medicinal Products,
—   for the preparation of the statement of revenue and expenditure and the execution of the budget of the Agency,
—   for all staff matters.

3.   Each year, the Executive Director shall submit to the Management Board for approval, while making a distinction between the Agency's activities concerning medicinal products for human use and those concerning veterinary medicinal products :

—   a draft report covering the activities of the Agency in the previous year, including information about the number of applications evaluated within the Agency, the time taken for the completion of the evaluation and the medicinal products authorised, rejected or withdrawn,
—   a draft programme of work for the coming year,
—   the draft annual accounts for the previous year,
—   the draft budget for the coming year.

4.   The Executive Director shall approve all financial expenditure of the Agency.

Article 56

1.   The Management Board shall consist of two representatives from each Member State, two representatives of the Commission and two representatives appointed by the European Parliament. One representative shall have specific responsibilities relating to medicinal products for human use and one relating to veterinary medicinal products.

Each representative may arrange to be replaced by an alternate.

2.   The term of office of the representatives shall be three years. It shall be renewable.

3.   The Management Board shall elect its Chairman for a term of three years and shall adopt its rules of procedure.

Decisions of the Management Board shall be adopted by a majority of two thirds of its members.

4.   The Executive Director shall provide the Secretariat of the Management Board.

5.   Before 31 January each year, the Management Board shall adopt the general report on the activities of the Agency for the previous year and its programme of work for the coming year and forward them to the Member States, the Commission, the Council and the European Parliament.

CHAPTER 2

Financial provisions

Article 57

1.   The revenues of the Agency shall consist of a contribution from the Community and the fees paid by undertakings for obtaining and maintaining a Community marketing authorisation and for other services provided by the Agency.

2.   The expenditure of the Agency shall include the staff, administrative, infrastructure and operational expenses and expenses resulting from contracts entered into with third parties.

3.   By 15 February each year at the latest, the Director shall draw up a preliminary draft budget covering the operational expenditure and the programme of work anticipated for the following financial year, and shall forward this preliminary draft to the Management Board together with an establishment plan.

4.   Revenue and expenditure shall be in balance.

5.   The Management Board shall adopt the draft budget and forward it to the Commission which on that basis shall establish the relevant estimates in the preliminary draft general budget of the European Communities, which it shall put before the Council pursuant to Article 203 of the Treaty.

6.   The Management Board shall adopt the Agency's final budget before the beginning of the financial year, adjusting it where necessary to the Community subsidy and the Agency's other resources.

7.   The Director shall implement the Agency's budget.

8.   Monitoring of the commitment and payment of all the Agency's expenditure and of the establishment and recovery of all the Agency's revenue shall be carried out by the financial controller appointed by the Management Board.

9.   By 31 March each year at the latest, the Director shall forward to the Commission, the Management Board and the Court of Auditors the accounts for all the Agency's revenue and expenditure in respect of the preceding financial year.

The Court of Auditors shall examine them in accordance with Article 206a of the Treaty.

10.   The Management Board shall give a discharge to the Director in respect of the implementation of the budget.

11.   After the Court of Auditors has delivered its opinion, the Management Board shall adopt the internal financial provisions specifying, in particular, the detailed rules for establishing and implementing the Agency's budget.

Article 58

The structure and the amount of the fees referred to in Article 57(1) shall be established by the Council acting under the conditions provided for by the Treaty on a proposal from the Commission, following consultation of organisations representing the interests of the pharmaceutical industry at Community level.

CHAPTER 3

General provisions governing the Agency

Article 59

The Agency shall have legal personality. In all Member States it shall benefit from the widest powers granted by law to legal persons. In particular it may acquire and dispose of real property and chattels and institute legal proceedings.

Article 60

1.   The contractual liability of the Agency shall be governed by the law applicable to the contract in question. The Court of Justice of the European Communities shall have jurisdiction to give judgment pursuant to any arbitration clause contained in a contract concluded by the Agency.

2.   In the case of non-contractual liability, the Agency shall, in accordance with the general principles common to the laws of the Member States, make good any damage caused by it or its servants in the performance of their duties.

The Court of Justice shall have jurisdiction in any dispute relating to compensation for such damages.

3.   The personal liability of its servants towards the Agency shall be governed by the relevant conditions applying to the staff of the Agency.

Article 61

The Protocol on the Privileges and Immunities of the European Communities shall apply to the Agency.

Article 62

The staff of the Agency shall be subject to the rules and regulations applicable to officials and other staff of the European Communities.

In respect of its staff, the Agency shall exercise the powers which have been devolved to the appointing authority.

The Management Board, in agreement with the Commission, shall adopt the necessary implementing provisions.

Article 63
Members of the Management Board, members of Committees and officials and other servants of the Agency shall be required, even after their duties have ceased, not to disclose information of the kind covered by the obligation of professional secrecy.

Article 64
The Commission may, in agreement with the Management Board and the relevant Committee, invite representatives of international organisations with interests in the harmonisation of regulations applicable to medicinal products to participate as observers in the work of the Agency.

Article 65
The Management Board shall, in agreement with the Commission, develop appropriate contacts between the Agency and the representatives of the industry, consumers and patients and the health professions.

Article 66
The Agency shall take up its responsibilities on 1 January 1995.

TITLE V

GENERAL AND FINAL PROVISIONS

Article 67
All decisions to grant, refuse, vary, suspend, withdraw or revoke a marketing authorisation which are taken in accordance with this Regulation shall state in detail the reasons on which they are based. Such decisions shall be notified to the party concerned.

Article 68
1.   An authorisation to place on the market a medicinal product coming within the scope of this Regulation shall not be refused, varied, suspended, withdrawn or revoked except on the grounds set out in this Regulation.

2.   An authorisation to place on the market a medicinal product coming within the scope of this Regulation shall not be granted, refused, varied, suspended, withdrawn or revoked except in accordance with the procedures set out in this Regulation.

Article 69
Without prejudice to Article 68, and without prejudice to the Protocol on the Privileges and Immunities of the European Communities, each Member State shall determine the penalties to be applied for the infringement of the provisions of this Regulation. The penalties must be sufficient to promote compliance with those measures.

Member States shall forthwith inform the Commission of the institution of any infringement proceedings.

Article 70

Additives covered by Council Directive 70/524/EEC of 23 November 1970 concerning additives in feedingstuffs[1], where they are intended to be administered to animals in accordance with that Directive, shall not be considered as veterinary medicinal products for the purposes of this Regulation.

Within three years of the entry into force of this Regulation the Commission shall produce a report on whether the level of harmonisation achieved by this Regulation and by Council Directive 90/167/EEC of 26 March 1990 laying down the conditions governing the preparation, placing on the market and use of medicated feedingstuffs in the Community[2] is equivalent to that provided for in Council Directive 70/524/EEC, accompanied if necessary by the proposals to modify the status of the coccidiostats and other medicinal substances covered by that Directive.

The Council shall decide on the Commission proposal no later than one year after their submission.

Article 71

Within six years of the entry into force of this Regulation, the Commission shall publish a general report on the experience acquired as a result of the operation of the procedures laid down in this Regulation, in Chapter III of Directive 75/319/EEC and in Chapter IV of Directive 81/851/EEC.

Article 72

Where the procedure laid down in this Article is to be followed the Commission shall be assisted by :

— the Standing Committee on Medicinal Products for Human Use, in the case of matters relating to medicinal products for human use,
— the Standing Committee on Veterinary Medicinal Products, in the case of matters relating to veterinary medicinal products.

The representative of the Commission shall submit to the Committee a draft of the measures to be taken. The Committee shall deliver its opinion on the draft within a time limit which the Chairman may lay down according to the urgency of the matter. The opinion shall be delivered by the majority laid down in Article 148(2) of the Treaty in the case of decisions which the Council is required to adopt on a proposal from the Commission. The votes of the representatives of the Member States within the Committee shall be weighted in the manner set out in that Article. The Chairman shall not vote.

The Commission shall adopt the measures envisaged if they are in accordance with the opinion of the Committee.

If the measures envisaged are not in accordance with the opinion of the Committee, or if no opinion is delivered, the Commission shall, without delay, submit to the Council a proposal relating to the measures to be taken. The Council shall act by a qualified majority.

---

1   OJ L270 14.12.70 p1.
2   OJ L92 7.4.90 p42.

If on the expiry of a period of three months from the date of referral to the Council, the Council has not acted, the proposed measures shall be adopted by the Commission.

Article 73

Where the procedure laid down in this Article is to be followed the Commission shall be assisted by :

— the Standing Committee on Medicinal Products for Human Use, in the case of matters relating to medicinal products for human use,
— the Standing Committee on Veterinary Medicinal Products, in the case of matters relating to veterinary medicinal products.

The representative of the Commission shall submit to the Committee a draft of the measures to be taken. The Committee shall deliver its opinion on the draft within a time limit which the Chairman may lay down according to the urgency of the matter. The opinion shall be delivered by the majority laid down in Article 148(2) of the Treaty in the case of decisions which the Council is required to adopt on a proposal from the Commission. The votes of the representatives of the Member States within the Committee shall be weighted in the manner set out in that Article. The Chairman shall not vote.

The Commission shall adopt the measures envisaged if they are in accordance with the opinion of the Committee.

If the measures envisaged are not in accordance with the opinion of the Committee, or if no opinion is delivered, the Commission shall, without delay, submit to the Council a proposal relating to the measures to be taken. The Council shall act by a qualified majority.

If on the expiry of a period of three months from the date of referral to the Council, the Council has not acted, the proposed measures shall be adopted by the Commission, save where the Council has decided against the said measures by a simple majority.

Article 74

This Regulation shall enter into force on the day following the decision taken by the competent authorities on the headquarters of the Agency.

Subject to the first subparagraph Titles I, II, III and V shall enter into force on 1 January 1995.

This Regulation shall be binding in its entirety and directly applicable in all Member States.

Done at Brussels, 22 July 1993.

For the Council

The President

M. OFFECIERS-VAN DE WIELE

ANNEX

PART A

Medicinal products developed by means of one of the following biotechnological processes :

—   recombinant DNA technology,
—   controlled expression of genes coding for biologically active proteins in prokaryotes and eukaryotes including transformed mammalian cells,
—   hybridoma and monoclonal antibody methods.

Veterinary medicinal products, including those not derived from biotechnology, intended primarily for use as performance enhancers in order to promote the growth of treated animals or to increase yields from treated animals.

PART B

Medicinal products developed by other biotechnological processes which, in the opinion of the Agency, constitute a significant innovation.

Medicinal products administered by means of new delivery systems which, in the opinion of the Agency, constitute a significant innovation.

Medicinal products presented for an entirely new indication which, in the opinion of the Agency, is of significant therapeutic interest.

Medicinal products based on radio-isotopes which, in the opinion of the Agency, are of significant therapeutic interest.

New medicinal products derived from human blood or human plasma.

Medicinal products the manufacture of which employs processes which, in the opinion of the Agency, demonstrate a significant technical advance such as two-dimensional electrophoresis under micro-gravity.

Medicinal products intended for administration to human beings, containing a new active substance which, on the date of entry into force of this Regulation, was not authorised by any Member State for use in a medicinal product intended for human use.

Veterinary medicinal products intended for use in food-producing animals containing a new active substance which, on the date of entry into force of this Regulation, was not authorised by any Member State for use in food-producing animals.

APPENDIX 6

COUNCIL DIRECTIVE (EEC) 93/39
of 14 June 1993

amending Directives 65/65/EEC, 75/318/EEC and 75/319/EEC in respect of medicinal products[1]

THE COUNCIL OF THE EUROPEAN COMMUNITIES,

Having regard to the Treaty establishing the European Economic Community, and in particular Article 100a thereof,

Having regard to the proposal from the Commission [2],

In co-operation with the European Parliament [3],

Having regard to the opinion of the Economic and Social Committee[4] ,

Whereas it is important to adopt measures with the aim of progressively establishing the internal market over a period expiring on 31 December 1992; whereas the internal market shall comprise an area without internal frontiers in which the free movement of goods, persons, services and capital is ensured;

Whereas Article 15(2) of Second Council Directive 75/319/EEC of 20 May 1975 on the approximation of provisions laid down by law, regulation or administrative action relating to proprietary medicinal products[5] provides that the Commission shall submit to the Council a proposal containing appropriate measures leading towards the abolition of any remaining barriers to the free movement of proprietary medicinal products;

Whereas, in the interest of public health and of the consumer of medicinal products, it is necessary that decisions on the authorisation to place medicinal products on the market be exclusively based on the criteria of quality, safety and efficacy; whereas these criteria have been extensively harmonised by Council Directive 65/65/EEC of 26 January 1965 on the approximation of provisions laid down by law, regulation or administration action relating to medicinal products[6] , by Council Directive 75/319/EEC, and by Council Directive 75/318/EEC of 20 May 1975 on the approximation of the laws of the Member States relating to analytical, pharmacotoxicological and clinical standards and protocols in respect of the testing of medicinal products [7]; whereas, however, Member States should exceptionally be able to prohibit the use on their territory of medicinal products which infringe objectively defined concepts of public order or public morality;

Whereas, with the exception of those medicinal products which are subject to the centralised Community authorisation procedure established by Council Regulation (EEC) No 2309/93 of 22 July 1993 laying down Community procedures for the authorisation and supervision of medicinal products for human and veterinary use

---

1.   OJ L214 24.8.93 p22.
2.   OJ C330 31.12.90 p18 and OJ C310 30.11.91 p22.
3.   OJ C183 15.7.91 p187 and OJ C150 31.5.93.
4.   OJ C269 14.10.91 p84.
5.   OJ L147 9.6.75 p13.
6.   OJ No 22 9.2.65 p369/65.
7.   OJ L147 9.6.75 p1.

and establishing a European Agency for the Evaluation of Medicinal Products[1] an authorisation to place a medicinal product on the market in one Member State ought in principle to be recognised by the competent authorities of the other Member States unless there are serious grounds for supposing that the authorisation of the medicinal product concerned may present a risk to public health; whereas, in the event of a disagreement between Member States about the quality, the safety or the efficacy of a medicinal product, a scientific evaluation of the matter should be undertaken by the Committee for Proprietary Medicinal Products attached to the European Agency for the Evaluation of Medicinal Products, leading to a single decision on the area of disagreement binding on the Member States concerned; whereas this decision should be adopted by a rapid procedure ensuring close co-operation between the Commission and the Member States;

Whereas in order better to protect public health and avoid any unnecessary duplication of effort during the examination of application for authorisation to place medicinal products on the market, Member States should systematically prepare assessment reports in respect of each medicinal product which is authorised by them, and exchange the reports upon request; whereas, furthermore, a Member State should be able to suspend the examination of an application for authorisation to place a medicinal product on the market which is currently under active consideration in another Member State with a view to recognising the decision reached by the latter Member State;

Whereas following the establishment of the internal market, specific controls to guarantee the quality of medicinal products imported from third countries can be waived only if appropriate arrangements have been made by the Community to ensure that the necessary controls are carried out in the exporting country;

Whereas it is desirable to codify and improve the co-operation and exchange of information between Member States relating to the supervision of medicinal products and in particular the monitoring of adverse reactions under practical conditions of use through the national pharmacovigilance systems,

HAS ADOPTED THIS DIRECTIVE:

[*Text of Directive not reproduced here*][2]

---

1.   See page 1 of OJ L214 24.8.93.
2.   Directive (EEC) 93/39 consists exclusively of amendments which have already been incorporated into the relevant legislation. The preamble is reproduced by way of background information.

APPENDIX 7

COUNCIL DIRECTIVE (EEC) 93/41
of 14 June 1993

repealing Directive 87/22/EEC on the approximation of national measures relating to the placing on the market of high-technology medicinal products, particularly those derived from biotechnology[1]

THE COUNCIL OF THE EUROPEAN COMMUNITIES,

Having regard to the Treaty establishing the European Economic Community, and in particular Article 100a thereof,

Having regard to the proposal from the Commission[2],

In co-operation with the European Parliament[3],

Having regard to the opinion of the Economic and Social Committee[4],

Whereas the provisions of Directive 87/22/EEC[5] have now been superseded by the provisions of Council Regulation (EEC) No 2309/93 of 22 July 1993 laying down Community procedures for the authorisation and supervision of medicinal products for human and veterinary use and establishing a European Agency for the Evaluation of Medicinal Products[6] and by Council Directive 88/182/EEC of 22 March 1988 amending Directive 83/189/EEC laying down a procedure for the provision of information in the field of technical standards and regulations[7];

Whereas provision has been made in Directive 93/39/EEC[8] for the continued management of marketing authorisations which have been granted by Member States following the opinion of the Committee for Proprietary Medicinal Products given in accordance with Directive 87/22/EEC;

Whereas, furthermore, provision has been made in Directive 93/40/EEC[9] for the continued management of marketing authorisation which have been granted by Member States following the opinion of the Committee for Veterinary Medicinal products given in accordance with Directive 87/22/EEC;

Whereas Directive 87/22/EEC should therefore be repealed;

Whereas in the interests of legal certainty, provision should be made for the continued examination of applications for marketing authorisation which have been referred to the Committee for Proprietary Medicinal Products or the Committee for Veterinary Medicinal Products in accordance with Directive 87/22/EEC before 1 January 1995,

---

1.   OJ L214 24.8.93 p40.
2.   OJ C58 8.3.90 p1.
3.   OJ C183 15.7.91 p145 and OJ C150 31.5.93.
4.   OJ C269 14.10.91 p84.
5.   OJ L15 17.1.87 p38.
6.   See OJ L214 24.8.93 p1.
7.   OJ L81 26.3.88 p75.
8.   See OJ L214 24.8.93 p22.
9.   See OJ L214 24.8.93 p31.

HAS ADOPTED THIS DIRECTIVE :

Article 1

With effect from 1 January 1995, Directive 87/22/EEC is hereby repealed.

Article 2

Applications for marketing authorisations which have been referred to the Committee for Proprietary Medicinal Products or to the Committee for Veterinary Medicinal Products before 1 January 1995 in accordance with Article 2 of Directive 87/22/EEC and in respect of which the Committee concerned has not given an opinion by 1 January 1995 shall be considered in accordance with Regulation (EEC) No 2309/93.

Article 3

Member States shall take all appropriate measures to comply with this Directive with effect from 1 January 1995. They shall forthwith inform the Commission thereof.

When Member States adopt these provisions, they shall contain a reference to this Directive or shall be accompanied by such reference at the time of their official publication. The methods of making such a reference shall be laid down by the Member States.

Article 4

This Directive is addressed to the Member States.

Done at Luxembourg, 14 June 1993.

For the Council

The President

J. TRØJBORG

APPENDIX 8

COUNCIL DIRECTIVE (EEC) 92/73
of 22 September 1992

**widening the scope of Directives 65/65/EEC and 75/319/EEC on the
approximation of provisions laid down by law, regulation or administrative action
relating to medicinal products and laying down additional provisions on
homeopathic medicinal products[1]**

THE COUNCIL OF THE EUROPEAN COMMUNITIES,

Having regard to the Treaty establishing the European Economic Community, and in particular Article 100a thereof,

Having regard to the proposal from the Commission[2],

In co-operation with the European Parliament[3],

Having regard to the opinion of the Economic and Social Committee[4],

Whereas differences currently existing between the provisions laid down by law, regulation or administrative action in the Member States may hinder trade in homeopathic medicinal products within the Community and lead to discrimination and distortion of competition between manufacturers of these products;

Whereas the essential aim of any rules governing the production, distribution and use of medicinal products must be to safeguard public health;

Whereas, despite considerable differences in the status of alternative medicines in the Member States, patients should be allowed access to the medicinal products of their choice, provided all precautions are taken to ensure the quality and safety of the said products;

Whereas the anthroposophic medicinal products described in an official pharmacopoeia and prepared by a homeopathic method are to be treated, as regards registration and marketing authorisation, in the same way as homeopathic medicinal products;

Whereas the provisions of Directive 65/65/EEC[5] and the Second Directive 75/319/EEC[6], are not always appropriate for homeopathic medicinal products;

Whereas homeopathic medicine is officially recognised in certain Member States but is only tolerated in other Member States;

Whereas, even if homeopathic medicinal products are not always officially recognised, they are nevertheless prescribed and used in all Member States;

---

1. OJ L297 13.10.92 p8.
2. OJ C108 1.5.90 p10 and OJ C244 19.9.91 p8.
3. OJ C183 15.7.91 p322 and OJ C241 21.9.92.
4. OJ C332 31.12.90 p29.
5. OJ No 22 9.2.65 p369/65.
6. OJ L147 9.6.75 p13.

Whereas it is desirable in the first instance to provide users of these medicinal products with a very clear indication of their homeopathic character and with sufficient guarantees of their quality and safety;

Whereas the rules relating to the manufacture, control and inspection of homeopathic medicinal products must be harmonised to permit the circulation throughout the Community of medicinal products which are safe and of good quality;

Whereas, having regard to the particular characteristics of these medicinal products, such as the very low level of active principles they contain and the difficulty of applying to them the conventional statistical methods relating to clinical trials, it is desirable to provide a special, simplified registration procedure for those traditional homeopathic medicinal products which are placed on the market without therapeutic indications in a pharmaceutical form and dosage which do not present a risk for the patient;

Whereas, however, the usual rules governing the authorisation to market medicinal products should be applied to homeopathic medicinal products placed on the market with therapeutic indications or in a form which may present risks which must be balanced against the desired therapeutic effect; whereas, in particular, those Member States which have a homeopathic tradition should be able to apply particular rules for the evaluation of the results of tests and trials intended to establish the safety and efficacy of these medicinal products provided that they notify them to the Commission,

HAS ADOPTED THIS DIRECTIVE :

CHAPTER I

Scope

Article 1

1.   For the purposes of this Directive, "homeopathic medicinal product" shall mean any medicinal product prepared from products, substances or compositions called homeopathic stocks in accordance with a homeopathic manufacturing procedure described by the *European Pharmacopoeia* or, in absence thereof, by the pharmacopoeias currently used officially in the Member States.

2.   A homeopathic medicinal product may also contain a number of principles.

Article 2

1.   The provisions of this Directive shall apply to homeopathic medicinal products for human use, to the exclusion of homeopathic medicinal products prepared in accordance with a magistral or an officinal formula as defined in Article 1(4) and (5) of Directive 65/65/EEC and of homeopathic medicinal products which satisfy the criteria laid down in Article 2(4) of the said Directive.

2.   The medicinal products referred to in paragraph 1 shall be identified by a reference on their labels, in clear and legible form, to their homeopathic nature.

CHAPTER II

Manufacture, control and inspection

Article 3

The provisions of Chapter IV of Directive 75/319/EEC shall apply to the manufacture, control, import and export of homeopathic medicinal products.

Article 4

The supervision measures and the sanctions provided for in Chapter V of Directive 75/319/EEC shall apply to homeopathic medicinal products, together with Articles 31 and 32 of the same Directive.

However, the proof of therapeutic efficacy referred to in Article 28(1)(b) of the same Directive shall not be required for homeopathic medicinal products registered in accordance with Article 7 of this Directive or, where appropriate, admitted in accordance with Article 6(2).

Article 5

Member States shall communicate to each other all the information necessary to guarantee the quality and safety of homeopathic medicinal products manufactured and marketed within the Community, and in particular the information referred to in Articles 30 and 33 of Directive 75/319/EEC.

CHAPTER III

Placing on the market

Article 6

1.   Member States shall ensure that homeopathic medicinal products manufactured and placed on the market within the Community are registered or authorised in accordance with Articles 7, 8 and 9. Each Member State shall take due account of registrations and authorisations previously granted by another Member State.

2.   A Member State may refrain from establishing a special, simplified registration procedure for the homeopathic medicinal products referred to in Article 7. A Member State applying this provision shall inform the Commission accordingly. The Member State concerned shall, by 31 December 1995 at the latest, allow the use in its territory of homeopathic medicinal products registered by other Member States in accordance with Articles 7 and 8.

3.   Advertising of the homeopathic medicinal products referred to in paragraph 2 of this Article and in Article 7(1) shall be subject to the provisions of Directive 92/28/EEC of 31 March 1992 on the advertising of medicinal products for human use[1], with the exception of Article 2(1) of that Directive.

However, only the information specified in Article 7(2) may be used in the advertising of such medicinal products.

Moreover, each Member State may prohibit in its territory any advertising of the homeopathic medicinal products referred to in paragraph 2 and in Article 7(1).

---

1.   OJ L113 30.4.92 p13.

Article 7

1.   Only homeopathic medicinal products which satisfy all of the following conditions may be subject to a special, simplified registration procedure :

—   they are administered orally or externally,
—   no specific therapeutic indication appears on the labelling of the medicinal product or in any information relating thereto,
—   there is a sufficient degree of dilution to guarantee the safety of the medicinal product; in particular, the medicinal product may not contain either more than one part per 10 000 of the mother tincture or more than 1/100th of the smallest dose used in allopathy with regard to active principles whose presence in an allopathic medicinal product results in the obligation to submit a doctor's prescription.

At the time of registration, Member States shall determine the classification for the dispensing of the medicinal product.

2.   In addition to the clear mention of the words "homeopathic medicinal product", the labelling and, where appropriate, package insert for the medicinal products referred to in paragraph 1 shall bear the following, and no other, information :

—   the scientific name of the stock or stocks followed by the degree of dilution, making use of the symbols of the pharmacopoeia used in accordance with Article 1(1),
—   name and address of the person responsible for placing the product on the market and, where appropriate, of the manufacturer,
—   method of administration and, if necessary, route,
—   expiry date, in clear terms (month, year),
—   pharmaceutical form,
—   contents of the sales presentation,
—   special storage precautions, if any,
—   a special warning if necessary for the medicinal product,
—   manufacturer's batch number,
—   registration number,
—   "homeopathic medicinal product without approved therapeutic indications",
—   a warning advising the user to consult a doctor if the symptoms persist during the use of the medicinal product .

3.   Notwithstanding paragraph 2, Member States may require the use of certain types of labelling in order to show :

—   the price of the medicinal product,
—   the conditions for refunds by social security bodies.

4.   The criteria and rules of procedure provided for in Articles 5 to 12 of Directive 65/65/EEC shall apply by analogy to the special, simplified registration procedure for homeopathic medicinal products, with the exception of the proof of therapeutic efficacy.

Article 8

An application for special, simplified registration submitted by the person responsible for placing the product on the market may cover a series of medicinal products derived from the same homeopathic stock or stocks. The following documents shall be included with the application in order to demonstrate, in particular, the pharmaceutical quality and the batch-to-batch homogeneity of the products concerned :

— scientific name or other name given in a pharmacopoeia of the homeopathic stock or stocks, together with a statement of the various routes of administration, pharmaceutical forms and degree of dilution to be registered,
— dossier describing how the homeopathic stock or stocks is/are obtained and controlled, and justifying its/their homeopathic nature, on the basis of an adequate bibliography,
— manufacturing and control file for each pharmaceutical form and a description of the method of dilution and potentisation,
— manufacturing authorisation for the medicinal product concerned,
— copies of any registrations or authorisations obtained for the same medicinal product in other Member States;
— one or more specimens or mock-ups of the sales presentation of the medicinal products to be registered,
— data concerning the stability of the medicinal product.

Article 9

1.   Homeopathic medicinal products other than those referred to in Article 7 of this Directive shall be authorised and labelled in accordance with Articles 4 to 21 of Directive 65/65/EEC including the provisions concerning proof of therapeutic effect and Articles 1 to 7 of Directive 75/319/EEC.

2.   A Member State may introduce or retain in its territory specific rules for the pharmacological and toxicological tests and clinical trials of homeopathic medicinal products other than those referred to in Article 7(1) in accordance with the principles and characteristics of homeopathy as practised in that Member State.

In this case, the Member State concerned shall notify the Commission of the specific rules in force.

CHAPTER IV

Final provisions

Article 10

1.   Member States shall take the measures necessary to comply with this Directive by 31 December 1993. They shall forthwith inform the Commission thereof.

When Member States adopt the said measures, they shall contain a reference to this Directive or be accompanied by such reference when they are officially published. The procedure for making such reference shall be adopted by the Member States.

2.   Applications for registration or for marketing authorisation for medicinal products covered by this Directive lodged after the date set in paragraph 1 shall comply with the provisions of this Directive.

3.   Not later than 31 December 1995, the Commission shall present a report to the European Parliament and the Council concerning the application of this Directive.

Article 11

This Directive is addressed to the Member States.

Done at Brussels, 22 September 1992.

For the Council

The President

R. NEEDHAM

APPENDIX 9

COMMISSION DIRECTIVE (EEC) 91/356
of 13 June 1991

laying down the principles and guidelines of good manufacturing practice for medicinal products for human use[1]

THE COMMISSION OF THE EUROPEAN COMMUNITIES,

Having regard to the Treaty establishing the European Economic Community,

Having regard to Council Directive 75/319/EEC of 20 May 1975 on the approximation of provisions laid down by law, regulation or administrative action relating to proprietary medicinal products[2], as last amended by Directive 89/381/EEC[3], and in particular Article 19a thereof,

Whereas all medicinal products for human use manufactured or imported into the Community, including medicinal products intended for export, should be manufactured in accordance with the principles and guidelines of good manufacturing practice;

Whereas, in accordance with national legislation, Member States may require compliance with these principles of good manufacturing practice during the manufacture of products intended for use in clinical trials;

Whereas the detailed guidelines mentioned in Article 19a of Directive 75/319/EEC have been published by the Commission after consultation with the pharmaceutical inspection services of the Member States in the form of a *"Guide to good manufacturing practice for medicinal products"*;

Whereas it is necessary that all manufacturers should operate an effective quality management of their manufacturing operations, and that this requires the implementation of a pharmaceutical quality assurance system;

Whereas officials representing the competent authorities should report on whether the manufacturer complies with good manufacturing practice and that these reports should be communicated upon reasoned request to the competent authorities of another Member State;

Whereas the principles and guidelines of good manufacturing practice should primarily concern personnel, premises and equipment, documentation, production, quality control, contracting out, complaints and product recall, and self inspection;

Whereas the principles and guidelines envisaged by this Directive are in accordance with the opinion of the Committee for the Adaptation to Technical Progress of the Directives on the Removal of Technical Barriers to Trade in the Proprietary Medicinal Products Sector set up by Article 2b of Council Directive 75/318/EEC of 20 May 1975 on the approximation of the laws of Member States relating to analytical, pharmaco-toxicological and clinical standards and protocols

---

1.   OJ L193 17.7.91 p30.
2.   OJ L147 9.6.75 p13.
3.   OJ L181 28.6.89 p44.

in respect of the testing of proprietary medicinal products[1], as last amended by Directive 89/341/EEC[2],

HAS ADOPTED THIS DIRECTIVE :

CHAPTER I

GENERAL PROVISIONS

Article 1

This Directive lays down the principles and guidelines of good manufacturing practice for medicinal products for human use whose manufacture requires the authorisation referred to in Article 16 of Directive 75/319/EEC.

Article 2

For the purposes of this Directive, the definition of medicinal products set out in Article 1(2) of Council Directive 65/65/EEC[3], shall apply.

In addition,

- "manufacturer" shall mean any holder of the authorisation referred to in Article 16 of Directive 75/319/EEC,
- "qualified person" shall mean the person referred to in Article 21 of Directive 75/319/EEC,
- "pharmaceutical quality assurance" shall mean the sum total of the organised arrangements made with the object of ensuring that medicinal products are of the quality required for their intended use,
- "good manufacturing practice" shall mean the part of quality assurance which ensures that products are consistently produced and controlled to the quality standards appropriate to their intended use.

Article 3

By means of the repeated inspections referred to in Article 26 of Directive 75/319/EEC, the Member States shall ensure that manufacturers respect the principles and guidelines of good manufacturing practice laid down by this Directive.

For the interpretation of these principles and guidelines of good manufacturing practice, the manufacturers and the agents of the competent authorities shall refer to the detailed guidelines referred to in Article 19a of Directive 75/319/EEC. These detailed guidelines are published by the Commission in the *"Guide to good manufacturing practice for medicinal products"* and in its Annexes (Office for Official Publications of the European Communities, *The rules governing medicinal products in the European Community,* Volume IV).

Article 4

The manufacturer shall ensure that the manufacturing operations are carried out in accordance with good manufacturing practice and with the manufacturing authorisation.

---

1. OJ L147 9.6.75 p1.
2. OJ L142 25.5.89 p11.
3. OJ No 22 9.2.65 p369/65.

For medicinal products imported from third countries, the importer shall ensure that the medicinal products have been manufactured by manufacturers duly authorised and conforming to good manufacturing practice standards, at least equivalent to those laid down by the Community.

Article 5

The manufacturer shall ensure that all manufacturing operations subject to an authorisation for marketing are carried out in accordance with the information given in the application for marketing authorisation as accepted by the competent authorities.

The manufacturer shall regularly review their manufacturing methods in the light of scientific and technical progress. When a modification to the marketing authorisation dossier is necessary, the application for modification must be submitted to the competent authorities.

CHAPTER II

PRINCIPLES AND GUIDELINES OF GOOD MANUFACTURING PRACTICE

Article 6
Quality management

The manufacturer shall establish and implement an effective pharmaceutical quality assurance system, involving the active participation of the management and personnel of the different services involved.

Article 7
Personnel

1.   At each manufacturing site, the manufacturer shall have competent and appropriately qualified personnel at his disposal in sufficient number to achieve the pharmaceutical quality assurance objective.

2.   The duties of managerial and supervisory staff, including the qualified person(s), responsible for implementing and operating good manufacturing practice shall be defined in job descriptions. Their hierarchical relationships shall be defined in an organisation chart. Organisation charts and job descriptions shall be approved in accordance with the manufacturer's internal procedures.

3.   Staff referred to in paragraph 2 shall be given sufficient authority to discharge their responsibilities correctly.

4.   Personnel shall receive initial and continuing training including the theory and application of the concept of quality assurance and good manufacturing practice.

5.   Hygiene programmes adapted to the activities to be carried out shall be established and observed. These programmes include procedures relating to health, hygiene and clothing of personnel.

Article 8
Premises and equipment

1.   Premises and manufacturing equipment shall be located, designed, constructed, adapted and maintained to suit the intended operations.

2.   Lay out, design and operation must aim to minimise the risk of errors and permit effective cleaning and maintenance in order to avoid contamination, cross contamination and, in general, any adverse effect on the quality of the product.

3.   Premises and equipment intended to be used for manufacturing operations which are critical for the quality of the products shall be subjected to appropriate qualification.

Article 9
Documentation

1.   The manufacturer shall have a system of documentation based upon specifications, manufacturing formulae and processing and packaging instructions, procedures and records covering the various manufacturing operations that they perform. Documents shall be clear, free from errors and kept up to date. Pre-established procedures for general manufacturing operations and conditions shall be available, together with specific documents for the manufacture of each batch. This set of documents shall make it possible to trace the history of the manufacture of each batch. The batch documentation shall be retained for at least one year after the expiry date of the batches to which it relates or at least five years after the certification referred to in Article 22(2) of Directive 75/319/EEC whichever is the longer.

2.   When electronic, photographic or other data processing systems are used instead of written documents, the manufacturer shall have validated the systems by proving that the data will be appropriately stored during the anticipated period of storage. Data stored by these systems shall be made readily available in legible form. The electronically stored data shall be protected against loss or damage of data (e.g. by duplication or back-up and transfer onto another storage system).

Article 10
Production

The different production operations shall be carried out according to pre-established instructions and procedures and in accordance with good manufacturing practice. Adequate and sufficient resources shall be made available for the in-process controls.

Appropriate technical and/or organisational measures shall be taken to avoid cross contamination and mix-ups.

Any new manufacture or important modification of a manufacturing process shall be validated. Critical phases of manufacturing processes shall be regularly revalidated.

Article 11
Quality control

1.   The manufacturer shall establish and maintain a quality control department. This department shall be placed under the authority of a person having the required qualifications and shall be independent of the other departments.

2.   The quality control department shall have at its disposal one or more quality control laboratories appropriately staffed and equipped to carry out the necessary examination and testing of starting materials, packaging materials and intermediate and finished products testing. Resorting to outside laboratories may be authorised

in accordance with Article 12 of this Directive after the authorisation referred to in Article 5b of Directive 75/319/EEC has been granted.

3.   During the final control of finished products before their release for sale or distribution, in addition to analytical results, the quality control department shall take into account essential information such as the production conditions, the results of in-process controls, the examination of the manufacturing documents and the conformity of the products to their specifications (including the final finished pack).

4.   Samples of each batch of finished products shall be retained for at least one year after the expiry date. Unless in the Member States of manufacture a longer period is required, samples of starting materials (other than solvents, gases and water) used shall be retained for at least two years after the release of the product. This period may be shortened if their stability, as mentioned in the relevant specification, is shorter. All these samples shall be maintained at the disposal of the competent authorities.

For certain medicinal products manufactured individually or in small quantities, or when their storage could raise special problems, other sampling and retaining conditions may be defined in agreement with the competent authority.

Article 12
Work contracted out

1.   Any manufacturing operation or operation linked with the manufacture which is carried out under contract, shall be the subject of a written contract between the contract giver and the contract acceptor.

2.   The contract shall clearly define the responsibilities of each party and in particular the observance of good manufacturing practice by the contract acceptor and the manner in which the qualified person responsible for releasing each batch shall undertake his full responsibilities.

3.   The contract acceptor shall not subcontract any of the work entrusted to him by the contract giver without the written authorisation of the contract giver.

4.   The contract acceptor shall respect the principles and guidelines of good manufacturing practice and shall submit to inspections carried out by the competent authorities as provided for by Article 26 of Directive 75/319/EEC.

Article 13
Complaints and product recall

The manufacturer shall implement a system for recording and reviewing complaints together with an effective system for recalling promptly and at any time the medicinal products in the distribution network. Any complaint concerning a defect shall be recorded and investigated by the manufacturer. The competent authority shall be informed by the manufacturer of any defect that could result in a recall or abnormal restriction on the supply. In so far as possible, the countries of destination shall also be indicated. Any recall shall be made in accordance with the requirements referred to in Article 33 of Directive 75/319/EEC.

Article 14
Self-inspection

The manufacturer shall conduct repeated self-inspections as part of the quality assurance system in order to monitor the implementation and respect of good manufacturing practice and to propose any necessary corrective measures. Records of such self-inspections and any subsequent corrective action shall be maintained.

CHAPTER III

FINAL PROVISIONS

Article 15

Member States shall bring into force the laws, regulations and administrative provisions necessary to comply with this Directive not later than 1 January 1992. They shall forthwith inform the Commission thereof.

When Member States adopt these provisions, these shall contain a reference to this Directive or shall be accompanied by such reference at the time of their official publication. The procedure for such reference shall be adopted by Member States.

Article 16

This Directive is addressed to the Member States.

Done at Brussels, 13 June 1991.

For the Commission

Martin BANGEMANN

Vice-President

APPENDIX 10

COUNCIL DIRECTIVE (EEC) 92/25
of 31 March 1992

on the wholesale distribution of medicinal products for human use[1]

THE COUNCIL OF THE EUROPEAN COMMUNITIES,

Having regard to the Treaty establishing the European Economic Community, and in particular Article 100a thereof,

Having regard to the proposal from the Commission[2],

In co-operation with the European Parliament[3],

Having regard to the opinion of the Economic and Social Committee[4],

Whereas it is important to adopt measures with the aim of progressively establishing the internal market over a period expiring on 31 December 1992; whereas the internal market is to comprise an area without internal frontiers in which the free movement of goods, persons, services and capital is ensured;

Whereas the wholesale distribution of medicinal products is at present subject to different provisions in the various Member States; whereas many operations involving the wholesale distribution of medicinal products for human use may cover several Member States simultaneously;

Whereas it is necessary to exercise control over the entire chain of distribution of medicinal products, from their manufacture or import into the Community through to supply to the public, so as to guarantee that such products are stored, transported and handled in suitable conditions; whereas the requirements which must be adopted for this purpose will considerably facilitate the withdrawal of defective products from the market and allow more effective efforts against counterfeit products;

Whereas any person involved in the wholesale distribution of medicinal products should be in possession of a special authorisation; whereas pharmacists and persons authorised to supply medicinal products directly to the public, and who confine themselves to this activity, should be exempt from obtaining this authorisation; whereas it is however necessary, in order to control the complete chain of distribution of medicinal products, that pharmacists and persons authorised to supply medicinal products to the public keep records showing transactions in products received;

Whereas authorisation must be subject to certain essential conditions and it is the responsibility of the Member State concerned to ensure that such conditions are met; whereas each Member State must recognise authorisations granted by other Member States;

---

1.   OJ L113 30.4.92 p1.
2.   OJ C58 8.3.90 p16 and OJ C207 8.8.91 p11.
3.   OJ C183 15.7.91 p139 and OJ C67 16.3.92.
4.   OJ C269 14.10.91 p84.

Whereas certain Member States impose on wholesalers who supply medicinal products to pharmacists and on persons authorised to supply medicinal products to the public certain public service obligations; whereas those Member States must be able to continue to impose those obligations on wholesalers established within their territory; whereas they must also be able to impose them on wholesalers in other Member States on condition that they do not impose any obligation more stringent than those which they impose on their own wholesalers and provided that such obligations may be regarded as warranted on grounds of public health protection and are proportionate in relation to the objective of such protection,

HAS ADOPTED THIS DIRECTIVE :

Article 1

1. This Directive covers the wholesale distribution in the Community of medicinal products for human use to which Chapters II to V of Council Directive 65/65/EEC of 26 January 1965 on the approximation of provisions laid down by law, regulation or administrative action relating to medicinal products[1] apply.

2. For the purposes of this Directive :

— *wholesale distribution of medicinal products* shall mean all activities consisting of procuring, holding, supplying or exporting medicinal products, apart from supplying medicinal products to the public; such activities are carried out with manufacturers or their depositories, importers, other wholesale distributors or with pharmacists and persons authorised or entitled to supply medicinal products to the public in the Member State concerned,

— *public service obligation* shall mean the obligation placed on wholesalers to guarantee permanently an adequate range of medicinal products to meet the requirements of a specific geographical area and to deliver the supplies requested within a very short time over the whole of the area in question.

Article 2

Without prejudice to Article 3 of Directive 65/65/EEC, Member States shall take all appropriate action to ensure that only medicinal products in respect of which a marketing authorisation has been granted in accordance with Community law are distributed on their territory.

Article 3

1. Member States shall take all appropriate measures to ensure that the wholesale distribution of medicinal products is subject to the possession of an authorisation to engage in activity as a wholesaler in medicinal products, stating the place for which it is valid.

2. Where persons authorised or entitled to supply medicinal products to the public may also, under national law, engage in wholesale business, such persons shall be subject to the authorisation provided for in paragraph 1.

3. Possession of an authorisation, as mentioned in Article 16 of Second Council Directive 75/319/EEC of 20 May 1975 on the approximation of provisions laid down by law, regulation or administrative action relating to proprietary medicinal products[2], shall include authorisation to distribute by wholesale the

---

1. OJ No 22 9.2.65 p369/65.
2. OJ L147 9.6.75 p13.

medicinal products covered by that authorisation. Possession of an authorisation to engage in activity as a wholesaler in medicinal products shall not give dispensation from the obligation to possess a manufacturing authorisation and to comply with the conditions set out in that respect, even where the manufacturing or import business is secondary.

4.   At the request of the Commission or any Member State, Member States shall supply all appropriate information concerning the individual authorisations which they have granted under paragraph 1.

5.   Checks on the persons and establishments authorised to engage in the activity of wholesaler in medicinal products and the inspection of their premises shall be carried out under the responsibility of the Member State which granted the authorisation.

6.   The Member State which granted the authorisation referred to in paragraph 1 shall suspend or revoke that authorisation if the conditions of authorisation cease to be met. It shall forthwith inform the other Member States and the Commission thereof.

7.   Should a Member State consider that, in respect of a person holding an authorisation granted by another Member State under the terms of paragraph 1, the conditions of authorisation are not, or are no longer, met, it shall forthwith inform the Commission and the other Member State involved. The latter shall take the measures necessary and shall inform the Commission and the first Member State of the decisions taken and the reasons for those decisions.

Article 4

1.   Member States shall ensure that the time taken for the procedure for examining the application for the authorisation referred to in Article 3(1) does not exceed 90 days from the day on which the competent authority of the Member State concerned receives the application.

The competent authority may, if need be, require the applicant to supply all necessary information concerning the conditions of authorisation. Where the authority exercises this option, the period laid down in this paragraph shall be suspended until the requisite additional data have been supplied.

2.   All decisions to refuse, suspend or revoke the authorisation referred to in Article 3(1) shall state in detail the reasons on which they are based. A decision shall be notified to the party concerned, who shall at the same time be informed of the redress available to him under the laws in force and of the time limit allowed for access to such redress.

Article 5

In order to obtain the authorisation referred to in Article 3(1), applicants must fulfil the following minimum requirements :

(a)   they must have suitable and adequate premises, installations and equipment so as to ensure proper conservation and distribution of the medicinal products;

(b)   they must have staff, and in particular a qualified person designated as responsible, meeting the conditions provided for by the legislation of the Member State concerned;

(c)   they must undertake to fulfil the obligations incumbent on them under the terms of Article 6.

Article 6

Holders of the authorisation referred to in Article 3(1) must fulfil the following minimum requirements :

(a) they must make the premises, installations and equipment referred to in Article 5(a) accessible at all times to the persons responsible for inspecting them;

(b) they must obtain their supplies of medicinal products only from persons who are themselves in possession of the authorisation referred to in Article 3(1) or who are exempt from obtaining such authorisation under the terms of Article 3(3);

(c) they must supply medicinal products only to persons who are themselves in possession of the authorisation referred to in Article 3(1) or who are authorised or entitled to supply medicinal products to the public in the Member State concerned;

(d) they must have an emergency plan which ensures effective implementation of any recall from the market ordered by the competent authorities or carried out in co-operation with the manufacturer or holder of the marketing authorisation for the product concerned;

(e) they must keep records either in the form of purchase/sales invoices, or on computer, or in any other form giving for any transaction in medicinal products received or dispatched at least the following information :
 — date,
 — name of the medicinal product,
 — quantity received or supplied,
 — name and address of the supplier or consignee, as appropriate;

(f) they must keep the records referred to under (e) available to the competent authorities, for inspection purposes, for a period of five years;

(g) they must comply with the principles and guidelines of good distribution practice for medicinal products as laid down in Article 10.

Article 7

With regard to the supply of medicinal products to pharmacists and persons authorised or entitled to supply medicinal products to the public, Member States shall not impose upon the holder of an authorisation referred to in Article 3(1) which has been granted by another Member State, any obligation, in particular public service obligations, more stringent than those they impose on persons whom they have themselves authorised to engage in equivalent activities.

The said obligations should, moreover, be justified, in keeping with the Treaty, on grounds of public health protection and be proportionate in relation to the objective of such protection.

Article 8

For all supplies of medicinal products to a person authorised or entitled to supply medicinal products to the public in the Member State concerned, the authorised wholesaler must enclose a document that makes it possible to ascertain :

— the date,
— the name and pharmaceutical form of the medicinal product,
— the quantity supplied,
— the name and address of the supplier and consignor.

Member States shall take all appropriate measures to ensure that persons authorised or entitled to supply medicinal products to the public are able to provide information that makes it possible to trace the distribution path of every medicinal product.

Article 9

The provisions of this Directive shall not prevent the application of more stringent requirements laid down by Member States in respect of the wholesale distribution of :

—   narcotic or psychotropic substances within their territory,
—   medicinal products derived from blood governed by Directive 89/381/EEC[1],
—   immunological medicinal products governed by Directive 89/342/EEC[2],
—   radiopharmaceuticals governed by Directive 89/343/EEC[3].

Article 10

The Commission shall publish guidelines on good distribution practice. To this end it shall consult the Committee for Proprietary Medicinal Products and the Pharmaceutical Committee.

Article 11

1.   Member States shall bring into force the laws, regulations and administrative provisions necessary to comply with this Directive by 1 January 1993.

They shall forthwith inform the Commission thereof.

2.   When these measures are adopted by the Member States, they shall contain a reference to this Directive or shall be accompanied by such reference on the occasion of their official publication. The methods of making such a reference shall be laid down by the Member States.

Article 12

This Directive is addressed to the Member States.

Done at Brussels, 31 March 1992.

For the Council

The President

Vitor MARTINS

---

1.   OJ L181 28.6.89 p44.
2.   OJ L142 25.5.89 p14.
3.   OJ L142 25.5.89 p16.

APPENDIX 11

COUNCIL DIRECTIVE (EEC) 92/26
of 31 March 1992

concerning the classification for the supply of medicinal products for human use[1]

THE COUNCIL OF THE EUROPEAN COMMUNITIES,

Having regard to the Treaty establishing the European Economic Community and in particular Article 100a thereof,

Having regard to the proposal from the Commission[2],

In co-operation with the European Parliament[3],

Having regard to the opinion of the Economic and Social Committee[4],

Whereas measures aimed at progressively establishing the internal market over a period expiring on 31 December 1992 need to be taken; whereas the internal market is to comprise an area without internal frontiers in which the free movement of goods, persons, services and capital is ensured;

Whereas the conditions for the supply of medicinal products for human use to the public vary appreciably from one Member State to another; whereas medicinal products sold without prescriptions in certain Member States can be obtained only on medical prescription in other Member States;

Whereas Directive 91/28/EEC[5] specifies what medicinal products may be advertised to the public; whereas, in view of the development of means of communication, the conditions governing the supply of medicinal products to the public should be harmonised.

Whereas, moreover, persons moving around within the Community have the right to carry a reasonable quantity of medicinal products lawfully obtained for their personal use; whereas it must also be possible for a person established in one Member State to receive from another Member State a reasonable quantity of medicinal products intended for his personal use; whereas it is important therefore to harmonise the conditions governing the supply of medicinal products to the public;

Whereas, in addition, under the new system of registration of medicinal products in the Community, certain medicinal products will be the subject of a Community marketing authorisation; whereas, in this context, the classification for the supply of medicinal products covered by a Community marketing authorisation needs to be established; whereas it is therefore important to set the criteria on the basis of which Community decisions will be taken;

Whereas it is therefore appropriate, as an initial step, to harmonise the basic principles applicable to the classification for the supply of medicinal products in

---

1. OJ L113 30.4.92 p5.
2. OJ C58 8.3.90 p18.
3. OJ C183 15.7.91 p178 and OJ C67 16.3.92.
4. OJ C225 10.9.90 p21.
5. See page 13 of OJ L113 30.4.92.

the Community or in the Member State concerned, while taking as a starting point the principles already established on this subject by the Council of Europe as well as the work of harmonisation completed within the framework of the United Nations, concerning narcotic and psychotropic substances;

Whereas this Directive is without prejudice to the national social security arrangements for reimbursement or payment for medicinal products on prescription,

HAS ADOPTED THIS DIRECTIVE :

Article 1

1.   This Directive concerns the classification for the supply of medicinal products for human use in the Community into :

—   medicinal products subject to medical prescription,
—   medicinal products not subject to medical prescription.

2.   For the purposes of this Directive, the definition of "medicinal product" in Article 1 of Council Directive 65/65/EEC of 26 January 1965 on the approximation of provisions laid down by law, regulation or administrative action relating to medicinal products[1] as last amended by Directive 89/343/EEC[2], shall apply. In addition, "medicinal prescription" shall mean any prescription issued by a professional person qualified to prescribe medicinal products.

Article 2

1.   When a marketing authorisation is granted, the competent authorities shall specify the classification of the medicinal product into :

—   a medicinal product subject to medical prescription,
—   a medicinal product not subject to medical prescription.

To this end, the criteria laid down in Article 3(1) shall apply.

2.   The competent authorities may fix sub-categories for medicinal products which are available on medical prescription only. In that case, they shall refer to the following classification :

(a)   medicinal products on renewable or non-renewable medical prescription;
(b)   medicinal products subject to special medical prescription;
(c)   medicinal products on restricted medical prescription, reserved for use in certain specialised areas.

Article 3

1.   Medicinal products shall be subject to medical prescription where they :

—   are likely to present a danger either directly or indirectly, even when used correctly, if utilised without medical supervision, or
—   are frequently and to a very wide extent used incorrectly, and as a result are likely to present a direct or indirect danger to human health, or

---

1.   OJ No 22 9.6.65 p369/65.
2.   OJ L142 25.5.89 p14.

—   contain substances or preparations thereof the activity and/or side effects of which require further investigation, or
—   are normally prescribed by a doctor to be administered parenterally.

2.   Where Member States provide for the sub-category of medicinal products subject to special medical prescription, they shall take account of the following factors :

—   the medicinal product contains, in a non-exempt quantity, a substance classified as a narcotic or a psychotropic substance within the meaning of the international conventions in force (United Nations Conventions of 1961 and 1971), or
—   the medicinal product is likely, if incorrectly used, to present a substantial risk of medicinal abuse, to lead to addiction or be misused for illegal purposes, or
—   the medicinal product contains a substance which, by reason of its novelty or properties, could be considered as belonging to that group as a precautionary measure.

3.   Where Member States provide for the sub-category of medicinal products subject to restricted prescription, they shall take account of the following factors :

—   the medicinal product, because of its pharmaceutical characteristics or novelty or in the interests of public health, is reserved for treatments which can only be followed in a hospital environment,
—   the medicinal product is used in the treatment of conditions which must be diagnosed in a hospital environment or in institutions with adequate diagnostic facilities, although administration and follow-up may be carried out elsewhere, or
—   the medicinal product is intended for outpatients but its use may produce very serious side-effects requiring a prescription drawn up as required by a specialist and special supervision throughout the treatment.

4.   A competent authority may waive application of paragraphs 1, 2 and 3 having regard to :

(a)   the maximum single dose, the maximum daily dose, the strength, the pharmaceutical form, certain types of packaging; and/or
(b)   other circumstances of use which it has specified.

5.   If a competent authority does not designate medicinal products into sub-categories referred to in Article 2(2), it shall nevertheless take into account the criteria referred to in paragraphs 2 and 3 of this Article in determining whether any medicinal product shall be classified as a prescription-only medicine.

Article 4
Medicinal products not subject to prescription shall be those which do not meet the criteria listed in Article 3.

Article 5
1.   The competent authorities shall draw up a list of the medicinal products subject on their territory to medical prescription, specifying, if necessary, the category of classification. They shall update this list annually.

2.   On the occasion of the five-yearly renewal of the marketing authorisation or when new facts are brought to their notice, the competent authorities shall examine

and, as appropriate, amend the classification of a medicinal product, by applying the criteria listed in Article 3.

Article 6

1. Within two years of adoption of this Directive, the Member States shall communicate the list referred to in Article 5(1) to the Commission and to the other Member States, when requested by the latter.

2. Each year, Member States shall communicate to the Commission and to the other Member States the changes that have been made to the list referred to in paragraph 1.

3. Within four years of the adoption of this Directive, the Commission shall submit a report to the Council on the application of this Directive. This report will be accompanied, if necessary, by appropriate proposals.

Article 7

Member States shall bring into force the laws, regulations and administrative provisions necessary to comply with this Directive before 1 January 1993. They shall forthwith inform the Commission thereof.

When Member States adopt these measures, they shall contain a reference to this Directive or shall be accompanied by such reference on the occasion of their official publication. The methods of making such a reference shall be laid down by the Member States.

Article 8

This Directive is addressed to the Member States.

Done at Brussels, 31 March 1992.

For the Council

The President

Vitor MARTINS

APPENDIX 12

COUNCIL DIRECTIVE (EEC) 92/27
of 31 March 1992

on the labelling of medicinal products for human use and on package leaflets[1]

THE COUNCIL OF THE EUROPEAN COMMUNITIES,

Having regard to the Treaty establishing the European Economic Community, and in particular Article 100a thereof,

Having regard to the Proposal from the Commission[2],

In co-operation with the European Parliament[3],

Having regard to the Opinion of the Economic and Social Committee[4],

Whereas measures aimed at progressively establishing the internal market over a period expiring on 31 December 1992 need to be taken; whereas the internal market is to comprise an area without internal frontiers in which the free movement of goods, persons, services and capital is ensured;

Whereas Council Directive 65/65/EEC of 26 January 1965 on the approximation of provisions laid down by law, regulations or administrative action relating to medicinal products[5], as last amended by Directive 89/343/EEC[6], establishes a list of particulars to be given on the immediate packaging and the outer packaging of medicinal products for human use; whereas this list should be supplemented and details given of how labelling is to be presented;

Whereas Second Council Directive 75/319/EEC of 20 May 1975 on the approximation of provisions laid down by law, regulation or administrative action relating to proprietary medicinal products[7], as last amended by Directive 89/381/EEC[8], establishes a non-exhaustive list of particulars to be included in package leaflets; whereas this list should be supplemented and details given of how such leaflets are to be presented;

Whereas the provisions on labelling and on package leaflets should be brought together in a single text;

Whereas the provisions governing the information supplied to users should provide a high degree of consumer protection, in order that medicinal products may be used correctly on the basis of full and comprehensible information;

Whereas the marketing of medicinal products whose labelling and package leaflets comply with this Directive should not be prohibited or impeded on grounds connected with the labelling or package leaflet,

---

1.   OJ L113 30.4.92 p8
2.   OJ C58 8.3.90 p21.
3.   OJ C183 15.7.91 p213.
4.   OJ C225 10.9.90 p24.
5.   OJ No 22 9.2.65 p369/65.
6.   OJ L142 25.5.89 p14.
7.   OJ L147 9.6.75 p13.
8.   OJ L81 28.6.89 p44.

HAS ADOPTED THIS DIRECTIVE :

CHAPTER I

Scope and definitions

Article 1
1.   This Directive deals with the labelling of medicinal products for human use and leaflets inserted in packages of such products, to which Chapters II, III, IV and V of Directive 65/65/EEC apply.

2.   For the purposes of this Directive :

—   *name of the medicinal product* means the name given to a medicinal product, which may be either an invented name or a common or scientific name, together with a trade mark or the name of the manufacturer; the invented name shall not be liable to confusion with the common name,
—   *common name* means the international non-proprietary name recommended by the World Health Organisation, or, if one does not exist, the usual common name,
—   *strength of the medicinal product* means the content of the active ingredient expressed quantitatively per dosage unit, per unit of volume or weight according to the dosage form,
—   *immediate packaging* means the container or other form of packaging immediately in contact with the medicinal product,
—   *outer packaging* means the packaging into which is placed the immediate packaging,
—   *labelling* means information on the immediate or outer packaging,
—   *package leaflet* means a leaflet containing information for the user which accompanies the medicinal product,
—   *manufacturer* means the holder of the authorisation referred to in Article 16 of Directive 75/319/EEC on behalf of whom the qualified person has performed the specific obligations laid down in Article 22 of that Directive.

CHAPTER II

Labelling of medicinal products

Article 2
1.   The following particulars shall appear on the outer packaging of medicinal products or, where there is no outer packaging, on the immediate packaging :

(a)   the name of the medicinal product followed by the common name where the product contains only one active ingredient and if its name is an invented name; where a medicinal product is available in several pharmaceutical forms and/or several strengths, the pharmaceutical form and/or the strength (baby, child or adult as appropriate) must be included in the name of the medicinal product;
(b)   a statement of the active ingredients expressed qualitatively and quantitatively per dosage unit or according to the form of administration for a given volume or weight, using their common names;
(c)   the pharmaceutical form and the contents by weight, by volume or by number of doses of the product;
(d)   a list of those excipients known to have a recognised action or effect and included in the guidelines published pursuant to Article 12. However, if the

product is injectable, or a topical or eye preparation, all excipients must be stated;

(e)   the method and, if necessary, the route of administration;

(f)   a special warning that the medicinal product must be stored out of reach of children;

(g)   a special warning, if this is necessary for the medicinal product concerned;

(h)   the expiry date in clear terms (month/year);

(i)   special storage precautions, if any;

(j)   special precautions for disposal of unused medicinal products or waste materials derived from such products, if appropriate;

(k)   the name and address of the holder of the authorisation for placing the medicinal product on the market;

(l)   the number of the authorisation for placing the medicinal product on the market;

(m)   the manufacturer's batch number;

(n)   in the case of self-medication, instructions on the use of the medicinal products.

2.   The outer packaging may include symbols or pictograms designed to clarify certain information mentioned in paragraph 1 and other information compatible with the summary of the product characteristics which is useful for health education, to the exclusion of any element of a promotional nature.

Article 3

1.   The particulars laid down in Article 2 shall appear on immediate packagings other than those referred to in paragraphs 2 and 3.

2.   The following particulars at least shall appear on immediate packagings which take the form of blister packs and are placed in an outer packaging that complies with the requirements laid down in Article 2 :

—   the name of the medicinal product as laid down in Article 2(a),

—   the name of the holder of the authorisation for placing the product on the market,

—   the expiry date,

—   the batch number.

3.   The following particulars at least shall appear on small immediate packaging units on which the particulars laid down in Article 2 cannot be displayed :

—   the name of the medicinal product and, if necessary, the strength and the route of administration,

—   the method of administration,

—   the expiry date,

—   the batch number,

—   the contents by weight, by volume or by unit.

Article 4

1.   The particulars referred to in Articles 2 and 3 shall be easily legible, clearly comprehensible and indelible.

2.   The particulars listed in Article 2 shall appear in the official language or languages of the Member State where the product is placed on the market. This provision shall not prevent these particulars from being indicated in several languages, provided that the same particulars appear in all the languages used.

Article 5

1.   Member States may not prohibit or impede the placing on the market of medicinal products within their territory on grounds connected with labelling where such labelling complies with the requirements of this Chapter.

2.   Notwithstanding paragraph 1, Member States may require the use of certain forms of labelling making it possible to indicate :

—   the price of the medicinal product,
—   the reimbursement conditions of social security organisations,
—   the legal status for supply to the patient, in accordance with Directive 92/26/EEC[1],
—   identification and authenticity.

CHAPTER III

User package leaflet

Article 6

The inclusion in the packaging of all medicinal products of a package leaflet for the information of users shall be obligatory unless all the information required by Article 7 is directly conveyed on the outer packaging or on the immediate packaging.

Article 7

1.   The package leaflet shall be drawn up in accordance with the summary of the product characteristics; it shall include, in the following order :

(a)   for the identification of the medicinal product :
—   the name of the medicinal product, followed by the common name if the product contains only one active ingredient and if its name is an invented name; where a medicinal product is available in several pharmaceutical forms and/or several strengths, the pharmaceutical form and/or the strength (for example, baby, child, adult) must be included in the name of the medicinal product,
—   a full statement of the active ingredients and excipients expressed qualitatively and a statement of the active ingredients expressed quantitatively, using their common names, in the case of each presentation of the product,
—   the pharmaceutical form and the contents by weight, by volume or by number of doses of the product, in the case of each presentation of the product,
—   the pharmaco-therapeutic group, or type of activity in terms easily comprehensible for the patient,
—   the name and address of the holder of the authorisation for placing the medicinal product on the market and of the manufacturer;

(b)   the therapeutic indications;

(c)   a list of information which is necessary before taking the medicinal product :
—   contra-indications,
—   appropriate precautions for use,

---

1.   See page 5 of OJ L113 30.4.92.

     — forms of interaction with other medicinal products and other forms of interaction (for example, alcohol, tobacco, foodstuffs) which may affect the action of the medicinal product,
     — special warnings.

this list must :
     — take into account the particular condition of certain categories of users (e.g. children, pregnant or breastfeeding women, the elderly, persons with specific pathological conditions),
     — mention, if appropriate, potential effects on the ability to drive vehicles or to operate machinery,
     — detail those excipients, knowledge of which is important for the safe and effective use of the medicinal product and included in the guidelines published pursuant to Article 12;

(d)   the necessary and usual instructions for proper use, in particular :
     — the dosage,
     — the method and, if necessary, route of administration,
     — the frequency of administration, specifying if necessary the appropriate time at which the medicinal product may or must be administered,

and, as appropriate, depending on the nature of the product :
     — the duration of treatment, where it should be limited,
     — the action to be taken in the case of an overdose (for example, symptoms, emergency procedures),
     — the course of action to take when one or more doses have not been taken,
     — indication, if necessary, of the risk of withdrawal effects;

(e)   a description of the undesirable effects which can occur under normal use of the medicinal product and, if necessary, the action to be taken in such a case; the patient should be expressly invited to communicate any undesirable effect which is not mentioned in the leaflet to his doctor or to his pharmacist;

(f)   a reference to the expiry date indicated on the label, with :
     — a warning against using the product after this date,
     — where appropriate, special storage precautions,
     — if necessary, a warning against certain visible signs of deterioration;

(g)   the date on which the package leaflet was last revised.

2.   Notwithstanding paragraph 1(b), the competent authorities may decide that certain therapeutic indications shall not be mentioned in the package leaflet, where the dissemination of such information might have serious disadvantages for the patient.

3.   The package leaflet may include symbols or pictograms designed to clarify certain information mentioned in paragraph 1 and other information compatible with the summary of the product characteristics which is useful for health education, to the exclusion of any element of a promotional nature.

Article 8

The package leaflet must be written in clear and understandable terms for the patient and be clearly legible in the official language or languages of the Member State where the medicinal product is placed on the market. This provision does not prevent the package leaflet being printed in several languages, provided that the same information is given in all the languages used.

Article 9

Member States shall not prohibit or impede the marketing or medicinal products within their territory on grounds relating to the package leaflet if the latter complies with the requirements of this Chapter.

CHAPTER IV

General and final provisions

Article 10

1.   One or more specimens or mock-ups of the outer packaging and the immediate packaging of a medicinal product, together with the draft package leaflet, shall be submitted to the authorities competent for authorising marketing when the authorisation for placing the medicinal product on the market is requested.

2.   The competent authorities shall refuse the authorisation for placing the medicinal product on the market if the labelling or the package leaflet do not comply with the provisions of this Directive or if they are not in accordance with the particulars listed in the summary of product characteristics referred to in Article 4b of Directive 65/65/EEC.

3.   All proposed changes to an aspect of the labelling or the package leaflet covered by this Directive and not connected with the summary of characteristics shall be submitted to the authorities competent for authorising marketing. If the competent authorities have not opposed a proposed change within 90 days following the introduction of the request, the applicant may put the change into effect.

4.   The fact that the competent authorities do not refuse an authorisation to place the medicinal product on the market pursuant to paragraph 2 or a change to the labelling or the package leaflet pursuant to paragraph 3 does not alter the general legal liability of the manufacturer or as appropriate the holder of the authorisation to place the medicinal product on the market.

5.   The competent authorities may exempt labels and package leaflets for specific medicinal products from the obligation that certain particulars shall appear and that the leaflet must be in the official language or languages of the Member State where the product is placed on the market, when the product is not intended to be delivered to the patient for self-administration.

Article 11

1.   Where the provisions of this Directive are not complied with, and a notice served on the person concerned has remained without effect, the competent authorities of the Member States may suspend the authorisation to place the medicinal product on the market, until the labelling and the package leaflet of the medicinal product in question have been made to comply with the requirements of this Directive.

2.   All decisions taken pursuant to paragraph 1 shall state in detail the reasons on which they are based. They shall be notified to the party concerned, who shall

at the same time be informed of the remedies available to him under the laws in force and of the time limit allowed for the exercise of such remedies.

Article 12

1.   As necessary, the Commission shall publish guidelines concerning in particular :

—   the formulation of certain special warnings for certain categories of medicinal products,
—   the particular information needs relating to self-medication,
—   the legibility of particulars on the labelling and package leaflet,
—   methods for the identification and authentication of medicinal products,
—   the list of excipients which must feature on the labelling of medicinal products and the way these excipients must be indicated.

2.   These guidelines shall be adopted in the form of a Directive addressed to the Member States, in accordance with the procedure laid down in Article 2c of Directive 75/318/EEC.

Article 13

Articles 13 to 20 of Directive 65/65/EEC and Articles 6 and 7 of Directive 75/319/EEC are hereby repealed.

Article 14

Member States shall take the measures necessary to comply with this Directive before 1 January 1993. They shall forthwith inform the Commission thereof.

When Member States adopt these measures, they shall contain a reference to this Directive or shall be accompanied by such reference on the occasion of their official publication. The methods of making such a reference shall be laid down by the Member States.

From 1 January 1994, Member States shall refuse an application for authorisation to place a medicinal product on the market or for the renewal of an existing authorisation, where the labelling and the package leaflet do not comply with the requirements of this Directive.

Article 15

This Directive is addressed to the Member States.

Done at Brussels, 31 March 1992.

For the Council

The President

Vitor MARTINS

APPENDIX 13

COUNCIL DIRECTIVE (EEC) 92/28
of 31 March 1992

on advertising of medicinal products for human use[1]

THE COUNCIL OF THE EUROPEAN COMMUNITIES,

Having regard to the Treaty establishing the European Economic Community, and in particular Article 100a thereof,

Having regard to the proposal from the Commission[2],

In co-operation with the European Parliament[3],

Having regard to the opinion of the Economic and Social Committee[4],

Whereas Directive 84/450/EEC[5] harmonised the laws, regulations and administrative provisions of the Member States concerning misleading advertising; whereas this Directive is without prejudice to the application of measures adopted pursuant to that Directive;

Whereas all Member States have adopted further specific measures concerning the advertising of medicinal products; whereas there are disparities between these measures; whereas these disparities are likely to have an impact on the establishment and functioning of the internal market, since advertising disseminated in one Member State is likely to have effects in other Member States;

Whereas Council Directive 89/552/EEC of 3 October 1989 on the co-ordination of certain provisions laid down by law, regulation or administrative action in Member States concerning the pursuit of television broadcasting activities[6] prohibits the television advertising of medicinal products which are available only on medical prescription in the Member State within whose jurisdiction the television broadcaster is located; whereas this principle should be made of general application by extending it to other media;

Whereas advertising to the general public, even of non-prescription medicinal products, could affect public health, were it to be excessive and ill-considered; whereas advertising of medicinal products to the general public, where it is permitted, ought therefore to satisfy certain essential criteria which ought to be defined;

Whereas, furthermore, distribution of samples free of charge to the general public for promotional ends must be prohibited;

Whereas the advertising of medicinal products to persons qualified to prescribe or supply them contributes to the information available to such persons; whereas, nevertheless, this advertising should be subject to strict conditions and effective

---

1. OJ L113 30.4.92 p13.
2. OJ C163 4.7.90 p10 and OJ C207 8.8.91 p25.
3. OJ C183 15.7.91 p227 and OJ C67 16.3.92.
4. OJ C60 8.3.91 p40.
5. OJ L250 19.9.84 p17.
6. OJ L298 17.10.89 p23.

monitoring, referring in particular to the work carried out within the framework of the Council of Europe;

Whereas medical sales representatives have an important role in the promotion of medicinal products; whereas, therefore, certain obligations should be imposed upon them, in particular the obligation to supply the person visited with a summary of product characteristics;

Whereas persons qualified to prescribe medicinal products must be able to carry out these functions objectively without being influenced by direct or indirect financial inducements;

Whereas it should be possible within certain restrictive conditions to provide samples of medicinal products free of charge to persons qualified to prescribe or supply them so that they can familiarise themselves with new products and acquire experience in dealing with them;

Whereas persons qualified to prescribe or supply medicinal products must have access to a neutral, objective source of information about products available on the market; whereas it is nevertheless for the Member States to take all measures necessary to this end, in the light of their own particular situation;

Whereas advertising of medicinal products should be subject to effective, adequate monitoring; whereas reference in this regard should be made to the monitoring mechanisms set up by Directive 84/450/EEC;

Whereas each undertaking which manufactures or imports medicinal products should set up a mechanism to ensure that all information supplied about a medicinal product conforms with the approved conditions of use,

HAS ADOPTED THIS DIRECTIVE :

CHAPTER I

Scope, definitions and general principles

Article 1

1.   This Directive concerns the advertising in the Community of medicinal products for human use covered by Chapters II to V of Council Directive 65/65/EEC of 26 January 1965 on the approximation of provisions laid down by law, regulation or administrative action relating to medicinal products[1].

2.   For the purposes of this Directive :

—   the definitions of the name of the medicinal product and of the common name shall be those laid down in Article 1 of Directive 92/27/EEC[2];

—   the summary of product characteristics shall be the summary approved by the competent authority which granted the marketing authorisation in accordance with Article 4b of Directive 65/65/EEC.

3.   For the purposes of this Directive, advertising of medicinal products shall include any form of door-to-door information, canvassing activity or inducement

---

1.   OJ No 22 9.2.65 p369/65. Directive last amended by Directive 89/341/EEC (OJ L142 25.5.89 p11).
2.   See page 8 of OJ L113 30.4.92.

designed to promote the prescription, supply, sale or consumption of medicinal products; it shall include in particular :

—   the advertising of medicinal products to the general public,
—   advertising of medicinal products to persons qualified to prescribe or supply them,
—   visits by medical sales representatives to persons qualified to prescribe medicinal products,
—   the supply of samples,
—   the provision of inducements to prescribe or supply medicinal products by the gift, offer or promise of any benefit or bonus, whether in money or in kind, except when their intrinsic value is minimal,
—   sponsorship of promotional meetings attended by persons qualified to prescribe or supply medicinal products,
—   sponsorship of scientific congresses attended by persons qualified to prescribe or supply medicinal products and in particular payment of their travelling and accommodation expenses in connection therewith.

4.   The following are not covered by this Directive :

—   the labelling of medicinal products and the accompanying package leaflets, which are subject to the provisions of Directive 92/27/EEC;
—   correspondence, possibly accompanied by material of a non-promotional nature, needed to answer a specific question about a particular medicinal product;
—   factual, informative announcements and reference material relating, for example, to pack changes, adverse-reaction warnings as part of general drug precautions, trade catalogues and price lists, provided they include no product claims;
—   statements relating to human health or diseases, provided there is no reference, even indirect, to medicinal products.

Article 2

1.   Member States shall prohibit any advertising of a medicinal product in respect of which a marketing authorisation has not been granted in accordance with Community law.

2.   All parts of the advertising of a medicinal product must comply with the particulars listed in the summary of product characteristics.

3.   The advertising of a medicinal product :

—   shall encourage the rational use of the medicinal product, by presenting it objectively and without exaggerating its properties,
—   shall not be misleading.

CHAPTER II

Advertising to the general public

Article 3

1.   Member States shall prohibit the advertising to the general public of medicinal products which :

—   are available on medical prescription only, in accordance with Directive 92/26/EEC[1],
—   contain psychotropic or narcotic substances, within the meaning of the international conventions,
—   may not be advertised to the general public in accordance with paragraph 2.

2.   Medicinal products may be advertised to the general public which, by virtue of their composition and purpose, are intended and designed for use without the intervention of a medical practitioner for diagnostic purposes or for the prescription or monitoring of treatment, with the advice of the pharmacist, if necessary.

Member States shall prohibit the mentioning in advertising to the general public of therapeutic indications such as :

—   tuberculosis,
—   sexually transmitted diseases,
—   other serious infectious diseases,
—   cancer and other tumoral diseases,
—   chronic insomnia,
—   diabetes and other metabolic illnesses.

3.   Member States shall also be able to ban on their territory advertising to the general public of medicinal products the cost of which may be reimbursed.

4.   The prohibition referred to in paragraph 1 shall not apply to vaccination campaigns carried out by the industry and approved by the competent authorities of the Member States.

5.   The prohibition referred to in paragraph 1 shall apply without prejudice to Articles 2, 3 and 14 of Directive 89/552/EEC.

6.   Member States shall prohibit the direct distribution of medicinal products to the public by the industry for promotional purposes; they may, however, authorise such distribution in special cases for other purposes.

Article 4

1.   Without prejudice to Article 3, all advertising to the general public of a medicinal product shall :

(a)   be set out in such a way that it is clear that the message is an advertisement and that the product is clearly identified as a medicinal product;

(b)   include the following minimum information :
—   the name of the medicinal product, as well as the common name if the medicinal product contains only one active ingredient,
—   the information necessary for correct use of the medicinal product,

---

1.   See page 5 of OJ L113 30.4.92.

> — an express, legible invitation to read carefully the instructions on the package leaflet or on the outer packaging, according to the case.

2.   Member States may decide that the advertising of a medicinal product to the general public may, notwithstanding paragraph 1, include only the name of the medicinal product if it is intended solely as a reminder.

Article 5

The advertising of a medicinal product to the general public shall not contain any material which :

(a)   gives the impression that a medical consultation or surgical operation is unnecessary, in particular by offering a diagnosis or by suggesting treatment by mail;

(b)   suggests that the effects of taking the medicine are guaranteed, are unaccompanied by side effects or are better than, or equivalent to, those of another treatment or medicinal product;

(c)   suggests that the health of the subject can be enhanced by taking the medicine;

(d)   suggests that the health of the subject could be affected by not taking the medicine; this prohibition shall not apply to the vaccination campaigns referred to in Article 3(4);

(e)   is directed exclusively or principally at children;

(f)   refers to a recommendation by scientists, health professionals or persons who are neither of the foregoing but who, because of their celebrity, could encourage the consumption of medicinal products;

(g)   suggests that the medicinal product is a foodstuff, cosmetic or other consumer product;

(h)   suggests that the safety or efficacy of the medicinal product is due to the fact that it is natural;

(i)   could, by a description or detailed representation of a case history, lead to erroneous self diagnosis;

(j)   refers, in improper, alarming or misleading terms, to claims of recovery;

(k)   uses, in improper, alarming or misleading terms, pictorial representations of changes in the human body caused by disease or injury, or of the action of a medicinal product on the human body or parts thereof;

(l)   mentions that the medicinal product has been granted a marketing authorisation.

CHAPTER III

Advertising to health professionals

Article 6

1.   Any advertising of a medicinal product to persons qualified to prescribe or supply such products shall include :

— essential information compatible with the summary of product characteristics;

— the supply classification of the medicinal product.

Member States may also require such advertising to include the selling price or indicative price of the various presentations and the conditions for reimbursement by social security bodies.

2.   Member States may decide that the advertising of a medicinal product to persons qualified to prescribe or supply such products may, notwithstanding paragraph 1, include only the name of the medicinal product, if it is intended solely as a reminder.

Article 7

1.   Any documentation relating to a medicinal product which is transmitted as part of the promotion of that product to persons qualified to prescribe or supply it shall include as a minimum the particulars listed in Article 6(1) and shall state the date on which it was drawn up or last revised.

2.   All the information contained in the documentation referred to in paragraph 1 shall be accurate, up-to-date, verifiable and sufficiently complete to enable the recipient to form his or her own opinion of the therapeutic value of the medicinal product concerned.

3.   Quotations as well as tables and other illustrative matter taken from medical journals or other scientific works for use in the documentation referred to in paragraph 1 shall be faithfully reproduced and the precise sources indicated.

Article 8

1.   Medical sales representatives shall be given adequate training by the firm which employs them and shall have sufficient scientific knowledge to be able to provide information which is precise and as complete as possible about the medicinal products which they promote.

2.   During each visit, medical sales representatives shall give the persons visited, or have available for them, summaries of the product characteristics of each medicinal product they present together, if the legislation of the Member State so permits, with details of the price and conditions for reimbursement referred to in Article 6(1).

3.   Medical sales representatives shall transmit to the scientific service referred to in Article 13(1) any information about the use of the medicinal products they advertise, with particular reference to any adverse reactions reported to them by the persons they visit.

Article 9

1.   Where medicinal products are being promoted to persons qualified to prescribe or supply them, no gifts, pecuniary advantages or benefits in kind may be supplied, offered or promised to such persons unless they are inexpensive and relevant to the practice of medicine or pharmacy.

2.   Hospitality at sales promotion must always be reasonable in level and secondary to the main purpose of the meeting and must not be extended to other than health professionals.

3.   Persons qualified to prescribe or supply medicinal products shall not solicit or accept any inducement prohibited under paragraph 1 or contrary to paragraph 2.

4.   Existing measures or trade practices in Member States relating to prices, margins and discounts shall not be affected by this Article.

Article 10

The provisions of Article 9(1) shall not prevent hospitality being offered, directly or indirectly, at events for purely professional and scientific purposes; such hospitality must always be reasonable in level and remain subordinate to the main scientific objective of the meeting; it must not be extended to persons other than health professionals.

Article 11

1.   Free samples shall be provided on an exceptional basis only to persons qualified to prescribe them and on the following conditions :

(a)   a limited number of samples for each medicinal product each year on prescription;
(b)   any supply of samples must be in response to a written request, signed and dated, from the recipient;
(c)   those supplying samples must maintain an adequate system of control and accountability;
(d)   each sample shall be identical with the smallest presentation on the market;
(e)   each sample shall be marked free medical sample - not for resale or bear another legend of analogous meaning;
(f)   each sample shall be accompanied by a copy of the summary of product characteristics;
(g)   no samples of medicinal products containing psychotropic or narcotic substances within the meaning of international conventions may be supplied.

2.   Member States may also place further restrictions on the distribution of samples of certain medicinal products.

CHAPTER IV

Monitoring of advertising

Article 12

1.   Member States shall ensure that there are adequate and effective methods to monitor the advertising of medicinal products. Such methods, which may be based on a system of prior vetting, shall in any event include legal provisions under which persons or organisations regarded under national law as having a legitimate interest in prohibiting any advertisement inconsistent with this Directive may take legal action against such advertisement, or bring such advertisement before an administrative authority competent either to decide on complaints or to initiate appropriate legal proceedings.

2.   Under the legal provisions referred to in paragraph 1, Member States shall confer upon the courts or administrative authorities powers enabling them, in cases where they deem such measures to be necessary taking into account all the interests involved and in particular the public interest :

—   to order the cessation of, or to institute appropriate legal proceedings for an order for the cessation of, misleading advertising, or
—   if misleading advertising has not yet been published but publication is imminent, to order the prohibition of, or to institute appropriate legal proceedings for an order for the prohibition of, such publication, even without proof of actual loss or damage or of intention or negligence on the part of the advertiser.

Member States shall also make provision for the measures referred to in the first subparagraph to be taken under an accelerated procedure :

—　　either with interim effect, or
—　　with definitive effect,

on the understanding that it is for each Member State to decide which of the two options to select.

Furthermore, Member States may confer upon the courts or administrative authorities powers enabling them, with a view to eliminating the continuing effects of misleading advertising the cessation of which has been ordered by a final decision :

—　　to require publication of that decision in full or in part and in such form as they deem adequate,
—　　to require in addition the publication of a corrective statement.

3.　　Under the legal provisions referred to in paragraph 1, Member States shall ensure that any decision taken in accordance with paragraph 2 shall state in detail the reasons on which it is based and shall be communicated in writing to the person concerned, mentioning the redress available at law and the time limit allowed for access to such redress.

4.　　This Article shall not exclude the voluntary control of advertising of medicinal products by self-regulatory bodies and recourse to such bodies, if proceedings before such bodies are possible in addition to the judicial or administrative proceedings referred to in paragraph 1.

Article 13

1.　　The marketing authorisation holder shall establish within his undertaking a scientific service in charge of information about the medicinal products which he places on the market.

2.　　The person responsible for placing the product on the market shall :

—　　keep available for, or communicate to, the authorities or bodies responsible for monitoring advertising of medicinal products a sample of all advertisements emanating from his undertaking together with a statement indicating the persons to whom it is addressed, the method of dissemination and the date of first dissemination,
—　　ensure that advertising of medicinal products by his undertaking conforms to the requirements of this Directive,
—　　verify that medical sales representatives employed by his undertaking have been adequately trained and fulfil the obligations imposed upon them by Article 8(2) and (3),
—　　supply the authorities or bodies responsible for monitoring advertising of medicinal products with the information and assistance they require to carry out their responsibilities,
—　　ensure that the decisions taken by the authorities or bodies responsible for monitoring advertising of medicinal products are immediately and fully complied with.

Article 14

Member States shall take the appropriate measures to ensure that all the provisions of this Directive are applied in full and shall determine in particular what penalties shall be imposed should the provisions adopted in the execution of this Directive be infringed.

Article 15

1.   Member States shall take the measures necessary in order to comply with this Directive with effect from 1 January 1993. They shall forthwith inform the Commission thereof.

2.   When Member States adopt the said measures, such measures shall contain a reference to this Directive or be accompanied by such reference on the occasion of their official publication. The methods of making such a reference shall be laid down by the Member States.

Article 16

This Directive is addressed to the Member States.

Done at Brussels, 31 March 1992.

For the Council

The President

Vitor MARTINS

APPENDIX 14

COUNCIL REGULATION (EEC) 1768/92
of 18 June 1992

concerning the creation of a supplementary protection certificate for medicinal products[1]

THE COUNCIL OF THE EUROPEAN COMMUNITIES,

Having regard to the Treaty establishing the European Economic Community, and in particular Article 100a thereof,

Having regard to the proposal from the Commission[2],

In co-operation with the European Parliament[3],

Having regard to the opinion of the Economic and Social Committee[4],

Whereas pharmaceutical research plays a decisive role in the continuing improvement in public health;

Whereas medicinal products, especially those that are the result of long, costly research will not continue to be developed in the Community and in Europe unless they are covered by favourable rules that provide for sufficient protection to encourage such research;

Whereas at the moment the period that elapses between the filing of an application for a patent for a new medicinal product and authorisation to place the medicinal product on the market makes the period of effective protection under the patent insufficient to cover the investment put into the research;

Whereas this situation leads to a lack of protection which penalises pharmaceutical research;

Whereas the current situation is creating the risk of research centres situated in the Member States relocating to countries that already offer greater protection;

Whereas a uniform solution at Community level should be provided for, thereby preventing the heterogeneous development of national laws leading to further disparities which would be likely to create obstacles to the free movement of medicinal products within the Community and thus directly affect the establishment and the functioning of the internal market;

Whereas, therefore, the creation of a supplementary protection certificate granted, under the same conditions, by each of the Member States at the request of the holder of a national or European patent relating to a medicinal product for which marketing authorisation has been granted is necessary; whereas a Regulation is therefore the most appropriate legal instrument;

Whereas the duration of the protection granted by the certificate should be such as to provide adequate effective protection; whereas, for this purpose, the holder of

---

1.   OJ L182 2.7.92 p1.
2.   OJ C114 8.5.90 p10.
3.   OJ C19 28.1.91 p94 and OJ C150 15.6.92.
4.   OJ C69 18.3.91 p22.

both a patent and a certificate should be able to enjoy an overall maximum of fifteen years of exclusivity from the time the medicinal product in question first obtains authorisation to be placed on the market in the Community;

Whereas all the interests at stake, including those of public health, in a sector as complex and sensitive as the pharmaceutical sector must nevertheless be taken into account; whereas, for this purpose, the certificate cannot be granted for a period exceeding five years; whereas the protection granted should furthermore be strictly confined to the product which obtained authorisation to be placed on the market as a medicinal product;

Whereas a fair balance should also be struck with regard to the determination of the transitional arrangements; whereas such arrangements should enable the Community pharmaceutical industry to catch up to some extent with its main competitors who, for a number of years, have been covered by laws guaranteeing them more adequate protection, while making sure that the arrangements do not compromise the achievement of other legitimate objectives concerning the health policies pursued both at national and Community level;

Whereas the transitional arrangements applicable to applications for certificates filed and to certificates granted under national legislation prior to the entry into force of this Regulation should be defined;

Whereas special arrangements should be allowed in Member States whose laws introduced the patentability of pharmaceutical products only very recently;

Whereas provision should be made for appropriate limitation of the duration of the certificate in the special case where a patent term has already been extended under a specific national law,

HAS ADOPTED THIS REGULATION :

Article 1
Definitions

For the purposes of this Regulation :

(a)   "medicinal product" means any substance or combination of substances presented for treating or preventing disease in human beings or animals and any substance or combination of substances which may be administered to human beings or animals with a view to making a medical diagnosis or to restoring, correcting or modifying physiological functions in humans or in animals;

(b)   "product" means the active ingredient or combination of active ingredients of a medicinal product;

(c)   "basic patent" means a patent which protects a product as defined in (b) as such, a process to obtain a product or an application of a product, and which is designated by its holder for the purpose of the procedure for grant of a certificate;

(d)   "certificate" means the supplementary protection certificate.

Article 2
Scope

Any product protected by a patent in the territory of a Member State and subject, prior to being placed on the market as a medicinal product, to an administrative authorisation procedure as laid down in Council Directive 65/65/EEC[1] or Directive 81/851/EEC[2] may, under the terms and conditions provided for in this Regulation, be the subject of a certificate.

Article 3
Conditions for obtaining a certificate

A certificate shall be granted if, in the Member State in which the application referred to in Article 7 is submitted and at the date of that application :

(a)   the product is protected by a basic patent in force;
(b)   a valid authorisation to place the product on the market as a medicinal product has been granted in accordance with Directive 65/65/EEC or Directive 81/851/EEC, as appropriate;
(c)   the product has not already been the subject of a certificate;
(d)   the authorisation referred to in (b) is the first authorisation to place the product on the market as a medicinal product.

Article 4
Subject-matter of protection

Within the limits of the protection conferred by the basic patent, the protection conferred by a certificate shall extend only to the product covered by the authorisation to place the corresponding medicinal product on the market and for any use of the product as a medicinal product that has been authorised before the expiry of the certificate.

Article 5
Effects of the certificate

Subject to the provisions of Article 4, the certificate shall confer the same rights as conferred by the basic patent and shall be subject to the same limitations and the same obligations.

Article 6
Entitlement to the certificate

The certificate shall be granted to the holder of the basic patent or his successor in title.

Article 7
Application for a certificate

1.   The application for a certificate shall be lodged within six months of the date on which the authorisation referred to in Article 3(b) to place the product on the market as a medicinal product was granted.

2.   Notwithstanding paragraph 1, where the authorisation to place the product on the market is granted before the basic patent is granted, the application for a certificate shall be lodged within six months of the date on which the patent is granted.

---

1.   OJ No 22 9.12.65 p369. Last amended by Directive 89/341/EEC (OJ L142 25.5.89 p11).
2.   OJ L317 6.11.81 p1. Amended by Directive 90/676/EEC (OJ L373 31.12.90 p15).

Article 8
Content of the application for a certificate

1.   The application for a certificate shall contain :

(a)   a request for the grant of a certificate, stating in particular :
    (i)   the name and address of the applicant;
    (ii)   if he has appointed a representative, the name and address of the representative;
    (iii)   the number of the basic patent and the title of the invention;
    (iv)   the number and date of the first authorisation to place the product on the market, as referred to in Article 3(b) and, if this authorisation is not the first authorisation for placing the product on the market in the Community, the number and date of that authorisation;
(b)   a copy of the authorisation to place the product on the market, as referred to in Article 3(b), in which the product is identified, containing in particular the number and date of the authorisation and the summary of the product characteristics listed in Article 4a of Directive 65/65/EEC or Article 5a of Directive 81/851/EEC;
(c)   if the authorisation referred to in (b) is not the first authorisation for placing the product on the market as a medicinal product in the Community, information regarding the identity of the product thus authorised and the legal provision under which the authorisation procedure took place, together with a copy of the notice publishing the authorisation in the appropriate official publication.

2.   Member States may provide that a fee is to be payable upon application for a certificate.

Article 9
Lodging of an application for a certificate

1.   The application for a certificate shall be lodged with the competent industrial property office of the Member State which granted the basic patent or on whose behalf it was granted and in which the authorisation referred to in Article 3(b) to place the product on the market was obtained, unless the Member State designates another authority for the purpose.

2.   Notification of the application for a certificate shall be published by the authority referred to in paragraph 1. The notification shall contain at least the following information :

(a)   the name and address of the applicant;
(b)   the number of the basic patent;
(c)   the title of the invention;
(d)   the number and date of the authorisation to place the product on the market, referred to in Article 3(b), and the product identified in that authorisation;
(e)   where relevant, the number and date of the first authorisation to place the product on the market in the Community.

Article 10
Grant of the certificate or rejection of the application

1.   Where the application for a certificate and the product to which it relates meet the conditions laid down in this Regulation, the authority referred to in Article 9(1) shall grant the certificate.

2.   The authority referred to in Article 9(1) shall, subject to paragraph 3, reject the application for a certificate if the application or the product to which it relates does not meet the conditions laid down in this Regulation.

3.   Where the application for a certificate does not meet the conditions laid down in Article 8, the authority referred to in Article 9(1) shall ask the applicant to rectify the irregularity, or to settle the fee, within a stated time.

4.   If the irregularity is not rectified or the fee is not settled under paragraph 3 within the stated time, the authority shall reject the application.

5.   Member States may provide that the authority referred to in Article 9(1) is to grant certificates without verifying that the conditions laid down in Article 3(c) and (d) are met.

Article 11
Publication

1.   Notification of the fact that a certificate has been granted shall be published by the authority referred to in Article 9(1). The notification shall contain at least the following information :

(a)   the name and address of the holder of the certificate;
(b)   the number of the basic patent;
(c)   the title of the invention;
(d)   the number and date of the authorisation to place the product on the market referred to in Article 3(b) and the product identified in that authorisation;
(e)   where relevant, the number and date of the first authorisation to place the product on the market in the Community;
(f)   the duration of the certificate.

2.   Notification of the fact that the application for a certificate has been rejected shall be published by the authority referred to in Article 9(1). The notification shall contain at least the information listed in Article 9(2).

Article 12
Annual fees

Member States may require that the certificate be subject to the payment of annual fees.

Article 13
Duration of the certificate

1.   The certificate shall take effect at the end of the lawful term of the basic patent for a period equal to the period which elapsed between the date on which the application for a basic patent was lodged and the date of the first authorisation to place the product on the market in the Community reduced by a period of five years.

2.   Notwithstanding paragraph 1, the duration of the certificate may not exceed five years from the date on which it takes effect.

Article 14
Expiry of the certificate

The certificate shall lapse :

(a)   at the end of the period provided for in Article 13;

(b)   if the certificate-holder surrenders it;
(c)   if the annual fee laid down in accordance with Article 12 is not paid in time;
(d)   if and as long as the product covered by the certificate may no longer be placed on the market following the withdrawal of the appropriate authorisation or authorisations to place on the market in accordance with Directive 65/65/EEC or Directive 81/851/EEC. The authority referred to in Article 9(1) may decide on the lapse of the certificate either of its own motion or at the request of a third party.

Article 15
Invalidity of the certificate

1.   The certificate shall be invalid if :

(a)   it was granted contrary to the provisions of Article 3;
(b)   the basic patent has lapsed before its lawful term expires;
(c)   the basic patent is revoked or limited to the extent that the product for which the certificate was granted would no longer be protected by the claims of the basic patent or, after the basic patent has expired, grounds for revocation exist which would have justified such revocation or limitation.

2.   Any person may submit an application or bring an action for a declaration of invalidity of the certificate before the body responsible under national law for the renovation of the corresponding basic patent.

Article 16
Notification of lapse or invalidity

If the certificate lapses in accordance with Article 14(b), (c) or (d) or is invalid in accordance with Article 15, notification thereof shall be published by the authority referred to in Article 9(1).

Article 17
Appeals

The decisions of the authority referred to in Article 9(1) or of the body referred to in Article 15(2) taken under this Regulation shall be open to the same appeals as those provided for in national law against similar decisions taken in respect of national patents.

Article 18
Procedure

1.   In the absence of procedural provisions in this Regulation, the procedural provisions applicable under national law to the corresponding basic patent shall apply to the certificate, unless that law lays down special procedural provisions for certificates.

2.   Notwithstanding paragraph 1, the procedure for opposition to the granting of a certificate shall be excluded.

Article 19
Transitional provisions

1.   Any product which, on the date on which this Regulation enters into force, is protected by a valid basic patent and for which the first authorisation to place it

on the market as a medicinal product in the Community was obtained after 1 January 1985 may be granted a certificate.

In the case of certificates to be granted in Denmark and in Germany, the date of 1 January 1985 shall be replaced by that of 1 January 1988.

In the case of certificates to be granted in Belgium and in Italy, the date of 1 January 1985 shall be replaced by that of 1 January 1982.

2.   An application for a certificate as referred to in paragraph I shall be submitted within six months of the date on which this Regulation enters into force.

Article 20
This Regulation shall not apply to certificates granted in accordance with the national legislation of a Member State before the date on which this Regulation enters into force or to applications for a certificate filed in accordance with that legislation before the date of publication of this Regulation in the *Official Journal of the European Communities.*

Article 21
In those Member States whose national law did not on 1 January 1990 provide for the patentability of pharmaceutical products, this Regulation shall apply five years after the entry into force of this Regulation.

Article 19 shall not apply in those Member States.

Article 22
Where a certificate is granted for a product protected by a patent which, before the date on which this Regulation enters into force, has had its term extended or for which such extension was applied for, under national patent law, the term of protection to be afforded under this certificate shall be reduced by the number of years by which the term of the patent exceeds 20 years.

FINAL PROVISION

Article 23
Entry into force
This Regulation shall enter into force six months after its publication in the *Official Journal of the European Communities.*

This Regulation shall be binding in its entirety and directly applicable in all Member States.

Done at Luxembourg, 18 June 1992.

For the Council

The President

Vitor MARTINS

APPENDIX 15

COUNCIL DIRECTIVE (EEC) 89/105
of 21 December 1988

relating to the transparency of measures regulating the pricing of medicinal products for human use and their inclusion in the scope of national health insurance systems[1]

THE COUNCIL OF THE EUROPEAN COMMUNITIES,

Having regard to the Treaty establishing the European Economic Community, and in particular Article 100a thereof,

Having regard to the proposal from the Commission[2],

In co-operation with the European Parliament[3],

Having regard to the opinion of the Economic and Social Committee[4],

Whereas marketing authorisations for proprietary medicinal products issued pursuant to Council Directive 65/65/EEC of 26 January 1965 on the approximation of provisions laid down by law, regulation or administrative action relating to proprietary medicinal products[5] as last amended by Directive 87/21/EEC[6], may be refused only for reasons relating to the quality, safety or efficacy of the proprietary medicinal products concerned;

Whereas Member States have adopted measures of an economic nature on the marketing of medicinal products in order to control public health expenditure on such products; whereas such measures include direct and indirect controls on the prices of medicinal products as a consequence of the inadequacy or absence of competition in the medicinal products market and limitations on the range of products covered by national health insurance systems;

Whereas the primary objective of such measures is the promotion of public health by ensuring the availability of adequate supplies of medicinal products at a reasonable cost; whereas, however, such measures should also be intended to promote efficiency in the production of medicinal products and to encourage research and development into new medicinal products, on which the maintenance of a high level of public health within the Community ultimately depends;

Whereas disparities in such measures may hinder or distort intra-Community trade in medicinal products and thereby directly affect the functioning of the common market in medicinal products;

Whereas the objective of this Directive is to obtain an overall view of national pricing arrangements, including the manner in which they operate in individual cases and all the criteria on which they are based, and to provide public access to

---

1.   OJ L40 11.2.89 p8.
2.   OJ C17 23.1.87 p6 and OJ C129 18.5.88 p14.
3.   OJ C94 11.4.88 p62 and OJ C326 19.12.88.
4.   OJ C319 30.11.87 p47.
5.   OJ No 22 9.2.65 p369/65.
6.   OJ L15 17.1.87 p36.

them for all those involved in the market in medicinal products in the Member States; whereas this information should be public;

Whereas, as a first step towards the removal of these disparities, it is urgently necessary to lay down a series of requirements intended to ensure that all concerned can verify that the national measures do not constitute quantitative restrictions on imports or exports or measures having equivalent effect thereto; whereas, however, these requirements do not effect the policies of those Member States which rely primarily upon free competition to determine the price of medicinal products; whereas these requirements also do not affect national policies on price setting and on the determination of social security schemes, except as far as it is necessary to attain transparency within the meaning of this Directive;

Whereas the further harmonisation of such measures must take place progressively,

HAS ADOPTED THIS DIRECTIVE :

Article 1
1.   Member States shall ensure that any national measure, whether laid down by law, regulation or administrative action, to control the prices of medicinal products for human use or to restrict the range of medicinal products covered by their national health insurance systems complies with the requirements of this Directive.

2.   The definition of "medicinal products" laid down in Article 1 of Directive 65/65/EEC shall apply to this Directive.

3.   Nothing in this Directive shall permit the marketing of a proprietary medicinal product in respect of which the authorisation provided for in Article 3 of Directive 65/65/EEC has not been issued.

Article 2
The following provisions shall apply if the marketing of a medicinal product is permitted only after the competent authorities of the Member State concerned have approved the price of the product :

1.   Member States shall ensure that a decision on the price which may be charged for the medicinal product concerned is adopted and communicated to the applicant within 90 days of the receipt of an application submitted, in accordance with the requirements laid down in the Member State concerned, by the holder of a marketing authorisation. The applicant shall furnish the competent authorities with adequate information. If the information supporting the application is inadequate, the competent authorities shall forthwith notify the applicant of what detailed additional information is required and take their final decision within 90 days of receipt of this additional information. In the absence of such a decision within the above-mentioned period or periods, the applicant shall be entitled to market the product at the price proposed.
2.   Should the competent authorities decide not to permit the marketing of the medicinal product concerned at the price proposed by the applicant, the decision shall contain a statement of reasons based on objective and verifiable criteria. In addition, the applicant shall be informed of the remedies available to him under the laws in force and the time limits allowed for applying for such remedies.
3:      At least once a year, the competent authorities shall publish in an appropriate publication, and communicate to the Commission, a list of the

medicinal products the price of which has been fixed during the relevant period, together with the prices which may be charged for such products.

Article 3

Without prejudice to Article 4, the following provisions shall apply if an increase in the price of a medicinal product is permitted only after prior approval has been obtained from the competent authorities :

1. Member States shall ensure that a decision is adopted on an application submitted, in accordance with the requirements laid down in the Member State concerned, by the holder of a marketing authorisation to increase the price of a medicinal product and communicated to the applicant within 90 days of its receipt. The applicant shall furnish the competent authorities with adequate information including details of those events intervening since the price of the medicinal product was last determined which in his opinion justify the price increase requested. If the information supporting the application is inadequate, the competent authorities shall forthwith notify the applicant of what detailed additional information is required and take their final decision within 90 days of receipt of this additional information.
    In case of an exceptional number of applications, the period may be extended once only for a further 60 days. The applicant shall be notified of such extension before the expiry of the period.

    In the absence of such a decision within the above-mentioned period or periods, the applicant shall be entitled to apply in full the price increase requested.
2. Should the competent authorities decide not to permit the whole or part of the price increase requested, the decision shall contain a statement of reasons based on objective and verifiable criteria and the applicant shall be informed of the remedies available to him under the laws in force and the time limits allowed for applying for such remedies.
3. At least once a year, the competent authorities shall publish in an appropriate publication and communicate to the Commission, a list of the medicinal products for which price increases have been granted during the relevant period, together with the new price which may be charged for such products.

Article 4

1. In the event of a price freeze imposed on all medicinal products or on certain categories of medicinal products by the competent authorities of a Member State, that Member State shall carry out a review, at least once a year, to ascertain whether the macro-economic conditions justify that the freeze be continued unchanged. Within 90 days of the start of this review, the competent authorities shall announce what increases or decreases in prices are being made, if any.

2. In exceptional cases, a person who is the holder of a marketing authorisation for a medicinal product may apply for a derogation from a price freeze if this is justified by particular reasons. The application shall contain an adequate statement of these reasons. Member States shall ensure that a reasoned decision on any such application is adopted and communicated to the applicant within 90 days. If the information supporting the application is inadequate, the competent authorities shall forthwith notify the applicant of what detailed additional information is required and take their final decision within 90 days of receipt of this additional information. Should the derogation be granted, the competent authorities shall forthwith publish an announcement of the price increase allowed.

Should there be an exceptional number of applications, the period may be extended once only for a further 60 days. The applicant shall be notified of such extension before the expiry of the initial period.

Article 5

Where a Member State adopts a system of direct or indirect controls on the profitability of persons responsible for placing medicinal products on the market, the Member State concerned shall publish the following information in an appropriate publication and communicate it to the Commission :

(a)   the method or methods used in the Member State concerned to define profitability : return on sales and/or return on capital;
(b)   the range of target profit currently permitted to persons responsible for placing medicinal products on the market in the Member State concerned;
(c)   the criteria according to which target rates of profit are accorded to an individual responsible for placing medicinal products on the market, together with the criteria according to which they will be allowed to retain profits above their given targets in the Member State concerned;
(d)   the maximum percentage profit which any person responsible for placing medicinal products on the market is allowed to retain above his target in the Member State concerned.

This information shall be updated once a year or when significant changes are made.

Where, in addition to operating a system of direct or indirect controls on profits, a Member State operates a system of controls on the prices of certain types of medicinal products which are excluded from the scope of the profit control scheme, Articles 2, 3 and 4 shall, where relevant, apply to such price controls. However, the said Articles shall not apply where the normal operation of a system of direct or indirect controls on profits results exceptionally in a price being fixed for an individual medicinal product.

Article 6

The following provisions shall apply if a medicinal product is covered by the national health insurance system only after the competent authorities have decided to include the medicinal product concerned in a positive list of medicinal products covered by the national health insurance system.

1.   Member States shall ensure that a decision on an application submitted, in accordance with the requirements laid down in the Member State concerned, by the holder of a marketing authorisation to include a medicinal product in the list of medicinal products covered by the health insurance systems is adopted and communicated to the applicant within 90 days of its receipt. Where an application under this Article may be made before the competent authorities have agreed the price to be charged for the product pursuant to Article 2, or where a decision on the price of a medicinal product and a decision on its inclusion within the list of products covered by the health insurance system are taken after a single administrative procedure, the time limit shall be extended for a further 90 days. The applicant shall furnish the competent authorities with adequate information. If the information supporting the application is inadequate, the time limit shall be suspended and the competent authorities shall forthwith notify the applicant of what detailed additional information is required.

Where a Member State does not permit an application to be made under this Article before the competent authorities have agreed the price to be charged for the product pursuant to Article 2, the Member State concerned shall ensure that the overall period of time taken by the two procedures does not exceed 180 days. This time limit may be extended in accordance with Article 2 or suspended in accordance with the provisions of the preceding subparagraph.

2. Any decision not to include a medicinal product in the list of products covered by the health insurance system shall contain a statement of reasons based upon objective and verifiable criteria, including, if appropriate, any expert opinions or recommendations on which the decision is based. In addition, the applicant shall be informed of the remedies available to him under the laws in force and of the time limits allowed for applying for such remedies.

3. Before the date referred to in Article 11(1), Member States shall publish in an appropriate publication and communicate to the Commission the criteria which are to be taken into account by the competent authorities in deciding whether or not to include medicinal products on the lists.

4. Within one year of the date referred to in Article 11(1), Member States shall publish in an appropriate publication and communicate to the Commission a complete list of the products covered by their health insurance system, together with their prices fixed by the national competent authorities. This information shall be updated at least once every year.

5. Any decision to exclude a product from the list of products covered by the health insurance system shall contain a statement of reasons based on objective and verifiable criteria. Such decisions, including, if appropriate, any expert opinions or recommendations on which the decisions are based, shall be communicated to the person responsible, who shall be informed of the remedies available to him under the laws in force and the time limits allowed for applying for such remedies.

6. Any decision to exclude a category of medicinal products from the list of products covered by the health insurance system shall contain a statement of reasons based on objective and verifiable criteria and be published in an appropriate publication.

Article 7

The following provisions shall apply if the competent authorities of a Member State are empowered to adopt decisions to exclude individual or categories of medicinal products from the coverage of its national health insurance system (negative lists) :

1. Any decision to exclude a category of medicinal products from the coverage of the national health insurance system shall contain a statement of reasons based upon objective and verifiable criteria and be published in an appropriate publication.

2. Before the date referred to in Article 11(1), Member States shall publish in an appropriate publication and communicate to the Commission the criteria which are to be taken into account by the competent authorities in deciding whether or not to exclude an individual medicinal product from the coverage of the national health insurance system.

3. Any decision to exclude an individual medicinal product from the coverage of the national health insurance system shall contain a statement of reasons based on objective and verifiable criteria. Such decisions, including, if appropriate, any expert opinions or recommendations on which the decisions are based, shall be communicated to the person responsible, who shall be informed of the remedies available to him under the laws in force and the time limits allowed for applying for such remedies.

4.   Within one year of the date referred to in Article 11(1), the competent authorities shall publish in an appropriate publication and communicate to the Commission a list of the individual medicinal products which have been excluded from the scope of its health insurance system. This information shall be updated at least every six months.

Article 8

1.   Before the date referred to in Article 11(1), Member States shall communicate to the Commission any criteria concerning the therapeutic classification of medicinal products which are used by the competent authorities for the purposes of the national social security system.

2.   Before the date referred to in Article 11(1), Member States shall communicate to the Commission any criteria which are used by the competent authorities in verifying the fairness and transparency of the prices charged for transfers within a group of companies of active principles or intermediate products used in the manufacture of medicinal products or finished medicinal products.

Article 9

1.   In the light of experience, the Commission shall, not later than two years after the date referred to in Article 11(1), submit to the Council a proposal containing appropriate measures leading towards the abolition of any remaining barriers to, or distortions of, the free movement of proprietary medicinal products, so as to bring this sector closer into line within the normal conditions of the internal market.

2.   The Council shall decide on the Commission proposal not later than one year after its submission.

Article 10

1.   A Committee called the "Consultative Committee for the implementation of Directive 89/105/EEC relating to the transparency of measures regulating the pricing of medicinal products for human use and their inclusion in the scope of national health insurance systems" shall be set up and attached to the Commission.

2.   The tasks of the committee shall be to examine any question relating to the application of this Directive which is brought up by the Commission or at the request of a Member State.

3.   The committee shall consist of one representative from each Member State. There shall be one deputy for each representative. This deputy shall be entitled to participate in meetings of the committee.

4.   A representative of the Commission shall chair the committee.

5.   The committee shall adopt its rules of procedure.

Article 11

1.   Member States shall bring into force the laws, regulations and administrative provisions necessary to comply with this Directive by 31 December 1989 at the latest. They shall forthwith inform the Commission thereof.

2.   Before the date referred to in paragraph 1, Member States shall communicate to the Commission the texts of any laws, regulations or administrative

provisions relating to the pricing of medicinal products, the profitability of manufacturers of medicinal products and the coverage of medicinal products by the national health insurance system. Amendments and modifications to these laws, regulations or administrative provisions shall be communicated to the Commission forthwith.

Article 12

This Directive is addressed to the Member States.

Done at Brussels, 21 December 1988.

For the Council

The President

V. PAPANDREOU

APPENDIX 16

Commission communication on parallel imports of proprietary medicinal products for which marketing authorisations have already been granted[1]

In order progressively to establish the free movement of proprietary medicinal products, the Council has adopted four Directives[2] essentially relating to the conditions in which the Member States deliver marketing authorisations for these products.

Furthermore, in the "De Peijper" case[3], the Court of Justice of the European Communities, to which the matter was referred under Article 177 of the EEC Treaty, has delivered a judgment on parallel imports of medicinal products. This judgment gives the Commission interpretative rulings enabling it to exercise more stringent checks on the application of the rules of the Treaty on free movement of goods, in particular the provision of Articles 30 to 36 of the EEC Treaty.

Following this judgment, the Commission considered it necessary to supplement the existing Directives by transmitting to the Council on 2 June 1980 a proposal for a Directive[4] relating to parallel imports of proprietary medicinal products.

The Commission has taken note of the objections raised by the Economic and Social Committee to the proposal relating to parallel imports and the negative vote taken on that proposal by the European Parliament on 16 October 1981.

The Commission has therefore decided to withdraw its proposal, especially as its adoption by the Council appears improbable in the present circumstances.

The Commission is not, however, abandoning its responsibility to ensure that full effect is given to the provisions of the Treaty relating to the free movement of goods. The Parliament stressed during its discussion and in the text of its resolution its attachment to the principle of free movement. This is why the Commission wishes to indicate, on the occasion of this withdrawal, the way in which it intends to apply, under its own responsibility, the rules embodied in the Treaty as interpreted by the Court of Justice, in order to preserve the unity of the Community's internal market.

In case 104/75, the Court had to give a ruling on a set of health regulations relating to the marketing of medicinal products that prevented the marketing of a medicinal product introduced as a parallel import.

The Court first of all established that national rules or practices which result in imports being channelled in such a way that only certain traders can effect these imports, whereas others are prevented from doing so, are caught by the prohibition set out in Article 30 of the EEC Treaty.

The Court went on to reaffirm the Member States' right, in pursuance of Article 36 of the EEC Treaty, to decide, subject to the limitations imposed by the Treaty, on

---

1.   OJ C115 6.5.82 p5.
2.   Directive 65/65/EEC of 26 January 1965, OJ L22 9.2.65 p369, Directive 75/318/EEC of 20 May 1975, OJ L147 9.6.75 p1; Directive 75/319/EEC of 20 May 1975 OJ L147 9.6.75 p13; Directive 78/25/EEC of 12 December 1977, OJ L11 14.1.78 p18.
3.   CJEC 20 May 1976, Case 104/75, 1976 Report, p613.
4.   Proposal dated 2 June 1980 for a Directive amending Directives 65/65/EEC and 75/319/EEC (OJ C143 12.6.80 p8).

the level of protection they wish to afford for the health and life of persons, in particular the stringency of the checks to be carried out.

It nevertheless immediately stressed the general context in which this competence of the Member States was to be exercised :

"National rules or practices which do restrict imports of pharmaceutical products or are capable of doing so are only compatible with the Treaty to the extent to which they are necessary for the effective protection of health and life of humans.

National rules or practices do not fall within the exception specified in Article 36 if the health and life of humans can be as effectively protected by measures which do not restrict intra-Community trade so much.

In particular Article 36 cannot be relied on to justify rules or practices which, even though they are beneficial, contain restrictions which are explained primarily by a concern to lighten the administration's burden or reduce public expenditure, unless, in the absence of the said rules or practices, this burden or expenditure clearly would exceed the limits of what can reasonably be required."

In the case in point the competent national authorities intended to prevent a parallel importer from marketing a medicinal product that was similar to a medicinal product which had already been authorised and was produced by the same manufacturer for two reasons.

First, the parallel manufacturer was not able to provide the authorities with the complete file[1] relating to the quality, efficacy and safety of the product in general, which the manufacturer's authorised importer had already supplied to those same authorities with a view to obtaining a marketing authorisation for that medicinal product.

Secondly, the parallel importer could not, unlike the authorised importer, obtain from the manufacturer the reports on checks made on each manufacturing batch.

In the judgment on the "De Peijper" case, the Court ruled that "national rules or practices which make it possible for a manufacturer of the pharmaceutical product in question and his duly appointed representative, simply by refusing to produce the documents relating to the medicinal preparation in general or to a specific batch of that preparation, to enjoy a monopoly of the importing and marketing of the product, must be regarded as being unnecessarily restrictive, unless it is clearly proved that any other rules or practices would obviously be beyond the means which can be reasonably expected of an administration operating in a normal manner ... "

"It is only if the information or documents to be produced by the manufacturer or his duly appointed importer show that there are several variants of the medicinal preparation and that the differences between these variants have a therapeutic effect that there would be any justification for treating the variants as different medicinal preparations, for the purpose of authorising them to be placed on the market and as regards producing the relevant documents ..."

The Commission, in its role as guardian of the Treaty, will ensure that the rules and practices applied by Member States to parallel imports of medicinal products, and in particular proprietary medicinal products which account for the majority of intra-

---

1.   This file comprises inter alia a description of the manufacturer's production and control methods and the results of the analytical, toxico-pharmacological and clinical tests conducted on the medicinal product in general.

Community trading operations in medicinal products, will remain within limits compatible with Articles 30 to 36.

In particular, such measures must :

—   be strictly necessary from the health standpoint,

—   obstruct intra-Community trade as little as possible,

—   require the Member States to adopt an active and vigilant attitude towards pharmaceutical companies.

The Commission points out that the competent authorities in the Member States are not entitled to oppose the marketing of any medicinal product, the subject of parallel importation, that already has a marketing authorisation, on the grounds that the parallel importer is not able to obtain documents which only the manufacturer or his approved representative can have at their disposal.

In the absence of any harmonised rules governing the system of parallel imports, it is up to the Commission, in accordance with the procedure under Article 169, and to the interested parties, in accordance with the means of redress which they have at their disposal, to ensure that parallel imports of medicinal products are made possible under the conditions laid down by the rulings of the Court.

After consulting senior experts in public health matters from the Member States' administrations meeting in the Pharmaceutical Committee[1], the Commission had proposed a uniform system for parallel imports of proprietary medicinal products. Despite the withdrawal of its proposal, the Commission considers it useful to indicate safe ways of monitoring parallel imports which, subject to the rulings of the Court, seem to it to be justified for the purpose of protecting the health and life of humans pursuant to Article 36 of the Treaty.

The Commission points out that the competent authorities of the Member States already have at their disposal two important safeguards for health in the case of parallel imports of proprietary medicinal products.

On the one hand, the national rules governing the activities of importers, wholesalers and, where applicable, manufacturers of proprietary medicinal products apply equally to parallel importers. These rules usually cover professional competence and responsibilities, the technical premises and equipment required and the rules for the operation of such establishments, in particular the procedures relating to the preservation of documents to facilitate official checks and inspections.

On the other hand, the authorities competent to issue marketing authorisations for proprietary medicinal products already, as a rule, possess the dossier relating to the quality, efficacy and safety of the medicinal product in general, which has been supplied by the manufacturer or his approved importer and which states, in pursuance of Article 4(11) of Directive 65/65/EEC, the authorisations already obtained for the product in any other Member State. According to the Court, the competent administration of the importing Member State is clearly entitled to require the manufacturer, or his duly appointed importer, to state whether the manufacturer, or the group of manufacturers to which he belongs produces several variants of the same medicinal product for different Member States. If this is so, it is only if the documents submitted by the manufacturer show that there are differences having a therapeutic effect that there would be any justification for

---

1.   Set up by Council Decision 75/320/EC of 20 May 1975, OJ L147 9.6.75 p23.

treating the variants as different medicinal products for the purpose of marketing authorisation.

In addition to these safeguards, the authorities have a legitimate interest in being able to verify, at all times and beyond doubt, whether the batches of imported medicinal products are in conformity with the particulars contained in the dossier.

The Commission concedes that the parallel importer may be required to supply the competent authorities in the Member State into which the product is imported with certain information readily accessible to him when he wants to market for the first time a proprietary medicinal product already marketed by the manufacturer or his duly appointed representative.

This information must allow the competent authorities in the Member State into which the product is imported to check, within a reasonable period, that the proprietary medicinal product that is the subject of parallel importation is effectively covered by the marketing authorisation already granted to the manufacturer or his duly appointed representative. In the Commission's view, this period should not exceed 45 days from the time the parallel importer gives the following information to the competent authorities :

(a) name of the proprietary medicinal product in the Member State into which it is imported and in the Member State from which it comes;

(b) name or corporate name and permanent address of the person responsible for placing the product on the market in the Member State into which it is imported and in the Member State from which it comes, and where appropriate, of the manufacturer(s);

(c) name or corporate name and permanent address of the parallel importer;

(d) numbers of the marketing authorisations in the Member State into which the product is imported and in the Member State from which it comes;

(e) any other general information useful for the marketing of the proprietary medicinal product in the Member State into which it is imported, i.e.

— qualitative and quantitative composition in terms of active principles, by dosage unit or in percentage, using the international non-proprietary names recommended by the World Health Organisation where such names exist,

— pharmaceutical form and route of administration,

— therapeutic indications and normal dosage,

— contra-indications and main side-effects,

— storage precautions, if any;

(f) one or more specimens or mock-ups of the proprietary product in the form in which it will be marketed in the Member State into which it is imported, including the package leaflet, if any.

To enable the authorities to be effectively informed of the marketing of each batch of the product imported, the parallel importer should, in the Commission's view, register the origin, quantity and batch numbers of the imported medicinal products whenever he imports them, and hold this information at the disposal of the competent authorities.

The Commission points out that pursuant to Chapter IV of Directive 75/319/EEC each batch of proprietary medicinal products manufactured in a Member State is checked by the manufacturer who makes out a certificate and registers the operations carried out in documents that remain at the disposal of the agents of the competent authority for at least five years. Because these control reports are sent to him by the manufacturer, the duly appointed importer is exempt from repeating the controls in the Member State into which the product is imported.

Since the parallel importer does not have access to these control reports, the national authorities have to adopt a more active policy when they wish to verify the controls carried out by the manufacturer on a given batch. They can choose for this purpose one of the four approaches given in the De Peijper judgment, ie :

— they can obtain the manufacturing control reports by taking legislative or administrative measures compelling the manufacturer himself, or his duly appointed representative, to supply them;

— they can obtain these reports through the authorities in the country of manufacture;

— they can, whenever possible, lay down a presumption of conformity with the specifications of the medicament and it would be up to them, in appropriate cases, to rebut this presumption after verification of the conformity;

— as far as this presumption is fully impracticable, they can allow the parallel importer to provide proof of conformity by any means other than by documents to which he has no access.

The parallel importer is liable, in the same way as the person responsible for marketing, to the measures taken by the Member States to withdraw the products, to suspend or revoke the authorisation or to prohibit supply of the product, pursuant to Article 28 of Directive 75/319/EEC.

By appropriate co-operation between the Member State authorities, it would be possible to supplement, if necessary, the monitoring measures compatible with Article 36 of the Treaty, designed to check the conformity of medicinal products imported in parallel.

In the De Peijper judgment, the Court held that simple co-operation between the authorities of the Member States would enable them to obtain on a reciprocal basis the documents necessary for checking certain largely standardised and widely distributed products.

In addition to the obligations resulting from Article 5 of the EEC Treaty, the obligation for the competent authorities to communicate to each other such information as is appropriate to guarantee that the requirements for the marketing or manufacturing authorisations are fulfilled is specifically spelled out in Article 30 of Directive 75/319/EEC.

The Commission for its part is prepared to do everything it can to assist the Member States in exchanging the information they consider necessary to check the conformity of parallel imports of proprietary medicinal products.

The Commission considers that the Committee for Proprietary Medicinal Products, set up by Directive 75/319/EEC, provides a suitable forum for any exchanges of information between the representatives of the Member States responsible for marketing authorisations for proprietary medicinal products. The Commission also holds at the disposal of Member States a continuously updated list of the persons appointed by the competent authorities to supply at short notice any necessary information on marketing or manufacturing authorisations in application of Articles 30 and 33 of Directive 75/319/EEC.

APPENDIX 17

Communication from the Commission on the compatibility with Article 30 of the EEC Treaty of measures taken by Member States relating to price controls and reimbursement of medicinal products[1]

I. INTRODUCTION

Elimination of unjustified barriers has traditionally been done through individual infringement proceedings. In its "White Paper on completing the internal market" (COM(85) 310), however, the Commission announced that it would also take more systematic action, by publishing general communications setting out the legal situation, particularly in regard to Articles 30 to 36 of the EEC Treaty, for the whole of an economic sector or in relation to a particular type of barrier (paragraph 155). Amongst the priority sectors quoted in this respect is the pharmaceutical sector (paragraph 156).

II. GENERAL REMARKS

The market for medicinal products has certain characteristics that distinguish it very clearly from the markets for other consumer products. Firstly, the final consumer of a medicinal product has scarcely any influence on the choice of medicinal product, at least in the case of those prescribed by a doctor. Moreover, the demand for a medicinal product is normally related to the treatment of a particular complaint, and medicinal products cannot readily be substituted for others. Secondly, the market for medicinal products is characterised by the payment of medical expenses by social security institutions instead of by consumers.

In these circumstances, it is understandable that Member States should try to limit expenditure on pharmaceuticals, since the community bears the greater part of it. To this end, most Member States have taken measures to control prices of medicinal products and reimbursements of medicinal products by social security : these measures form part of the health policy of the Member States and aim to offer the best possible treatment to all citizens, without excessive cost to the public purse.

Such measures are in principle compatible with Community law, provided that their restrictive effect on the free movement of goods is not disproportionate in relation to the legitimate interest which it is sought to protect. It is important, in particular, that such measures should not involve any difference in treatment that places products imported from other Member States at a disadvantage, and that they should not render the sale of imported products economically unviable or more difficult than that of domestic products, or make certain import routes impossible or more costly than others.

The Court of Justice has had occasion to restate these principles, notably in two judgments handed down recently in references for preliminary rulings (judgments of the Court of 29 November 1983 in Case 181/82 "Roussel" (1983), ECR 3849 to 3871, and of 7 February 1984 in Case 238/82 "Duphar" (1984), ECR 523 to 545). These judgments offer the Commission interpretative guidelines which enable it to exercise stricter control of the application of the rules of the EEC Treaty on the free movement of goods, in particular Articles 30 to 36 thereof.

---

1.   OJ C310 4.12.86 p7.

As announced in its White Paper on the completion of the internal market (COM(85) 310), in 1986 the Commission will be transmitting to the Council a proposal for a directive on the transparency of prices for pharmaceutical products and reimbursements by social security. The communication does not prejudge proposals which the Commission may make on that occasion : it sets out Member States' obligations under the rules of the EEC Treaty itself, as interpreted by the Court of Justice, and as the Commission intends to apply them, under its own responsibility, in order to achieve a unified internal market in the Community.

III. PRICE CONTROL FOR MEDICINAL PRODUCTS

A. General

In the absence of Community provisions, Member States are free, each within their own territories, to adopt legislation to control prices of pharmaceutical products, provided that such legislation does not hinder the free movement of goods within the Community.

Article 30 of the EEC Treaty prohibits all measures having an effect equivalent to a quantitative restriction on trade between Member States. According to the well-established case-law of the Court, any measures which are capable of hindering, directly or indirectly, actually or potentially, trade between Member States are to be regarded as measures having such effect (see judgment of the Court of 11 July 1974 in Case 8/74 "Dassonville" (1974), ECR 837 to 865).

The Court had occasion to state that these principles apply to price control systems. It stressed in this aspect that whilst rules controlling prices applicable equally to domestic and imported products do not in themselves amount to a measure having an effect equivalent to a quantitative restriction, they may in fact produce such an effect when prices are fixed at such a level that the marketing of imported products becomes either impossible or more difficult than the marketing of national products (see judgment of the Court of 6 November 1979 in Cases 16 to 20/79 "Danis" (1979), ECR 3327 to 3342).

On the other hand, in the case of price controls providing for separate or different systems for imported and domestic products, the Court has indicated that such rules must be considered as a measure having an effect equivalent to a quantitative restriction wherever it is capable of hindering the sale of imported products in any way (see the above-mentioned judgment 181/82 "Roussel").

Furthermore, in Directive 70/50/EEC of 22 December 1969[1] the Commission points out the incompatibility with Article 30 of measures which :

—	lay down, for imported products only, minimum or maximum prices below or above which imports are prohibited, reduced or made subject to conditions liable to hinder importation,

—	lay down less favourable prices for imported products than for domestic products,

—	preclude any increase in the price of the imported product corresponding to the supplementary costs and charges inherent in importation,

---

1.	OJ L13 19.1.70 p29.

— fix the prices of products solely on the basis of the cost price or the quality of domestic products at such a level as to create a hindrance to import.

B. Determination of prices

The general principles to be observed here are grouped around two main aspects : realistic prices and transparency of prices. Each product must be able to have its own price, calculated on the basis of its real cost using a transparent method of calculation.

It is generally for manufacturers and importers to determine the prices of each of their products, which are then assessed by the authorities in accordance with measures designed to control the prices of proprietary pharmaceuticals.

If, when new products are placed on the market, Member States can justify asking firms for information to enable them to assess the components of the prices that such firms propose to charge, they must then allow pharmaceutical firms to take account of the various elements making up the cost of the products (research, raw materials, processing, advertising, transport, expenses and charges inherent in importing, etc).

In any case, the marketing authorisation (within the meaning of Council Directive 65/65/EEC of 26 January 1965[1]) for a pharmaceutical product may not in any circumstances be refused, suspended or revoked save on grounds relating to public health. This means, in particular, that a Member State may not refuse, suspend or revoke a marketing authorisation simply because it considers the price of a pharmaceutical product to be excessive (see judgment of the Court of 26 January 1984 in Case 301/82 "Clin-Midy" (1984), ECR 251 to 260).

C. Price freezes

1. Differentiated price freezes

Firstly, it is clear that Member States may not introduce price controls that are applicable solely to imported products; such measures always contravene Article 30 of the EEC Treaty in so far as they can be a hindrance to imported products, particularly when the prices fixed are not sufficient to cover the price of the product.

In the above-mentioned judgment 181/82 "Roussel", the Court ruled on a price control system that differentiated between domestic and imported products. After noting that "the legislation in question does not apply to domestic products and imported products alike but consists of different sets of rules for the two groups of products, laid down by different decrees and different also as regards their substantive content", the Court ruled that "legislation of that kind, which differentiates between the two groups of products, must be regarded as a measure having an effect equivalent to a quantitative restriction where it is capable of making more difficult, in any manner whatever, the sale of imported products". Article 30 of the EEC Treaty therefore precludes a Member State from introducing specific legislation which refers to the manufacturer's basic prices usually charged for pharmaceutical products intended for consumption within the territory of the Member State in which they are produced, where the legislation applicable to domestic production is based solely on a freeze of the level of prices at a given reference date (see the above-mentioned judgment 181/82 "Roussel").

---

1.   OJ L22 9.2.65 p369.

On the other hand, according to the Commission, a system that freezes the prices of domestic pharmaceutical products and margins on the importation and distribution of imported products should not in itself be regarded as incompatible with Article 30 of the EEC Treaty, in as much as such a system would enable importers either to increase the prices of their products in line with increases in costs in the Member State in which they were manufactured, or not to increase them in order to maintain their competitive position in relation to domestic products whose prices have been frozen.

2. Non-differentiated price freezes

According to the case-law of the Court, whilst rules imposing a price freeze which are applicable equally to domestic products and imported products do not amount in themselves to a measure having an effect equivalent to a quantitative restriction, they may in fact produce such an effect when prices are at such a level that the marketing of imported products becomes either impossible or more difficult than the marketing of national products (see the above-mentioned judgment "Danis") .

This is especially the case, according to the Court, where national rules, while preventing the increased prices of imported products from being passed on in sale prices, freeze prices at a level so low that — taking into account the general situation of imported products in relation to that of domestic products — traders wishing to import the products in question into the Member State concerned can do so only at a loss, or, having regard to the level at which prices for national products are frozen are impelled to give preference to the latter products (see the same judgment).

This is the case where measures fix the price of products solely on the basis of the cost price of domestic products at such a level as to create a hindrance to importation or preclude any increase in the price of the imported product corresponding to the supplementary costs and charges inherent in import (see Commission Directive 70/50/EEC) .

The Court of Justice has nevertheless acknowledged that Member States have the possibility of "combating inflation and adopting measures intended to control increases in the price of medicines, whatever their origin, on condition that they do so by means of measures which do not place imported medicines at a disadvantage" (see the above-mentioned judgment 181/82 "Roussel"). In this respect, the Commission reserves the right to verify the real nature of such aims in the public interest and to take action against measures which have other objectives or place imported products at a disadvantage.

Finally, the Commission considers that a Member State may not freeze prices of pharmaceutical products so as to preclude any influence, on the prices of imported products, of an increase in costs in the Member State in which they are produced or of a change in exchange rates.

3. Freezing of margins

On the one hand, the Commission would point out that in its Directive 70/50/EEC it considered that national measures which "fix profit margins or any other price components for imported products only or fix these differently for domestic products and for imported products, to the detriment of the latter", constitute measures having an effect equivalent to quantitative restrictions.

On the other hand, the fixing of maximum margins for the distribution and retail sale of both domestic and imported pharmaceutical products is not, in principle likely to hinder the free movement of goods in the Community, whether the margin is calculated on the price of the product or corresponds to a fixed amount.

Maximum margins fixed for the distribution and retail sale of pharmaceutical products may not, however, include import costs in the case of pharmaceutical products imported from another Member State. Such a system would tend to discourage imports from other Member States and encourage wholesalers and retailers to obtain supplies on the national market (see judgment of the Court of June 1985 in Case 116/84 "Roelstraete" (1985), ECR 1705).

According to the Commission, the freezing of importers' margins on imports is compatible with Article 30 of the EEC Treaty only on the dual condition that the measure allows importers to cover the costs and charges inherent in import (see the above-mentioned Directive 70/50/EEC) and that it is accompanied by a price freezing system for domestic products.

4. Revision of prices and derogations from freezes

The Commission would point out to Member States that fixed or frozen prices must be revised when economic conditions so require, following any changes in the market. However, when authorising price rises for domestic or imported pharmaceutical products, Member States may not base the change solely on the cost price of national products. In any case, the various components of the cost must be taken into consideration with a view to establishing prices that are sufficiently remunerative.

Finally, Member States may not link the grant of price rises or derogations from price freezes to conditions that can be met only by firms established within the territory of the State in question, such as conditions or undertakings relating to the development of research, job creation, investments within the territory of the State concerned or growth of exports and recovery of the trade balance.

IV. REIMBURSEMENTS FOR MEDICINAL PRODUCTS

A. General

According to the Court of Justice, measures adopted within the framework of a compulsory national healthcare scheme with the object of refusing insured persons the right to be supplied, at the expense of the insurance institution, with specifically named medicinal preparations are compatible with Article 30 of the EEC Treaty if the determination of the excluded medicinal preparations involves no discrimination regarding the origin of the products and is carried out on the basis of objective and verifiable criteria, such as the existence on the market of other, less expensive products having the same therapeutic effect, the fact that the preparations in question are freely marketed without the need for any medical prescription, or are products excluded from reimbursement for reasons of a pharmaco-therapeutic nature justified by the protection of public health, and provided that it is possible to amend the lists whenever compliance with the specified criteria so requires (see the above-mentioned judgment "Duphar").

These principles, set out for a negative list (listing medicinal products which are ineligible for reimbursement), apply mutatis mutandis to positive lists (listing medicinal products which are approved for reimbursement).

B. Application of objective criteria

The Court has essentially laid down a fundamental condition to be satisfied by the Member States to ensure that their reimbursement systems for medicinal products are compatible with Article 30 : the determination of medicinal products excluded in the case of a negative list or included in the case of a positive list must be carried out in accordance with objective criteria regardless of the origin of the products.

The Court has given three examples of objective criteria which could justify a decision to exclude a product from reimbursement:

— the existence on the market of other, less expensive products having the same therapeutic effect,

— the fact that the preparations in question are freely marketed without the need for any medical prescription,

— reasons of a pharmaco-therapeutic nature justified by the protection of public health.

These examples enable the Commission to state the conditions under which Member States may exclude certain medicinal products from reimbursement.

Medicinal products may be excluded from the list of reimbursable products on a group basis or individually, subject to certain conditions in each case.

1. Exclusion of categories of products

The definition of groups or categories of products which are approved or ineligible for reimbursement must be based on objective, general criteria of a therapeutic nature. When therapeutic classes are defined, for reimbursement purposes, they may not therefore be reduced to a single product or single active substance, which, by the approval of one class, would allow the reimbursement of a particular product and, by the prohibition of another class, would prevent another product having an equivalent therapeutic effect from being reimbursed.

When a therapeutic class is approved for reimbursement, all products in that class need not necessarily be reimbursable : in this case, individual products may not be excluded except as indicated below.

2. Exclusion of individual products

The exclusion from reimbursement or the refusal to allow reimbursement of specifically named medicinal products must be based on an assessment of the cost (financial) and benefit (therapeutic) of the treatment, in comparison with other treatments. The assessment may lead to the exclusion from reimbursement of medicinal products whose efficacy has not been proven in application of Community directives or whose cost is excessive, and to the exclusion of certain indications which could lead to unjustified social security expenditure.

In general, the Commission considers that the only financial criterion that may be taken into account to approve a particular medicinal product for reimbursement or to exclude it from reimbursement is the cost of treatment. Thus a medicinal product may be excluded from reimbursement owing to the existence on the market of one or more medicinal products having an equivalent therapeutic effect, provided that, for the assessment of the therapeutic effect, account is taken of the indications and side effects of each medicinal product. Account should be taken, when comparing treatment costs, of the dosage and presumed duration of the treatment until the therapeutic effect in question is achieved.

3. Notes

The exclusion from reimbursement of products freely marketed without a medical prescription is in line with the principles set out above (see the above-mentioned judgment 238/82 "Duphar").

The Commission regards the following as incompatible with the principles set out above :

—   the exclusion from reimbursement, for one or more therapeutic classes, of proprietary products only, regardless of price, or the approval for reimbursement of unbranded products only, regardless of price,

—   the exclusive approval for reimbursement, for each therapeutic class or for all therapeutic classes, of a predetermined number of medicinal products.

C. Procedural questions

According to the Court of Justice, the criteria used by Member States to exclude certain medicinal products from reimbursement must be verifiable by any importer. Furthermore, it must be possible to amend the lists of medicinal products approved for reimbursement or ineligible for reimbursement whenever compliance with the specified criteria so requires. Decisions relating to approval for reimbursement or exclusion from reimbursement must therefore satisfy certain formal and procedural conditions. In this connection also, a distinction should be made between the exclusion of classes of products and individual decisions relating to certain products.

1. Exclusion of categories of products

Decisions relating to the exclusion of certain categories of products, defined as set out above, must be published officially. If all products belonging to the categories of products for which reimbursement is approved are not reimbursed, the criteria used to determine which products are excluded or which are approved must likewise be published.

2. Exclusion of certain products

(a) Time limits
When they receive an application for the approval of a medicinal product for reimbursement, Member States are bound to make a decision within a reasonable period. In the Commission's view, this period should in no case exceed 120 days as allowed for the granting of a marketing authorisation (see Article 7 of the above-mentioned Directive 65/65/EEC).

(b) Grounds
Reasons must be given for decisions by virtue of which certain products are not approved for reimbursement. When the reason given for exclusion from reimbursement relates to the existence on the market of other products having an equivalent therapeutic effect, the decision must name these products, give their prices and details of the dosage and duration of treatment used to compare prices.

(c) Notification and means of redress

Decisions by virtue of which certain products are not approved for reimbursement must be notified to the firms concerned with an indication of the means of redress against such decisions and the time limits within which appeals must be made.

3. Revision of lists

As the Court has stated, Member States are bound to amend the lists of medicinal products ineligible for reimbursement whenever compliance with the specified criteria so requires. To this end, Member States must arrange for periodic revision of the positive and negative lists.

V. CONCLUSION

The Commission invites the Member States to examine their rules and administrative practices in the light of the principles set out in this Communication and, where necessary, to bring them into line with these principles. Without prejudice to its intention, mentioned above, to put to the Council in the near future a proposal for a Directive on transparency of prices for pharmaceutical products and reimbursements by social security schemes, the Commission reserves the right to commence proceedings under Article 169 of the EEC Treaty, or to pursue such proceedings which have already been opened, against Member States which in its view have failed to fulfil the obligations incumbent upon them in this sector under the EEC Treaty.

INDEX